SOFT CONTACT LENS

Symposium and Workshop
of the University of Florida,
Gainesville

SOFT CONTACT LENS

Symposium and Workshop of the University of Florida, Gainesville

EDITED BY

Antonio R. Gasset, M.D.

Assistant Professor of Ophthalmology, Department of Ophthalmology,
College of Medicine, University of Florida

Herbert E. Kaufman, M.D.

Professor of Ophthalmology and Pharmacology,
Chairman, Department of Ophthalmology, and Acting Dean,
College of Medicine, University of Florida

With 126 illustrations, including 8 color illustrations in 1 plate

The C. V. Mosby Company

Saint Louis/1972

Contributors

JAMES V. AQUAVELLA, M.D.

Attending Surgeon and Chief of Medical Staff, Park Avenue Hospital, Rochester, New York

VICTOR CHIQUIAR ARIAS, O.D.

Professor of Contactology, Department of Ophthalmology, Hospital General Del Centro Médico Nacional, Mexico City, Mexico

NEAL J. BAILEY, O.D., Ph.D.

Clinical Associate Professor, College of Optometry, The Ohio State University, Columbus, Ohio

JOSEPH A. BALDONE, M.D.

New Orleans, Louisiana

BERNARD BECKER, M.D.

Professor and Head, Department of Ophthalmology, Washington University School of Medicine, St. Louis, Missouri

CHESTER J. BLACK, M.D.

Head of Contact Lens Clinic, Cook County Hospital, Chicago, Illinois

STUART I. BROWN, M.D.

Clinical Associate Professor, Department of Ophthalmology, Cornell University Medical Center, New York, New York

JOSEPH A. CAPELLA, M.S.

Administrator and Research Director, Lions Eye Bank, Washington, D. C.

JOHN E. CARNEY, Sr.

Nashville, Tennessee

HENRY F. EDELHAUSER, Ph.D.

Associate Professor of Physiology and Ophthalmology, Medical College of Wisconsin, Milwaukee, Wisconsin

GERALD L. FELDMAN, Ph.D.

Nashville, Tennessee

MICHAEL A. FRIEDBERG, O.D.

Pittsburgh, Pennsylvania

ANTONIO R. GASSET, M.D.

Assistant Professor of Ophthalmology, Department of Ophthalmology, College of Medicine, University of Florida, Gainesville, Florida

G. PETER HALBERG, M.D.

Clinical Professor, Division of Ophthalmology, Downstate Medical Center, New York State University, Brooklyn, New York; Corresponding Secretary, Contact Lens Association of Ophthalmologists

JACK HARTSTEIN, M.D.

Assistant Professor of Clinical Ophthalmology, Washington University School of Medicine, St. Louis, Missouri

HERBERT E. KAUFMAN, M.D.

Professor of Ophthalmology and Pharmacology, Chairman, Department of Ophthalmology, and Acting Dean, College of

Medicine, University of Florida, Gainesville, Florida

HOWARD M. LEIBOWITZ, M.D.

Professor and Chairman, Department of Ophthalmology, Boston University School of Medicine; Ophthalmologist in Chief, Department of Ophthalmology, University Hospital, Boston, Massachusetts

HISAO MAGATANI, M.D.

Associate Professor, Department of Ophthalmology, Juntendo University School of Medicine, Tokyo, Japan

SAIICHI MISHIMA, M.D.

Professor and Chairman, Department of Ophthalmology, Tokyo University, School of Medicine, Tokyo, Japan

DENNIS R. MORRISON, Ph.D.

Postdoctoral Fellow, Department of Ophthalmology, College of Medicine, University of Florida, Gainesville, Florida

HAROLD I. MOSS, O.D.

Guest Lecturer in Contact Lenses, Pennsylvania College of Optometry, Philadelphia, Pennsylvania

AKIRA NAKAJIMA, M.D.

Professor and Chairman, Department of Ophthalmology, Juntendo University School of Medicine, Tokyo, Japan

KENNETH F. O'DRISCOLL, Ph.D.

Professor and Chairman, Department of Chemical Engineering, University of Waterloo, Waterloo, Ontario, Canada

DAVID B. PEARCE, M.D.

Department of Ophthalmology, New York Hospital—Cornell University Medical Center, New York, New York

RUSSELL E. PHARES, Jr., Ph.D.

Technical Director, Barnes-Hind Pharmaceuticals, Inc., Sunnyvale, California

STEVEN M. PODOS, M.D.

Assistant Professor of Ophthalmology, Washington University School of Medicine, St. Louis, Missouri

MAURICE G. POSTER, O.D.

Chief, Contact Lens Clinic, Optometric Center of New York, New York; Associate Clinical Professor, State College of Optometry, State University of New York, New York, New York

IDA SCHAEFER, B.S.

Laboratory Technician, Department of Ophthalmology, College of Medicine, University of Florida, Gainesville, Florida

EDWARD L. SHAW, M.D.

Resident, Department of Ophthalmology, College of Medicine, University of Florida, Gainesville, Florida

MICHAEL P. TRAGAKIS, M.D.

Department of Ophthalmology, New York Hospital—Cornell University Medical Center, New York, New York

MAIJA H. UOTILA, R.N.

Assistant in Ophthalmology, Department of Ophthalmology, College of Medicine, University of Florida, Gainesville, Florida

EMILY D. VARNELL, B.S.

Research Instructor, Department of Ophthalmology, College of Medicine, University of Florida, Gainesville, Florida

KEITH A. WHITHAM

Technician, Manhattan Eye, Ear, Nose, and Throat Hospital, New York, New York; Technical Coordinator, Griffin Laboratories, Inc., Buffalo, New York

GEORGE M. WODAK, S.G.A.O., F.A.C.L.P.

Head, Contact Lens Institute, Tel-Aviv, Israel

THOMAS O. WOOD, M.D.

Corneal Fellow, Department of Ophthalmology, College of Medicine, University of Florida, Gainesville, Florida

THOM J. ZIMMERMAN, M.D.

Resident, Department of Ophthalmology, College of Medicine, University of Florida, Gainesville, Florida

To all practitioners in the contact lens field

and

To Gloria, Carin, and Anthony

Preface

History may not repeat itself but historians do. After the introduction of the plastic corneal contact lens by Kevin Tuohy almost three decades ago, the ophthalmic community welcomed the lens with unwarranted enthusiasm and general acceptance only to criticize it and discontinue fitting it shortly thereafter.

Then, through the continuous and monumental work of a small group of people, improvement in technology and fitting produced a lens that was again accepted by the ophthalmic community. It was at this time of general acceptance, almost two decades after the plastic contact lens was first introduced on a black Friday, March 12, 1964, that the majority of the nation's newspapers and magazines printed articles with such titles as "U. S. Investigates Plastic Lenses—Blindness Linked."

This episode in the history of the contact lens industry was brought about by expert testimony before a hearing in the U. S. Senate and in a report to the FDA. As a result, the contact lens industry was thrown into a state of confusion. The facts were not readily available. Time was needed for the industry to investigate the charges, to repudiate false statements, and to determine whether or not acrylic acid did in fact leach out of the plastic lens material, causing blindness. Of course, with the passing of time, these allegations have proved false.

The use of cross-linked hydrophilic polymers for contact lenses was first reported by Wichterle and Lim in 1960. Since that time hydrophilic contact lenses have undergone great improvement. Ophthalmologists, optometrists, chemists, pharmaceutical companies, and contact lens manufacturers have efficiently cooperated in the most extensive testing ever carried out for any contact lens or even an ophthalmic drug. Once again, almost a decade after the development of hydrophilic contact lenses, on another black Friday, October 1, 1971, headlines in the *Wall Street Journal* read "Soft Contact Lens Hits Hard Obstacles as Doctors Debate Its Safety for Users." Historians have again failed to write the true history; as was true of hard plastic contact lenses, soft hydrophilic lenses are here to stay.

Heretofore, the development of soft contact lenses had benefited greatly from supervision by the FDA. Prior to the FDA action designating the hydrophilic contact lens as a drug rather than a device, much of the investigation was conducted in circles rather than in progression, with much criticism but little improvement. In retrospect, this FDA action can be considered as the single most important event that could have happened in the development of these lenses. It prevented the premature marketing of a product and resulted in an investigation that has brought to light uses far more important (such as therapy for and prevention of eye disease and blindness) than the more lucrative use as cosmetic lenses. It has forced manufacturers to make changes and improvements that otherwise would have taken years or perhaps never would have been achieved. It has benefited the patient, the practitioner, and, in the long run, even the manufacturer.

In view of the enormous amount of work invested in the evaluation of these lenses by so many investigators and, even more crucial, the need for these lenses in the treatment of corneal disease for which no other form of therapy is available, we hope that FDA approval of the remaining lenses will be forthcoming shortly. Present restrictions force the conscientious practitioner to select poor but readily available substitutes in the hope of at least partially treating conditions for which no other sight-preserving techniques are available.

In the beginning, hydrophilic lenses were available to only a selected group of investigators. A nationwide evaluation for safety and efficacy has already been conducted for two lenses: the Griffin Naturalens and the Bausch & Lomb Soflens. Data from more than 3,000 patients have been collected and reported, and data from hundreds of other patients have been published in subspecialty journals. To date there has been no compilation of these results or authoritative compendium of sound clinical judgment concerning the use of hydrophilic (soft) contact lenses. The purpose of this symposium and fitting manual is to fill these needs.

For clarity as well as freedom, much repetition has been allowed in order to record the differences between the main types of lenses as well as medical experiences with these lenses. With equal justification, some differences and possibly contrary opinions have been retained. Dr. Kaufman and I have tried not to interfere with any author's freedom of expression except when limitation of space or unnecessary repetition demanded curtailment. During the symposium, Sy Trager, Director of Clinical Research of Burton, Parsons and Company, Inc., Washington, D. C., presented an interesting and controversial paper, "Some Interesting Findings with Soft Lens Solutions and Various Hydrophilic Contact Lenses and Materials." However, at Mr. Trager's request, this paper was not submitted for publication.

This book assembles the judgment of a selected group of ophthalmologists and optometrists with extensive experience, expertise, and knowledge in the field of soft contact lenses for the correction of myopia, hyperopia, aphakia, keratoconus, bullous keratopathy, corneal ulcers, drying conditions, and glaucoma.

My colleagues should receive the majority of credit for this work, but the errors are my own.

Antonio R. Gasset

Contents

PART I

Lens composition

Chapter 1

Polymeric aspects of
soft contact lenses

Kenneth F. O'Driscoll, Ph.D.

Until recent years the fitter of contact lenses could safely ignore the material of which lenses were made, since they were all made from glasses—either inorganic or organic. The most common lenses have been of the latter category, being made essentially of poly(methylmethacrylate), which is a rather ordinary plastic, being glassy at temperatures up to the boiling point of water. However, the last decade has seen the beginning of materials whose major common attribute is their lack of glassy character. The fitter must now make choices between very different materials.

Presented here are some of the fundamental principles of polymer chemistry and physics as they pertain to these new materials. In doing so, I hope that fitters of "soft lenses" will come to recognize some of the important differences that these lenses have introduced into the *system* of the eye plus the lens. Only through such recognition and subsequent feedback can scientists further improve lens materials.

POLYMERIZATION

The word *polymer* is composed of Greek roots meaning 'many parts.' A synthetic polymer is usually found in the chemical reaction of polymerization wherein many small molecules (the *monomer*) are linearly added to each other (or condensed together) to form a polymeric chain of very high molecular weight. The average number of monomer molecules held together in a single polymer molecule is called the *degree of polymerization* (DP). Values of the DP for common high polymers range from perhaps 100 to 10,000. When a vinyl monomer such as methylmethacrylate is polymerized, the reaction is often initiated by a small amount of a free radical–forming reagent called (somewhat improperly) a "catalyst." A typical set of reactions for additional polymerization of a vinyl monomer would be as follows:

Initiation

Benzoyl peroxide   **Free radicals**   (1)

3

$$R^\cdot + C{=}C \underset{X}{|} \longrightarrow R{-}C{-}C^\cdot \underset{X}{|} \qquad (2)$$

Vinyl type of   **Start of**
monomer   **polymer chain**

A catalyst having a weak bond, such as benzoyl peroxide, fragments to give very reactive species called free radicals. One such free radical adds to the carbon-carbon double bond of a vinyl type of monomer (such as methylmethacrylate) and the polymer chain has begun.

Propagation

$$R{-}C{-}C{-}C{-}C^\cdot + C{=}C \longrightarrow R{-}({-}C{-}C{-})_2{-}C{-}C^\cdot \qquad (3)$$

$$R{-}({-}C{-}C{-})_n{-}C{-}C + C{=}C \rightarrow R{-}({-}C{-}C{-})_{n+1}{-}C{-}C^\cdot \qquad (4)$$

Polymer with a DP $= n + 1$ **Polymer with a DP $= n + 2$**

The nascent polymer chain continues its growth by successively adding more monomer units.

Transfer to species SH

$$R{-}({-}C{-}C{-})_{n-1}{-}C{-}C^\cdot + SH \longrightarrow R{-}({-}C{-}C{-}){-}H + S^\cdot \qquad (5)$$

$$S^\cdot + C{=}C \longrightarrow S{-}C{-}C^\cdot \qquad (6)$$

The growth of a particular chain might be interrupted by a transfer reaction. The particular transfer reagent, symbolically indicated as *SH*, might be a monomer molecule, solvent, impurity, catalyst, or other polymer molecule. In the latter case, the polymer is undergoing a *chain branching* reaction:

$$2\,R{-}({-}C{-}C{-})_n{-}C{-}C^\cdot \longrightarrow R{-}({-}C{-}C{-})_{2n+2}{-}R \qquad (7)$$

Ultimately two free radicals meet and mutually annihilate each other, thus terminating the growth of each particular radical.

It is particularly important to recognize that in the previously mentioned set of reactions the propagation or chain growth is competitive with the transfer and

POLYMERIC ASPECTS OF SOFT CONTACT LENSES

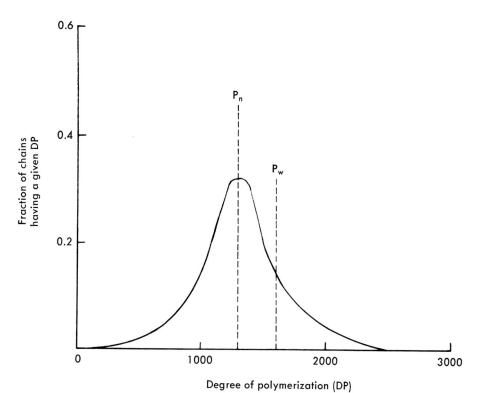

Fig. 1-1. Distribution of molecular weights.

termination reactions. This competition, occurring randomly at the molecular level, leads to a variety of degrees of polymerization for individual polymer molecules. This in turn leads to the concept of a *distribution of molecular weights* (or DP) for the polymer molecules produced in a given polymerization (Fig. 1-1). Unlike small molecules, a complete characterization of a given polymer sample can only be obtained if one specifies its average molecular weight and the breadth of the distribution. Even then, there must also be a specification with respect to the *linearity* of the polymer chain; if chain transfer to polymer has occurred (Formulas 5 and 6), the chain is said to be *branched* and nonlinear.

COPOLYMERIZATION

The above descriptions all apply to what might be called *homopolymers*, that is, polymers whose only one monomer has been used. If more than one monomer is used, *copolymerization* may be said to have occurred. Two types of copolymerizations are of importance: random and nonrandom.

In a random copolymerization of two monomers the copolymer chain produced can be represented as the result of a random coin-tossing process yielding heads, A, and tails, B, where one of the monomers is represented by A and the other by B. A typical chain might thus appear as

-A-A-A-B-B-A-B-B-B-B-A-B-A-B-A-A-A-   and so on.

The relative frequencies of A and B, as well as the sequence distributions, depend on the relative concentration of the monomers in the reaction and their unique chemical reactivities.

There are several types of nonrandom copolymerization. Of particular interest in this paper is the process known as *graft copolymerization*. A special case of the chain transfer reaction is shown in Formulas 5 and 6.

If monomer A is caused to polymerize in the presence of the polymer of a different monomer B, then the chain transfer to polymer B will cause the formation of a graft copolymer:

$$R^{\cdot} + (n + 1)A \longrightarrow R-(-A-)_n - A^{\cdot} \qquad (8)$$

$$R-(-A-)_n - A^{\cdot} + R-(-B-)_m - R \longrightarrow$$
$$R-(-A-)_{n+1} - H + R-(-B-)_x - \dot{B} - (-B-)_y - R$$

$$R-(-B-)_x - \dot{B} - (-B-)_y - R + (n + 1)A$$
$$\llcorner\!\!\rightarrow R-(-B-)_x - B-(-B-)_y - R$$
$$\diagdown (-A-)_n - A^{\cdot}$$

(where x + y + 1 = m)

The branched chain of growing polymer A on the chain of polymer B will then proceed as in Formulas 1-7.

Distinguishing between random and nonrandom copolymers is important because of the large difference in physical properties that can be obtained from two copolymers of identical composition but different arrangements of monomer units. To oversimply a bit, we can say that the random copolymer has properties that are intermediate between those of its parent homopolymers, whereas the nonrandom copolymer (as illustrated by a graft copolymer) may have some or all of the properties of its parents.

CROSS-LINKING

To stabilize the physical form of a polymeric material, it is sometimes desirable to introduce chemical bonds between different polymer chains. This may be done in the course of the polymerization reaction by copolymerizing with cross-linking monomer, or the formed polymer may be caused to cross-link by the action of some chemical or heat or some other energy source.

If a cross-linking monomer is copolymerized with an ordinary monomer, the reaction sequence includes the following unique steps:

$$2\ R^{\cdot} + (x + y)C{=}C + C{=}C \longrightarrow \qquad (9)$$
$$\qquad\qquad\quad | \qquad\quad |$$
$$\qquad\qquad\quad X \qquad\quad X$$
$$\qquad\qquad\qquad\qquad |$$
$$\qquad\qquad\qquad\qquad C{=}C$$

$$R-(-C-C-)_x-C-C-(-C-C-)_y-R$$

with X substituents, and a $C=C$ branch below the middle unit.

which when reacted with:

$$R-(-C-C-)_n-C-C^{\cdot}$$

yields a growing, branched polymer:

$$R-(-C-C-)_x-C-C-(-C-C-)_y-R$$

$$R-(-C-C-)_n-C-C-C-C^{\cdot}$$

which can further propagate.

Inclusion of a large number of cross-linking monomer units results in a network of polymer chains extending throughout the entire polymeric mass; in a sense, a highly cross-linked polymer sample, such as a rubber tire, is one molecule.

The foregoing descriptions of polymerization have used the addition polymerization of vinyl monomers as examples. For a full understanding of soft contact lenses the nature of the silicone lenses must also be included. These polymers are long-chain molecules also, but they are produced by *condensation* of silanols, which in turn are formed by hydrolysis of halosilanes:

$$Cl-\underset{R}{\overset{R}{Si}}-Cl \;+\; 2H_2O \;\longrightarrow\; HO-\underset{R}{\overset{R}{Si}}-OH \;+\; 2HCl$$

Halosilane   **Silanol**

$$n \; HO-\underset{R}{\overset{R}{Si}}-OH \;\longrightarrow\; HO-(-\underset{R}{\overset{R}{Si}}-O-)_n-H \;+\; (n-1)\,H_2O$$

Poly(siloxane)

The group R may be varied; — CH_3 is most common, and therefore these polymers are hydrophobic. It is possible to vary the group R, and by suitable choice one obtains a variety of copolymers, as well as cross-linking ability.

PHYSICAL PROPERTIES OF POLYMERS

The most important physical properties of a soft, polymeric contact lens can be grouped under the fundamental headings of solution behavior, flow (or rheology), and permeability. This relatively short list either explicitly or implicitly includes the important properties of lenses one could quickly list such as toughness, scratch resistance, flexibility, comfort, water content, oxygen or carbon dioxide diffusion rates, and so on. It does not include index of refraction for the simple reason that there is little variability possible among the many polymeric systems for this particular parameter. A refractive index value of 1.5 to 1.6 seems to cover most polymers; if a solvent (for example, water) is incorporated, the refractive index can be greatly changed, but only at the expense of changing other properties drastically.

Solution and swelling of polymers. If an un–cross-linked polymer is placed in a solvent capable of dissolving it, a viscous solution will result. If the solvent is a poor one, the polymer may imbibe some of the solvent and become plasticized. Solubility of a given polymer in a particular solvent can be improved by copolymerizing with another monomer whose homopolymer is quite soluble in the solvent (Fig. 1-2). Alternatively, graft copolymerization can also produce a marked change in solubility characteristics.

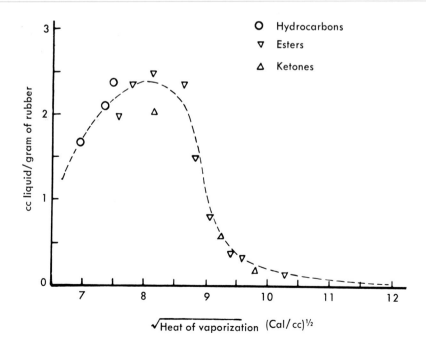

Fig. 1-2. Swelling of natural rubber in various solvents.

If a cross-linked polymer is placed in a good solvent, a solution is not produced. Instead, the polymer imbibes a limited (but sometimes large) amount of solvents, swells, and takes on the physical characteristics of a gel. The extent of swelling and the amount of solvent imbibed is rigorously determined by the physicochemical interactions between the solvent and the polymer, and by the extent of cross-linking. A measure of control over both of these factors exists in the polymerization (or copolymerization) process.

Rheological behavior. The single most important rheological characteristic of polymers is their tendency to flow or creep under a sustained load. The rate of creep for a given polymer may be decreased by lowering the temperature, by introducing monomer units that stiffen the polymer chain, or by cross-linking the polymer.

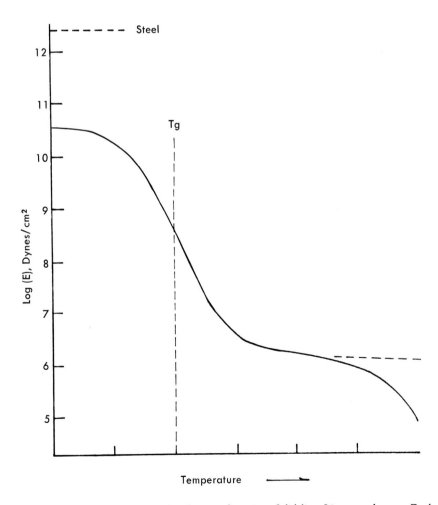

Fig. 1-3. Temperature dependence of polymer elasticity. *Solid line,* Linear polymer. *Dashed line,* Cross-linked polymer.

The stiffness of a polymeric material is often characterized by Young's modulus of elasticity, E, which is defined as the ratio of tensile stress to strain (or stretching load applied divided by dimensional change induced). The creep characteristic of polymers results in the modulus of elasticity being time dependent.

$$E = \frac{Force}{Change\ of\ length\ per\ unit\ of\ length}$$

Since the change of length will be an increase, E will decrease with time.

A plot characteristic of *all* linear, noncrystalline polymers (Fig. 1-3) shows graphically what our common experience indicates as the mechanical behavior of ordinary plastic materials. At low temperatures they are quite rigid and glassy, having a modulus of elasticity not too different from steel. As the temperature is raised, the modulus suddenly goes through a rapid change, or transitional region, in which the polymer has a leathery type of behavior. It is tough, but fairly flexible. This is called the "glass transition region," and may be characterized by a single temperature, T_g. With further increase in temperature, the polymer becomes rubbery in quality. The "rubbery plateau" is characterized by modulus, E, of about 10^7 dynes/cm.^{2}. If the polymer is heated beyond the rubbery state, it becomes molten and behaves like a very viscous liquid, losing all structural rigidity.

The temperatures range necessary for quantitative observation of these four distinct types of behavior may be quite large if all measurements are made by exactly the same technique. It was pointed out above that the measured modulus is a function of time; since it is also a function of temperature, this fact may be used to observe all regions. Fig. 1-4 shows plots of measurements of E for polymethylmethacrylate at a variety of temperatures as a function of time. Note that the time scale is logarithmic, and consider the task of the experimenter trying to obtain data that will yield equally spaced points on such a plot: the necessary time intervals might be after 1, 10, and 100 seconds, providing a hectic beginning to the experiment. The next reading might be 1,000 seconds, allowing time for a quick coffee break. This will be followed by a period of 10,000 seconds, which makes for a fairly leisurely afternoon. The problems of working in logarithmic time are thus seen to be quite different from those in linear time. It is fortunate, then, that the effects of time and temperature may be superimposed so that data may be gathered over a reasonable temperature interval without undue haste or excessive leisure.

Experiments that yield data such as those in Fig. 1-4 are known as creep or stress relaxation experiments. They may be performed by subjecting a sample to a constant load and measuring the changing strain or creep of the sample as a function of time, or maintaining a constant deformation or strain and following the decreasing amount of stress needed to maintain the strain. Either type of experiment may be performed quite simply in a crude fashion, but to obtain meaningful data, considerable refinement of technique is necessary. This refinement has sometimes taken the form of applying a time-variant load to the sample, in which case the frequency of application of the load determines the time scale of the measurement.

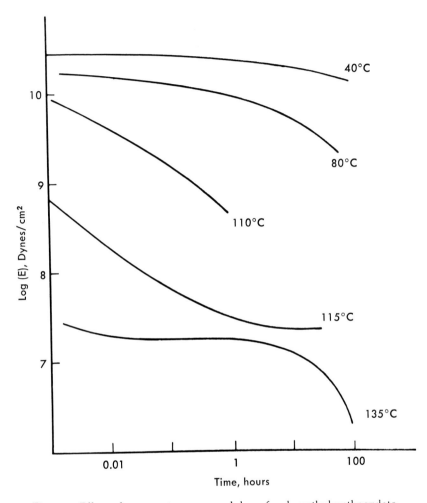

Fig. 1-4. Effect of temperature on modulus of polymethylmethacrylate.

The study of the phenomena involved in the various types of experiments is termed "rheology," which means the 'study of flow.' It is a particularly appropriate name since not only is the macroscopic flow of polymeric materials studied, but the microscopic interpretation of the observations is based on the flow of molecules past one another. In the glassy region, modulus is almost time independent, which is to say that there is no flow. The molecules are constrained by weak, short-range forces because of dipole interactions. These forces are too small to maintain most low molecular weight substances in a solid state, but the magnitude of the force per molecule becomes very great for high polymers. This results in the glassy state. As the polymer is warmed, it achieves sufficient kinetic energy to overcome a portion of these short-range forces and enters into the transition region, where short-range motions of segments of the polymer chains are possible. Ultimately, if the polymer is warmed enough, all the short-range forces will be overcome. The only constraint then placed upon the polymer is that of the chain entanglements. That these entanglements can hold the whole collection of chains together for fairly long time periods is readily apparent to anyone who has tried to untangle a snarled fishing line. But, just as the fishing line ultimately can be untangled, so, too, given time, can the polymer chains slide past one another and lose their entanglements. Since it is essentially a kinetic problem of the chains, it can be solved either by allowing them time or by giving them more kinetic energy, that is, raising the temperature. Thus the superposition of time and temperature effects mentioned above is seen to have a simple molecular explanation. Once the chains have slipped their entanglements, flow of the polymer mass is analogous to that of a liquid. The extreme lengths of the molecules makes this flow viscous.

If this viscous flow were allowed to occur, *no* polymer would have any structural integrity under stress for long time periods. Fortunately, cross-linking provides a perfect mechanism for preventing viscous flow. In a rheological sense cross-linking results in extending the rubbery plateau as shown by the dotted line in Fig. 1-3. High levels of cross-linking raise the value of E above that common to "rubber," whereas swelling of a cross-linked polymer by a solvent lowers E.

Permeability. The process of a small molecule passing from the exterior of one side of a membrane or film and emerging on the other side is termed "permeation." For permeation to occur in a material lacking the continuous holes or pores there must occur for the permeant the steps of solution in the membrane followed by diffusion through it. Permeability, P, for a given membrane-permeant is defined by

$$P = \frac{\text{Flow per unit time per unit area}}{\text{Permeant concentration difference across membrane divided by membrane thickness}} \tag{11}$$

The solubility, S, of the permeant in the film is given by

$$S = \frac{\text{Concentration of permeant in film's upper layer}}{\text{Concentration of permeant outside film}} \tag{12}$$

whereas the diffusivity, D, is given by Fick's first law

$$D = \frac{\text{Permeant flux across membrane}}{\text{Concentration gradient of permeant across membrane}} \tag{13}$$

One can show readily that

$$P = D \times S \tag{14}$$

Diffusion through a polymeric membrane that contains no pores or solvent occurs by an *activated* process that requires cooperative movements of many (10 to 20) segments of the polymer chain. This type of diffusion may be augmented if the membrane contains such a large amount of solvent that hydraulic flow occurs when a pressure is applied across the membrane. The flow changes exponentially with increase of water in hydrophilic materials according to recent work.

THEORY AND PRACTICE

There are basically two types of soft lenses that have been investigated so far: those achieving their softness because of the intrinsic properties of the material (low glass transition temperatures) and those whose softness is attributable to hydration of an otherwise glassy polymer. The best known example of the former are the silicone polymers, whereas the latter are exemplified by the Bausch & Lomb Soflens or the Griffin Naturalens. Since only the latter two are in commercial production, the following discussion is restricted to them.

The Bausch & Lomb lens is based on material originally developed by Professor O. Wichterle of the Macromolecular Research Institute in Prague. As originally described, it consisted of a homopolymer of hydroxyethylmethacrylate (HEMA) lightly cross-linked with ethylene glycol dimethacrylate (EDMA):

HEMA   **EDMA**

EDMA, when swollen in water, has an upper limit of about 45% water content (all percentages herein are based on wet weight).

The Griffin polymer is formed by polymerizing HEMA containing some EDMA and about 20% poly(N-vinylpyrrolidone) (PVP):

$$R-(-CH_2-CH-)_n-R$$

PVP

The PVP is probably present in the finished material as a graft copolymer with the lightly cross-linked poly(HEMA) and, as a result, cannot be extracted from the polymeric mass.

Besides the PVP content (and because of it) the most obvious (nonproprietary) difference between the Griffin and B & L materials is the higher water content of the Griffin lens. When soaked in normal saline, the Griffin materials contains 55% to 60% water (on a wet basis) compared to about 40% for the B & L material. Therefore, if one wishes to compare physical properties, the fundamentals stated above must all be related to the great difference in water content. In general, one would expect the Griffin lens (relative to the B & L lens) to be both more flexible and more susceptible to tearing for a given thickness because of a lower modulus of elasticity, and to have greater permeability because of the exponential dependence of flow on water content. (In actuality, minor modifications of both materials have undoubtedly been brought about by addition of small amounts of co-monomers in attempts to optimize these interdependent properties. Therefore, the first approximation of consideration of relative properties may need to be modified by the experience of practitioners.) The expectation of greater permeability of the Griffin lens is indeed sustained and it is a slightly weaker material, but any increased flexibility it may have does not seem to have adversely affected its optical properties, probably because of the careful design of the physical configuration of the lens, which was undertaken with its great flexibility in mind.

A number of properties of these hydrophilic materials that have been attributed to them by self-appointed experts need to be explicitly refuted. In particular, one may dogmatically state that there exists no *permanent* "pore" structure of a size large enough to permit the passage of a bacterium or virus particle. The

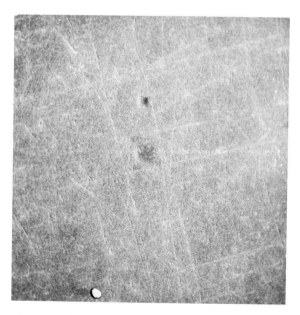

Fig. 1-5. Scanning electron microscope view of a gold-coated, fully hydrated Griffin lens. Indentations in the center are caused by focusing of electron beam. (× 1,000.)

segmented motion, described in the section on permeability, readily permits the diffusion of moderately large, water-soluble molecules (up to a molecular weight of about 500) but almost certainly prohibits the diffusion of contaminating bacteria into the lens. Fig. 1-5 shows a scanning electron microscope picture of a hydrated Griffin lens at a magnification sufficient to reveal any structure greater than 0.0001/cm. Obviously, none exists other than a few surface scratches.

Besides bacterial contamination, the "leaching out" of PVP during use has been attributed to the Griffin lens. Not only would any diffusive motion of the PVP be reduced to zero by the size of the PVP molecules (DP greater than 100) but also they are probably covalently bonded to the poly(HEMA) network because of chain transfer to the PVP occurring during the polymerization of HEMA.

Finally, visual acuity and wearing comfort that can be attained with the lens, as well as its strength and lasting qualities when used or abused by the patient, are strongly dependent on the relationship between the physical dimensions (or design) of the lens and the rheological properties of the polymer. It is inappropriate to view the lens as a single entity or a simple piece of material. The lens must be appreciated *in context as part of a system* that includes the eye, tears, lid action, and the lens and its design.

Future modifications of these materials and introduction of completely different ones are most probable. It is possible, given the necessary information from the manufacturer, for the fitter to use the principles set down here as a guide for his decision making, and, just as importantly, as the basis for feedback to the developers of material.

PART II
Corneal physiology under contact lenses

PART II
Corneal physiology under contact lenses

Chapter 2

Corneal physiology under
contact lenses

Saiichi Mishima, M.D.

Twenty years have passed since the classical work of G. K. Smelser,[1] who demonstrated unequivocally that the corneal opacity after wearing a tight-fitting contact lens was caused by prevention of corneal uptake of atmospheric oxygen. Ever since, technical improvements in the field of contact lens engineering and fitting seem to have overcome most of the early troubles related to corneal respiration. Further knowledge on the corneal metabolism and respiration has also been accumulated, and our understanding on the corneal physiology related to the contact lens has become deeper than ever. In recent years, precise data on the corneal respiration became available and experiments have been done on subtle corneal changes from contact lens wearing. At this point, it seems worthwhile to review these recent works and to try to understand how the cornea behaves under a contact lens. Such undertaking also seems valuable for understanding corneal behavior in relation to hydrophilic contact lenses.

CORNEAL METABOLISM AND RESPIRATION

Supply and metabolism of glucose. Since energy necessary for corneal integrity is derived from glucose metabolism, the supply of glucose is of prime importance. The following three possible routes of supply may be considered: (1) from the tears across the corneal epithelium, (2) from the limbal vessels, and (3) from the aqueous humor across the corneal endothelium. To find out which one of these routes plays the major role, one should know glucose concentrations in the structures concerned. Fig. 2-1 depicts such concentrations, which were calculated from the data of Reim and co-workers.[2] The very low concentration in the tears seems to rule out the tears as the major route of supply. Very low epithelial permeability to monosaccharides substantiates this conclusion.[3] The contribution of the limbal vessels may be calculated from diffusion coefficients of glucose in corneal stroma and its permeability across the endothelium. Maurice[4,5] concluded from such calculation that glucose supply from the limbal vessels extends only to the peripheral cornea about 1 mm. from the limbus (Fig. 2-2). Therefore the central cornea receives glucose almost exclusively from the aqueous humor.

The uptake of glucose from the aqueous humor was recently determined for rabbit cornea to be approximately 90 μg. per hour per cm.^{2}.[6] Such high rate of glucose uptake could by no means be explained only by diffusion, which was calculated by using assumed endothelial permeability to glucose and the concen-

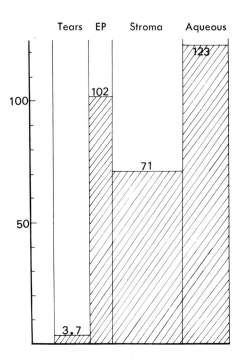

Fig. 2-1. Glucose concentration (mg./dl.) in tears, epithelium **(EP)**, corneal stroma, and aqueous humor. (From data of Reim, M., Lax, F., Lichte, H., and Turss, R.: Steady state levels of glucose in the different layers of the cornea, aqueous humor, blood and tears in vivo, Ophthalmologica **154:**39, 1967.)

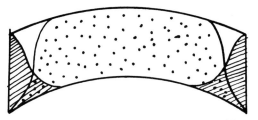

Fig. 2-2. Supply of glucose to cornea. *Dotted part,* From aqueous humor. *Hatched part,* From limbal vessels. (From Maurice, D. M.: Anatomia e fisiologia della cornea trapiantata. Simposia sulla cheratoplastica, Atti Soc. Ottalmol. Lombarda, Fasc. II, p. 97, 1963.)

tration gradient.[5] Recently, conclusive evidence was reported to show the presence of a facilitated or active transport of glucose across the corneal endothelium.[7,8] The high uptake rate could thus be explained only on the basis of the facilitated transport and the additional diffusional flux across the corneal endothelium.

The supply of glucose and its utilization are in balance under normal conditions, and glucose concentration in corneal tissue maintains a constant level, with part of it (glycogen) stored mostly in the epithelium. Since the epithelium comprises the major part of the corneal cellular element, most glucose is metabolized

Table 2-1. Oxygen uptake by the corneal layers of rabbit*

Corneal layer	O_2, 37° C.
Epithelium	4.8
Stroma	0.76
Endothelium	6.0
(μl. of O_2 per hour per mg. of dry weight)	

*From Kohra, T.: On the metabolism of the cornea, Acta Soc. Ophthal. Jap. **39:**1429, 1935.

in this cellular layer. Combustion of glucose occurs via two pathways.[9] The hexose-monophosphate shunt mechanism was shown to be active in the corneal epithelium, and the amount of glucose utilized by this direct oxidative mechanism was reported to be about 35% or even 70% of glucose used.[10-12] The rest is metabolized by glycolysis, which is linked under aerobic conditions to the tricarboxylic acid (TCA) cycle, giving carbon dioxide and water as final products. In the cornea, glycolysis is effective, and even under the presence of enough oxygen, some amount of lactate is accumulated.[9] Under anoxic conditions, only glycolysis takes place, leading to an accumulation of lactate. Since synthetic activity of glycogen is inhibited, the glycogen store is depleted.

Because of the mode of glucose supply mentioned above, covering the corneal surface with a contact lens will not interfere with the uptake of glucose by the cornea. However, it interferes with oxygen uptake, and the subsequent anaerobic condition alters the normal metabolic chain of the cornea.

Uptake of oxygen. Utilization of atmospheric oxygen by the cornea was first reported by Fischer.[13] A recent polarographic determination gave a rate of oxygen uptake by the living human cornea to be about 4.8 μl. per hour per cm.[2],[14] The respiration of the excised cornea was studied by Kohra[15] using the Warburg technique; and his results on rabbit cornea are summarized in Table 2-1. Many later investigators gave similar results for various species. One cm.[2] of human corneal epithelium has approximately 1 mg. of dry weight, and the result shown in Table 2-1 corresponds to an oxygen flux of 4.8 μl. per hour per cm.[2] at the corneal surface. The excellent correlation between in vivo and in vitro studies indicates that most of oxygen taken up from the atmosphere is consumed by the epithelium.

Supply of oxygen to the tissue occurs because oxygen is dissolved in it, depending on the partial pressure, and diffuses in the tissue according to the concentration gradient, that is, partial pressure gradient. The consumption and supply are in balance so that the oxygen pressure in the tissue must be at a steady state. Such a steady-state gradient of oxygen partial pressure in the cornea was calculated by Fatt and Bieber.[16] Their results are shown in Figs. 2-3 and 2-4.

When the eye is open, the precorneal tear film is in contact with the atmosphere and the oxygen partial pressure at the corneal surface is 155 mm. Hg. This pressure then decreases toward the deeper layers of the cornea. The anterior chamber receives oxygen from iris circulation and its oxygen partial pressure has been measured to be approximately 55 mm. Hg.[17-20] When the eye is closed, the corneal surface must receive oxygen from the conjunctival circulation and therefore the oxygen

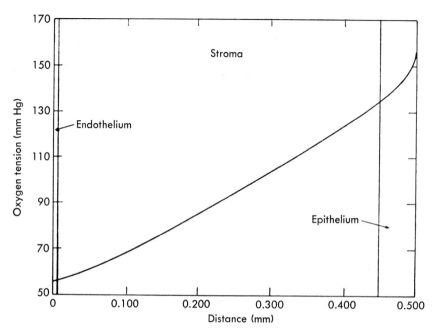

Fig. 2-3. Steady-state partial pressure of oxygen in the cornea when the eye is open. (From Fatt, I., and Bieber, M. T.: The steady state distribution of oxygen and carbon dioxide in the in vivo cornea. I. The open eye in air and the closed eye, Exp. Eye Res. **7:**103, 1968.)

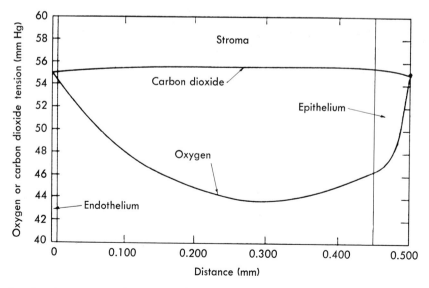

Fig. 2-4. Steady-state partial pressure of oxygen in the cornea when the eye is closed. (From Fatt, I., and Bieber, M. T.: The steady state distribution of oxygen and carbon dioxide in the in vivo cornea. I. The open eye in air and the closed eye, Exp. Eye Res. **7:**103, 1968.)

partial pressure of the corneal surface becomes equal to that of the conjunctival tissue (55 mm. Hg).

When the cornea is covered with a contact lens and its access to oxygen prevented, the oxygen partial pressure in the epithelium will be rapidly reduced to zero because of active consumption by the tissue. However, the oxygen pressure at the endothelial surface is not affected and remains at a normal level.[17] Under this condition, oxygen supplied to the epithelium from the anterior chamber is only[21] 0.36 μl. per hour per cm.[2] and this amount can by no means meet the requirement of the epithelium.[17]

Corneal changes in anoxia. The corneal epithelium takes up oxygen from the atmosphere, and the endothelium takes up oxygen from iris circulation via the aqueous humor. For contact lens wearing, therefore, anoxia to the corneal epithelium is of immediate concern.[21]

Smelser[1] demonstrated for the first time that atmospheric oxygen is necessary for the maintenance of the optical property of the cornea. He applied tight-fitting goggles on human subjects and filled the space in front of the eye with various gases. The halo from the epithelial edema was seen only when oxygen was absent. Corneal clouding after wearing of the contact lens was shown to be caused by corneal oxygen deprivation and holes in the contact lens to facilitate oxygen supply prevented the clouding. A biochemical study showed that atmospheric oxygen was necessary to prevent an accumulation of lactate in the cornea.[22] Contact lens wear in animals thus leads to an accumulation of lactate, disappearance of glycogen

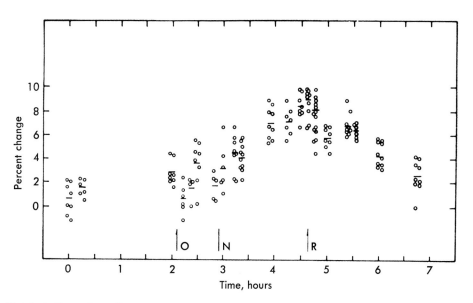

Fig. 2-5. Corneal swelling (percent change) due to anoxia to the corneal surface. **O,** Goggle on. **N,** Nitrogen in front of cornea. **R,** Goggle removed. Original corneal thickness was 0.49 mm. (From Mandell, R. B., Polse, K. A., and Fatt, I.: Corneal swelling caused by contact lens wear, Arch. Ophthal. **83:**3, 1970.)

store, swelling of the corneal epithelium, and finally to an impairment of corneal transparency.[23,24]

Since the aerobic metabolism is indispensable for the cornea to maintain its deturgescent state and hence its transparency, the above anaerobic alteration of the corneal metabolism leads to a corneal swelling.[25] When tight-fitting goggles were applied to human subjects and the space was filled with wet nitrogen, the cornea swelled by about 8%, and the swelling was reversed by removing the goggles (Fig. 2-5). What then is the critical oxygen partial pressure in preventing the corneal swelling and clouding? This question was studied by using similar goggles and gases having various levels of oxygen partial pressure.[26] This investigation indicated that the critical partial pressure to be 11.4 to 19 mm. Hg. If the oxygen partial pressure in the tear film is lower than this level, the cornea swells. This swelling up to about 8% may be explained mostly by epithelial swelling, which comprises about 10% of the total corneal thickness.

What then is the effect of the endothelial anoxia on the corneal thickness? Excised rabbit cornea was clamped in a Plexiglas chamber and incubated at a body temperature with the endothelial surface bathed by an artificial medium known to maintain normal corneal thickness under an aerobic condition.[27] When the medium was bubbled with nitrogen, while the corneal surface was covered with moist air, the cornea swelled at a much higher rate than in the case of the epithelial anoxia. Under total anoxia of the cornea, a similar swelling was observed, but this swelling could be stopped or even reversed by reoxygenating the endothelial surface to an oxygen pressure of 55 mm. Hg (Fig. 2-6). The aerobic condition of

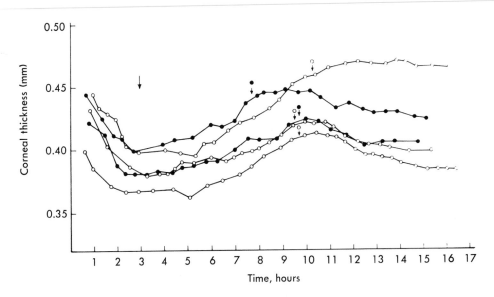

Fig. 2-6. Effect of endothelial anoxia to corneal swelling. *First arrow,* Beginning of anoxic condition. *Circles with small arrow,* Reoxygenation of endothelial surface. (From Mishima, S., Kaye, G. I., Takahasi, G. H., Kudo, T., and Trenberth, S. M.: The function of the corneal endothelium in the regulation of corneal hydration. In Longham, M. E., editor: The cornea, Baltimore, 1969, The Johns Hopkins Press, p. 207.)

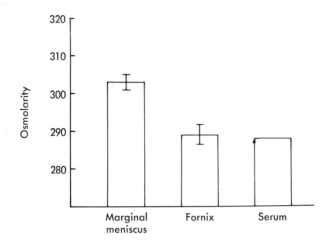

Fig. 2-7. Osmolarity (milliosmoles per liter) of tears. (From Mishima, S., Kubota, Z., and Farris, R. L.: Tear flow dynamics in normal and keratoconjunctivitis sicca cases, XXI Concilium Ophthal. Acta, part II, 1801, 1970.)

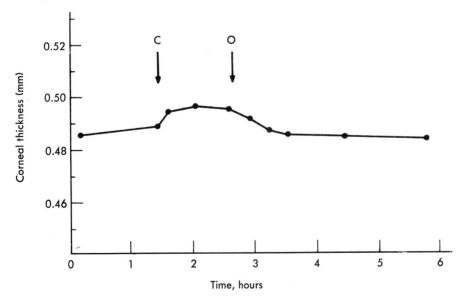

Fig. 2-8. Thickness change of human cornea on opening, **O,** and closing, **C,** the eye. (From Mishima, S.: Some physiological aspects of the precorneal tear film, Arch. Ophthal. **73:**233, 1965.)

Table 2-2. Tear osmolarity and the corneal thickness before and after contact lens wear*

	Before	After 8 hours of contact lens wear
Tear osmolarity (% NaCl)	0.91 ± 0.06†	0.92 ± 0.06
Corneal thickness	0.504 ± 0.023	0.530 ± 0.023

*From Farris, R. L., Kubota, Z., and Mishima, S.: Epithelial decompensation with corneal contact lens wear, Arch. Ophthal. **85**:651, 1971.
†Mean ± standard deviation.

the endothelium is thus shown to be indispensable for the prevention of the stromal swelling. Covering the corneal surface, however, has no effect on the oxygen supply to the endothelium and contact lens wearing will not cause serious stromal swelling.

HARD CONTACT LENSES AND THE CORNEA

Some corneal swelling is known to occur after wearing contact lenses, even if they are well fitted. Two possible reasons for this may be considered: (1) change of the tear osmolarity and (2) oxygen deprivation.

Tear osmolarity and the corneal thickness. When one wears corneal contact lenses for the first time, usually a lacrimation is induced and the tear osmolarity is lowered, leading to corneal swelling.[28] Such change of tear osmolarity is now considered. When the eye is open, an evaporation makes the tear osmolarity higher than when the eye is closed. A microcryoscopic determination indicated that the tears in the meniscus at the lid margin had higher osmolarity by about 5% than the tears in the fornix, which was isosmolar with the serum (Fig. 2-7).[29] The cornea was found to be thinner in open and thicker in closed eyes (Fig. 2-8); the difference of thickness is less than 4% and this difference can be explained by the difference of the tear osmolarity[30] shown above. Consequently, one may attribute any corneal swelling more than this range to other causes than the tear osmolarity (for example, most likely oxygen deprivation).

When patients are well adapted to wearing contact lenses, lacrimation is not extensive, since microcryoscopic determination failed to show any significant difference of the tear osmolarity before and after wearing contact lenses (Table 2-2).[31] Nevertheless, a significant increase of the corneal thickness was found, and this must be related to hypoxic conditions of the cornea.

Hypoxia and corneal changes. An increase in corneal thickness and occurrence of epithelial edema have taken place after wearing hard contact lenses.[32] Such changes are more pronounced in beginners and become less in patients adapted well to the lenses. Such adaptation was reported by many investigators and an example is shown in Fig. 2-9.[25,31,32]

To know if the increase in corneal thickness is related to oxygen deprivation, Farris and co-workers[31] made polarographic determinations of oxygen uptake by the cornea on patients, before and after contact lens wear. Even though these patients adapted well to the contact lenses, a significant increase of oxygen uptake

CORNEAL PHYSIOLOGY UNDER CONTACT LENSES

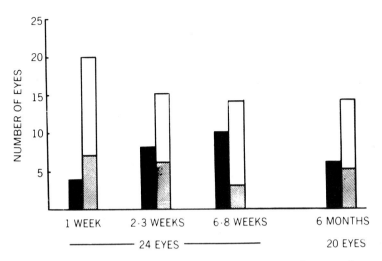

Fig. 2-9. Incidence of corneal thickness changes after 8 hours of contact lens wear. *Solid bars,* Less than 0.010 mm. *Hatched bars,* 0.010 to 0.019 mm. *Open bars,* More than 0.020 mm. (From Farris, R. L., Kubota, Z., Mishima, S.: Epithelial decompensation with corneal contact lens wear, Arch. Ophthal. **85:**651, 1971.)

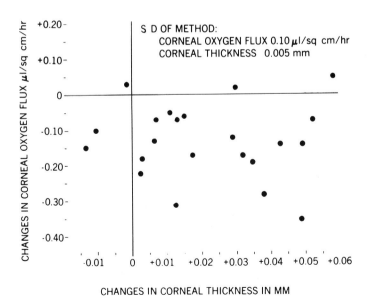

Fig. 2-10. Change of corneal thickness after 8 hours of contact lens wear and the oxygen uptake 10 minutes after lens removal. **S D,** Standard deviation. (From Farris, R. L., Kubota, Z., Mishima, S.: Epithelial decompensation with corneal contact lens wear, Arch. Ophthal. **85:**651, 1971.)

was found immediately after 8 hours of contact lens wear, indicating that a hypoxic condition of the cornea had been present. Ten minutes after the lens removal, however, a reduction of oxygen uptake was detected, suggesting a lowered activity of the corneal epithelium. A good correlation was found between the rate of oxygen uptake 10 minutes after the lens removal and the increase of corneal thickness (Fig. 2-10). One may therefore conclude that corneal swelling after wearing hard contact lenses is attributable to subnormal epithelial activity caused by oxygen deprivation. When pronounced increase of corneal thickness was found, the epithelium showed some edema; such corneal edema was previously shown to be associated with the subnormal oxygen uptake of the corneal epithelium.[33] After removal of the contact lens the edema disappears rapidly.

TEARS UNDER HARD CONTACT LENSES

If the hard contact lens covers the cornea without any movement, oxygen dissolved in the tears under the lens is consumed very rapidly. Table 2-3 shows such a typical hard contact lens; the amount of oxygen contained initially in the tear volume of about 2 μl. is calculated to be $1.1 \times 10^2 \mu$l., which will be consumed completely in 14 seconds. Lateral diffusion of oxygen from the edge of the contact lens was shown to be ineffective.[34] Therefore, frequent movement of the lens and subsequent tear exchange are mandatory for comfortable lens wearing. In this section the mechanism of tear exchange, rate of blinking, and oxygen partial pressure under the lens are considered.

Tear exchange. Fluorescein staining of tears under a hard contact lens reveals the presence of a tear reservoir around the lens corresponding to the beveled edge. With a slit lamp microscope, one can observe a flow of small particles in this tear reservoir, which is connected to the meniscus at the lid margin; this observation suggests that the tear reservoir around the lens is being constantly exchanged. At the time of blink movement, one can notice communication of the tear reservoir with the tears under the lens, where a vigorous stirring of small particles can be seen. The tear exchange seems to occur by a pumping of tears from the reservoir, with the pumping action being created by lens movement. Such lens movement and subsequent pressure change under the lens is depicted in Fig. 2-11. When a small hole is bored at the center of the lens and the change of the tear meniscus in the hole is observed, a pressure change under the lens becomes obvious. When

Table 2-3. Consumption of oxygen contained in the tears under the contact lens

Lens diameter	8 mm.
Base curve	7.6 mm.
Corneal curvature	7.65 mm.
Tear volume	About 2 μl.
Total O_2 (155 mm. Hg)	$1.1 \times 10^{-2} \mu$l.
Corneal area	55 mm.^{2}
Rate of consumption	$7.7 \times 10^{-4} \mu$l./sec.
O_2	Decrease to zero in 14 seconds

the upper lid drags the lens upward, it also moves the lens away from the cornea, creating a negative pressure under the lens. The tears in the reservoir around the lens are sucked into the space under the lens. When the eye is wide open, the lens moves down and toward the cornea, creating a positive pressure under the lens; and an excess of tears under the lens is then pushed out. At every blink movement, the above cycle of pumping action is repeated. For this mode of tear exchange, enough amount of tear reservoir at the beveled edge is very important,

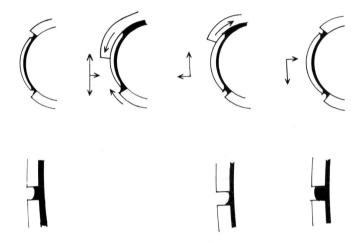

Fig. 2-11. Movement of corneal contact lens *(arrow)* on blink movement. Change of tear meniscus in the hole of the contact lens, corresponding to the blink movement.

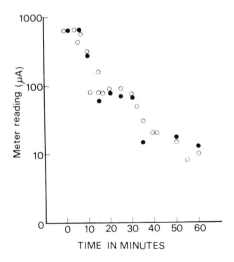

Fig. 2-12. Change of fluorescein concentration, by time, in the tears under contact lens *(solid circles)* and in the meniscus at lid margin *(open circles).* Concentration is expressed arbitrarily by meter reading.

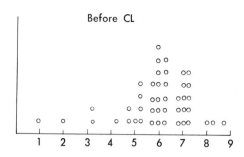

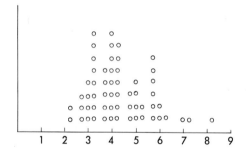

Fig. 2-13. Diagram of blink intervals before and after the contact lens wear **(CL).** *Abscissa,* Seconds.

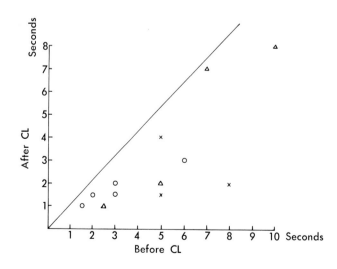

Fig. 2-14. Change of peak blink interval before and with contact lens wear. *Open circles,* 30 minutes of contact lens wear. *Crosses,* 1 to 2 hours. *Triangles,* 5 to 9 hours.

and in cases of reduced tears, that is, in dry eye conditions, the corneal contact lens creates troubles.[32]

One may ask then to what extent the tear exchange occurs in well-fitted contact lenses. For study of the effectiveness of the tear exchange, the tears were stained with fluorescein and the concentrations under the contact lens as well as at the lid margin were followed at intervals (Fig. 2-12). The same rate of concentration decay was obtained at both places, suggesting a fairly effective exchange of tears.

Blink intervals. The effectiveness of the tear exchange depends not only on the condition of the tears but also on the frequency of blink movement. The blink interval was, therefore, determined for subjects who were well adapted to their

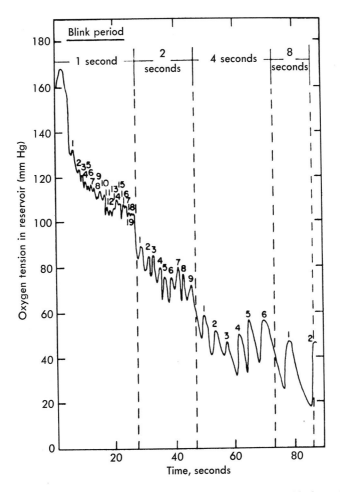

Fig. 2-15. Change of oxygen partial pressure under contact lens by blinking. Tear volume under lens, 5.8 μl. Area-volume ratio, 135.5. (From Fatt, I., and Hill, R. M.: Oxygen tension under a contact lens during blinking—a comparison of theory and experimental observation, Amer. J. Optom. **47:**50, 1970.)

corneal contact lenses. An example of the diagram of blink interval is given in Fig. 2-13. In this particular case, the peak interval is found at 6 seconds before and at 3.5 seconds with the contact lens; the blink interval is definitely shortened by wearing the contact lens. Such determination of the peak blink interval was done on 12 cases, and the results are plotted in Fig. 2-14. In all cases, the blink interval is shorter with the lens than without the lens; and the average blink interval before the lens was 4.8 seconds and with the lens 2.9 seconds. From the point of view of tear exchange, the shorter blink interval is beneficial.

Partial pressure of oxygen under hard contact lenses. The blink movement brings new tears under the contact lens and should raise the oxygen partial pressure available. During the blink interval, the partial pressure of oxygen under the contact lens reduces rapidly, and therefore it must be changing in a wavy fashion during the contact lens wear. The level of the oxygen pressure should depend on the volume of the tears under the lens, the amount of the tear exchange per blink, the area of the cornea concerned, the blink interval, and the rate of oxygen consumption by the cornea.[35,36] Fatt and Hill determined such undulation of oxygen pressure by applying a micropolarographic electrode to a contact lens.[36] One example is shown in Fig. 2-15, where lower steady-state oxygen level by prolonged blink interval is obvious. In Fig. 2-16 the oxygen pressure is plotted as a function of the blink interval, the corneal area, and the tear volume under the lens. In their experiments, the oxygen pressure corresponded to the amount of tear exchange of

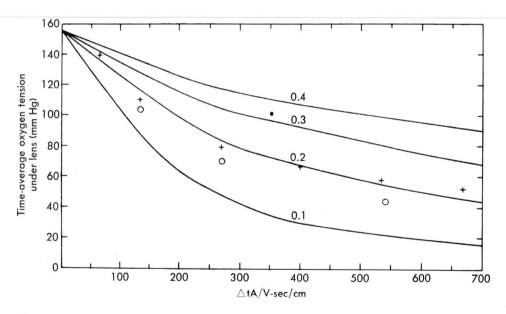

Fig. 2-16. Average steady-state oxygen pressure under contact lens and blink interval (Δt), area of contact lens (**A**), tear volume under lens (**V**). Numbers are rate of tear exchange per blink. Circles and crosses are experimental values. (From Fatt, I., and Hill, R. M.: Oxygen tension under a contact lens during blinking—a comparison of theory and experimental observation, Amer. J. Optom. 47:50, 1970.)

about 20% per each blink. In case of a typical corneal contact lens shown in Table 2-3, the oxygen pressure may be calculated to be about 45 to 50 mm. Hg for a blink interval of 3 seconds and tear exchange of 20% per blink. Therefore, in cases of well-fitted lenses and well-adapted persons, supply of oxygen to the cornea may be considered reasonably good. If, however, the blink interval is long or blink movement is too weak to produce enough tear exchange, a hypoxic condition of the cornea is the inevitable result and the patients must be looked after carefully.

HYDROPHILIC CONTACT LENSES AND OXYGEN

Most of the hydrophilic contact lenses are larger than the cornea and the lens is fixed at its periphery on the corneal limbus or the pericorneal conjunctiva. Under this condition tear exchange under the lens is not as effective as in hard contact

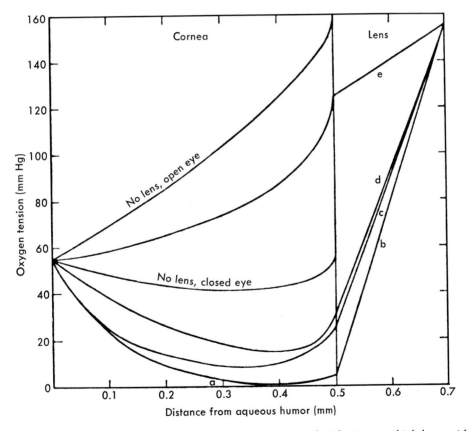

Fig. 2-17. Steady-state oxygen pressure in the cornea covered with 0.2 mm. thick lens, with different oxygen transmissibility. Eye is open. Oxygen transmissibility: **a,** 0; **b,** 0.04 × 10^{-10}; **c,** 1.0 × 10^{-10}; **d,** 3.0 × 10^{-10}; **e,** 50 × 10^{-10} cm^2 ml. O$_2$/sec. ml. mm. Hg. (From Fatt, I., Bieber, M. T., and Pye, S. D.: Steady state distribution of oxygen and carbon dioxide in the in vivo cornea of an eye covered by a gas-permeable contact lens, Amer. J. Optom. **46:**3, 1969.)

lenses, and therefore the cornea will become anoxic unless the lens allows oxygen to permeate through its material. The oxygen permeability of commercially available hydrophilic lenses was determined by Fatt and St. Helen[37] and also by Edelhauser.[38] They found that the material is indeed permeable to oxygen, although some difference between the materials was found.

One may now ask what the steady-state partial pressure of oxygen in the cornea will be when such hydrophilic contact lenses are worn. No direct determinations have been done, but the oxygen pressure level may be calculated by using the transmissibility of the lens material to oxygen and the known rate of corneal consumption. Such calculation was done by Fatt and others[39] and the data are given in Fig. 2-17 for the lens thickness of 0.2 mm. In the case of commercially available hydrophilic lenses, the oxygen pressure varies along a line between *c* and *d* in the figure. When the lens becomes thicker, the oxygen pressure in the cornea is, of course, reduced. However, one should remember that the data are for lenses tightly covering the cornea without any movement and that oxygen is

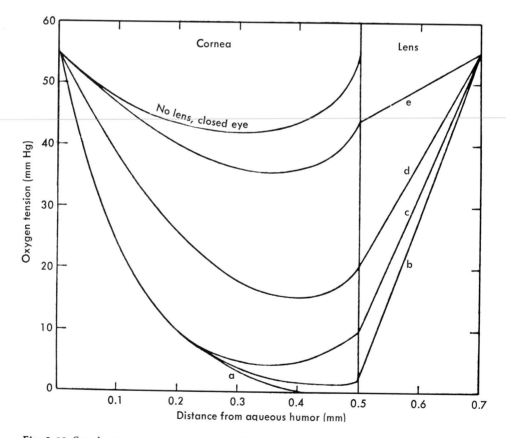

Fig. 2-18. Steady-state oxygen pressure in the cornea covered with 0.2 mm. thick lens, with different oxygen transmissibility. Eye is closed. Oxygen transmissibility is as in Fig. 2-17. (From Fatt, I., Bieber, M. T., and Pye, S. D.: Steady state distribution of oxygen and carbon dioxide in the in vivo cornea of an eye covered by a gas-permeable contact lens, Amer. J. Optom. **46:**3, 1969.)

supplied by diffusion only. In practice, there is a space between the lens and the cornea; the blink movement produces pumping action of the lens so that the tears are exchanged under the lens. Such pump action and the change of pressure under the lens subsequent to the blink movement can readily be seen by watching a small air bubble occasionally trapped under the lens. The pumping of the tears should increase oxygen supply to the cornea, and the oxygen pressure level in the cornea is expected to be reasonably high. Comfort of wearing hydrophilic contact lenses is therefore explained by good oxygen supply to the cornea, in addition to the hydrophilic nature of the material.

When the eye is closed, the oxygen pressure in the cornea can be reduced below the critical level of 11.4 to 19 mm. Hg (Fig. 2-18), if oxygen were to be supplied by diffusion only. Successful continuous wearing of hydrophilic lenses during sleep may be attributable to tear exchange under the lens subsequent to unconscious eye movement and blink movement occurring during the sleep. Be warned, however, that such mechanism of tear exchange may have individual variation and that uninterrupted wearing of lenses thicker than 0.2 mm. needs individual attention.

REFERENCES

1. Smelser, G. K.: Relation of factors involved in the maintenance of optical properties of cornea to contact-lens wear, Arch. Ophthal. **47**:328, 1952.
2. Reim, M., Lax, F., Lichte, H., and Turss, R.: Steady state levels of glucose in the different layers of the cornea, aqueous humor, blood and tears in vivo, Ophthalmologica **154**:39, 1967.
3. Mishima, S., Hattori, E., and Yamanouchi, H.: In vivo determination of the corneal permeability, Acta Soc. Ophthal. 75(suppl.):198, 1971.
4. Maurice, D. M.: Anatomia e fisiologia della cornea trapiantata. Simposia sulla cheratoplastica, Atti Soc. Ottalmol. Lombarda, Fasc. II, p. 97, 1963.
5. Maurice, D. M.: The cornea and sclera. In Davson, H., editor: The eye, ed. 2, New York, 1969, Academic Press Inc., vol. 1, p. 489.
6. Riley, M. V.: Glucose and oxygen utilization by the rabbit cornea, Exp. Eye Res. **8**:193, 1969.
7. Hale, P. N., and Maurice, D. M.: Sugar transport across the corneal endothelium, Exp. Eye Res. **8**:205, 1969.
8. Mishima, S., and Hayakawa, M.: The function of the corneal endothelium in relation to corneal dehydration and nutrition. Jerusalem Seminar on Prevention of Blindness, proceedings, 1971. (In press.)
9. Kinoshita, J. H.: Some aspects of the carbohydrate metabolism of the cornea, Invest. Ophthal. **1**:178, 1962.
10. Kinoshita, J. H., and Masurat, T.: The direct oxidative carbohydrate cycle of bovine corneal epithelium, Arch. Biochem. **53**:9, 1954.
11. Kinoshita, J. H., and Masurat, T.: Aerobic pathways of glucose metabolish in bovine corneal epithelium, Amer. J. Ophthal. **48**:47, 1959.
12. Kuhlman, R. E., and Resnik, R. A.: The oxydation of ^{14}C-labelled glucose and lactate by the rabbit cornea, Arch. Biochem. **85**:29, 1959.
13. Fisher, F. P.: Ueber den Gasaustausch der Hornhaut mit der Luft, Arch. Augenheilk. **102**:146, 1930.
14. Hill, R. N., and Fatt, I.: Oxygen uptake from a reservoir of limited volume by the human cornea in vivo, Science **142**:1295, 1963.
15. Kohra, T.: On the metabolism of the cornea, Acta Soc. Ophthal. Jap. **39**:1429, 1935.

16. Fatt, I., and Bieber, M. T.: The steady state distribution of oxygen and carbon dioxide in the in vivo cornea. I. The open eye in air and the closed eye, Exp. Eye Res. **7**:103, 1968.
17. Friedenwald, J. S., and Pierce, H. F.: Circulation of the aqueous. VI. Intraocular gas exchange, Arch. Ophthal. **17**:477, 1937.
18. Drenckhahn, D. O., and Lorenzen, U. K.: Der Sauerstoffdruck in der Vorderkammer des Auges und die Geschwindigkeit des Sauerstoffsattigung des Kammerwassers, Graefe Arch. Ophthal. **160**:378, 1958.
19. Kleifeld, O., and Neumann, H. G.: Die Sauerstoffgehalt des menschlichen Kammerwassers, Klin. Mbl. Augenheilk. **135**:224, 1959.
20. Kleifeld, O., and Hockwin, O.: Der Sauerstoffgehalt des menschlichen Kammerwassers nach Beatmung, Klin. Mbl. Augenheilk. **139**:513, 1961.
21. Hill, R. M., and Fatt, I.: Oxygen deprivation of the cornea by contact lenses and lid closure, Amer. J. Optom. **41**:678, 1954.
22. Langham, M. E.: Glycolysis in the cornea of the rabbit, J. Physiol. **126**:396, 1954.
23. Smelser, G. K., and Ozanics, V.: Structural changes in the corneas of guinea pigs after wearing contact lenses, Arch. Ophthal. **49**:335, 1953.
24. Smelser, G. K., and Chen, D. K.: Physiological changes in the cornea induced by contact lenses, Arch. Ophthal. **53**:676, 1955.
25. Mandell, R. B., Polse, K. A., and Fatt, I.: Corneal swelling caused by contact lens wear, Arch. Ophthal. **83**:3, 1970.
26. Polse, K. A., and Mandell, R. B.: Critical oxygen tension at the corneal surface, Arch. Ophthal. **84**:505, 1970.
27. Mishima, S., Kaye, G. I., Takahasi, G. H., Kudo, T., and Trenberth, S. M.: The function of the corneal endothelium in the regulation of corneal hydration. In Langham, M. E., editor: The cornea, Baltimore, 1969, The Johns Hopkins Press, p. 207.
28. Kinsey, V. E.: An explanation of the corneal haze and halos produced by contact lenses, Amer. J. Ophthal. **35**:691, 1952.
29. Mishima, S., Kubota, Z., and Farris, R. L.: Tear flow dynamics in normal and keratoconjunctivitis sicca cases, XXI Concilium Ophthal. Acta, part II, 1801, 1970.
30. Mishima, S.: Some physiological aspects of the precorneal tear film, Arch. Ophthal. **73**:233, 1965.
31. Farris, R. L., Kubota, Z., and Mishima, S.: Epithelial decompensation with corneal contact lens wear, Arch. Ophthal. **85**:651, 1971.
32. Girard, L. J.: Corneal contact lenses, ed. 2, St. Louis, 1970, The C. V. Mosby Co.
33. Hill, R. M., and Schoessler, J.: Epithelial edema: Respiratory characteristics of the lesion, Amer. J. Optom. **45**:241, 1968.
34. Hill, R. M.: Respiratory profiles of the corneal epithelium. 1. Control profiles and effects of the non-aperature lens, Amer. J. Optom. **43**:233, 1966.
35. Fatt, I.: Oxygen tension under a contact lens during blinking, Amer. J. Optom. **46**:662, 1969.
36. Fatt, I., and Hill, R. M.: Oxygen tension under a contact lens during blinking—a comparison of theory and experimental observation, Amer. J. Optom. **47**:50, 1970.
37. Fatt, I., and Helen, R. S.: Oxygen tension under an oxygen-permeable contact lens, Amer. J. Optom. **48**:545, 1971.
38. Edelhauser, H. F.: Oxygen, calcium, lactate, chloride, and sodium permeability of soft contact lenses. See Chapter 3.
39. Fatt, I., Bieber, M. T., and Pye, S. D.: Steady state distribution of oxygen and carbon dioxide in the in vivo cornea of an eye covered by a gas-permeable contact lens, Amer. J. Optom. **46**:3, 1969.

Chapter 3

Oxygen, calcium, lactate, chloride, and sodium permeability of soft contact lenses

Henry F. Edelhauser, Ph.D., and Dennis R. Morrison, Ph.D.

Recent popularity and the clinical testing of hydrophilic soft contact lenses has created a need for basic information on the lens permeability of essential metabolites and ions critical for corneal homeostasis. This basic information is necessary for evaluations of any influence that the lenses may have on the normal ion and metabolite exchanges that occur between the tears, lens, and cornea. Furthermore this information is needed as a basis for future evaluation and development of clinically acceptable soft contact lenses. Such evaluations may include lens permeability effects on bacterial contamination, new sterilization procedures, formation of ion deposits, and general effects on the interrelationships between the lens and normal tear parameters.

This study compares the oxygen, calcium, lactate, chloride, and sodium permeability of various hydrophilic contact lenses.

MATERIALS AND METHODS

The ion permeability studies were carried out by using a special perfusion apparatus previously described by Morrison and Edelhauser.[1] The diffusion of isotopically labeled metabolites and ions was determined as the material(s) permeated from one Lucite perfusion chamber to another through a soft lens clamped in a leak-free holder between the chambers. The Lucite chambers previously described[2] had a fluid circulation network using an air-lift siphon that permitted continuous circulation during sampling. Labeled materials were added to one of the two chambers, each filled with equal volumes of 0.9% saline. The following are the specific activities of the radioactive materials: ^{22}Na—3.3 μCi. per 0.1 ml.; ^{45}Ca—20 μCi. per 0.1 ml.; sodium lactate-l-^{14}C—2.5 μCi. per 0.1 ml.; ^{36}Cl—2.49 μCi. per 0.1 ml. Serial samples were removed from each chamber at hourly intervals and counted with either a liquid scintillation counter (Nuclear Chicago Unilux II) or a well-type gamma counter (Nuclear Chicago). The permeability constants were calculated from the previously described flux equation.[1]

Oxygen permeability rates were determined by using a previously described Lucite oxygen diffusion apparatus and a new glass diffusion system illustrated in Fig. 3-1. Oxygen, bubbled through one chamber, diffuses through the lens into the sealed second chamber. Samples are removed from the sealed chamber by a

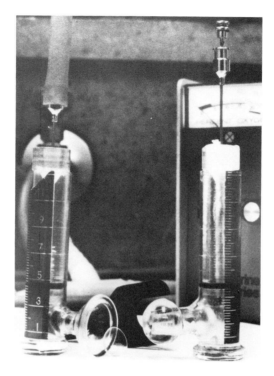

Fig. 3-1. Specially constructed glass oxygen diffusion chamber.

syringe. The dissolved oxygen is measured on a radiometer blood gas analyser, which reads out in mm. Hg P_{O_2}. As the samples are removed, the Lucite plunger (which seals the second chamber) is depressed to reduce the chamber volume by the exact volume that is being removed. This prevents the formation of a vacuum within the sealed chamber because of sample volume removal. The oxygen diffusion constants were calculated as previously described.[1]

Lens material. Four different types of hydrophilic soft contact lenses were compared in this study. HEMA (hydroxethylmethacrylate) copolymer lenses of constant thickness were supplied by Griffin Laboratories, Buffalo, New York. Similar lenses of PHP-1A copolymer were supplied by Physiological Polymers, Hollywood, California. Bausch and Lomb Soflens, fabricated with −3.0 to −5.0 diopters, and constant-thickness lenses from Titmus Company, Germany, were also used. The thickness of each lens was verified by pachometer measurements before and after each experiment. All of the lenses had a diameter of at least 12.5 mm. The effective surface areas for diffusion were calculated from the radius of curvature of the lens and the measured diameter.

RESULTS

The diffusion rates for the essential ions and sodium lactate are shown in Table 3-1. Green has previously shown that mammalian corneas require approx-

Table 3-1. Mean ± standard error diffusion constants of various substances through two hydrophilic contact lenses

Substance	Atomic or molecular weight	Diffusion constant (Df) $\left(\dfrac{\mu g. \text{ (or } \mu Eq.) \cdot cm.}{cm.^2 \cdot hr.} \right)$	
		Griffin (1×10^{-2})	PHP-1A (1×10^{-2})
Sodium (^{22}Na)	23	231.75 ± 1.68 (3)	167.65 ± 53.31 (3)
Chloride (^{36}Cl)	35	53.66 ± 3.89 (3)	56.63 ± 6.00 (3)
Calcium (^{45}Ca)*	40	0.38 ± 0.007 (4)	0.19 ± — (2)
Sodium lactate (^{14}C)	112	1.32 ± 0.14 (3)	1.21 ± 0.078 (3)

( ) in body of table represents number of lenses studied.

*Bausch & Lomb calcium Df (0.009 ± 0.001) × 10^{-2} $\dfrac{\mu g. \text{ cm.}}{cm.^2 \cdot hr.}$.

imately 0.4 μEq. per cm.^{2} of sodium ions, actively transported across the corneal epithelium, to maintain corneal hydration.[3] Our results indicate that the Griffin lens transmits almost five times this critical sodium flux and the PHP lens transmits almost four times the required sodium flux. Sodium ions were the most permeable of all the ions and metabolites tested. The PHP lenses were not as permeable to sodium as were the Griffin lenses.

Chloride fluxes were approximately equal through both the Griffin and PHP lenses, but substantially lower than the sodium fluxes through either lens.

Calcium ion fluxes through the lenses were considerably less than either the sodium or chloride fluxes. Although the calcium has a greater atomic weight, this significantly lower flux would not be expected from the differences in atomic weight alone. The divalent character of the calcium ion may be of primary importance in determining this flux. Of particular interest is the very low calcium permeability through the Bausch & Lomb Soflens (not shown in Table 3-1). The Bausch & Lomb lenses transmitted calcium at only 0.009 × 10^{-2} μg.cm./cm.^{2}·hr. as compared to the fluxes for the Griffin lens of 0.38 × 10^{-2} and PHP lenses of 0.19 × 10^{-2} μg.cm./cm.^{2}·hr. This extremely low calcium permeability through the Bausch & Lomb lenses cannot be justified by the low water and oxygen permeability previously reported for these lenses.[1]

Sodium lactate, a metabolic by-product of aerobic corneal metabolism, is diffusible through the Griffin and PHP lenses at approximately the same rate. These fluxes approximate the bulk flow of water that passes through these lenses.[1]

A comparison of the diffusion constant for a particular monovalent substance and its respective atomic or molecular weight (Fig. 3-2) indicates that the permeability of a substance through these lenses is a function of its atomic or molec-

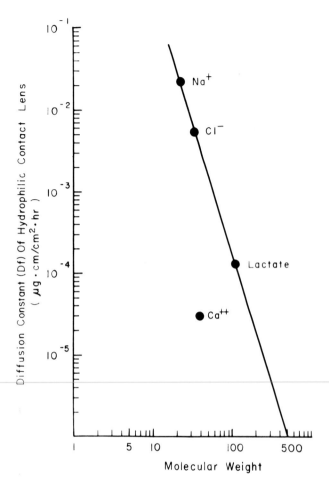

Fig. 3-2. Graph of molecular weight of a particular substance and its respective diffusion constant through Griffin hydrophilic soft contact lenses.

ular weight. Despite the large molecular weight, deposition of sodium lactate should not occur if adequate water flow through the lens is maintained.

The oxygen diffusion rates reported in this study were determined at partial pressure gradients across the lens of approximately 4:1. The results are compared with previously published diffusion constants for synthetic polymers[4] and several other lenses (Table 3-2). The diffusion rates shown have been converted from the reported values to equivalent rates with common units for comparison:

$$\frac{cm.^3}{sec.} \cdot \frac{cm.(thickness)}{cm.^2 \cdot mmHg}, \text{ which simplified is } \frac{cm.^2}{sec. \cdot mmHg}$$

The two types of silicone "soft" contact lenses previously investigated[1,5] have the greatest oxygen permeability of all the various soft contact lenses. A compar-

Table 3-2. Comparison of oxygen diffusion constants for various soft contact lenses and potential lens materials

Source	Material*	Reference	Diffusion constants $\left(cm. \cdot \dfrac{cm.}{cm.^2 \cdot mmHg} \right)$
Silicone rubber	S	Rogers[4]	100.0×10^{-9}
Silicone (Milton Roy)	LM	Morrison[1]	28.1×10^{-9}
Silicone (Meuller-Welt)	L	Fatt[5]	10.0×10^{-9}
Bionite (Griffin)	L	Morrison[1]	5.51×10^{-9}
Bionite (Griffin)	L	Fatt[5]	5.16×10^{-9}
Ewell	L	Fatt[5]	3.87×10^{-9}
Butterfield	L	Fatt[5]	2.63×10^{-9}
Physiological Polymers	L	Morrison[1]	2.44×10^{-9}
Physiological Polymers	LM	Seiderman[6]	1.8×10^{-9}
Soflens (Bausch & Lomb)	L	Morrison[1]	1.63×10^{-9}
Soflens (Bausch & Lomb)	L	Fatt[5]	2.87×10^{-9}
Teflon-FEP (Dow)	S	Seiderman[6]	1.05×10^{-9}
Teflon-TFE (Dow)	S	Seiderman[6]	0.91×10^{-9}
Titmus	L	Present study	0.62×10^{-9}

*L, Lens; LM, lens material; S, other synthetic material.

ison of our previous data with that of Fatt and St. Helen[5] confirms that the Griffin lenses are the most oxygen permeable of all the hydrophilic lenses tested. Other lenses, notably the PHP and Bausch & Lomb lenses, have lower rates of oxygen diffusion, in that order. By comparison, our present study indicated that the Titmus lenses had the lowest rate of oxygen diffusion (0.62×10^{-9} cm.^{2}/sec.$\cdot$mmHg) of any hydrophilic contact lens yet tested. Oxygen diffusion through the Titmus lenses appears to be even slower then the reported oxygen diffusion through Teflon.[6]

DISCUSSION

These results and previous reports[1,5,6] are all representative of the maximum diffusion capabilities of the lenses under ideal laboratory conditions. This information has established the basic guidelines for the diffusional characteristics of the various hydrogel contact lenses. The actual permeability of a particular metabolite or ion through one of these lenses may be less or altered under actual physiological conditions. Recent experiments[7] with patients wearing hydrophilic contact lenses have indicated that the effective oxygen diffusion through these lenses may be much less than expected under certain wearing conditions. It is not clear whether other factors, such as anterior surface drying of the lenses, effects on tear tonicity, tear pH, and precorneal tear film composition may alter the physical properties of these lenses during normal wear.

Apparently none of the hydrophilic lenses pass enough water to supply dissolved oxygen in quantities sufficient to maintain the metabolic requirements of the cornea. These studies agree that both the water and oxygen diffusion are related to the degree of hydration of the different lens. Although more than enough sodium ions get through the lenses to supply corneal requirements, the differences in sodium permeability between the lenses appears to be comparable to the difference in the degree of hydration.

An extrapolation of the graphic relationship between the diffusion constants and their atomic or molecular weights (Fig. 3-2) agrees with O'Driscoll's predictions[8] that the diffusion of materials with a molecular weight greater than 500 should be negligible through these lenses. The molecular weight of diffusing substances is not the only parameter that may affect the permeability of metabolites and ions through the lenses. Sodium lactate, with a molecular weight three times that of calcium, diffused much faster than did calcium. The molecular charge may have more influence on the permeability of a particular ion or substance than the molecular size.

Clinical testing of hydrophilic lenses have shown isolated occurrences of calcium deposition on the lens. The low rate of calcium permeability through these lenses may be a mitigating factor in these instances of calcium deposition. If the diffusion rate were the only factor that produced calcium deposits on these lenses, we would expect the Bausch & Lomb lenses to have frequent calcium buildups because of their extremely low calcium permeability. Since this has not been reported, it is probable that the rate of calcium diffusion through the lens is only one of the factors that can influence calcium deposition.

The comparison of all of the oxygen diffusion rates indicates that even the least permeable hydrophilic lens should be capable of transmitting sufficient oxygen to meet corneal requirements, provided that a reasonable oxygen partial pressure gradient exists across the lens. If enough oxygen is available at the anterior surface of the lens, sufficient quantities will diffuse through the lens. If minimal oxygen is available, that is, when the eyelids are closed, the amounts of oxygen that diffuse through the lens may be insufficient to supply the metabolic needs of the cornea.

It is not yet clear whether the mere physical presence of a hydrophilic lens will have subtle effects on the tear-cornea interrelationship. This baseline date should be useful in future investigations into the lens-tear-cornea relationships.

SUMMARY

The permeability characteristics of soft contact lenses are undoubtably important to the effects of the lenses on corneal physiology. The permeability may also be influential in determining the acceptable handling, sterility, and durability characteristics of these new lenses.

These diffusion studies show that the hydrogel lenses are adequately permeable to water, oxygen, sodium lactate, and essential tear ions. The various lens permeabilities confirm the observed hydrophilic properties of these hydrogel lenses. Permeability characteristics of a particular lens may be affected by the lens thickness and the state of hydration. The diffusion rate of a particular substance through a lens is not only influenced by the molecular weight, but probably involves the ionic charge of the molecule and other unknown factors. The actual molecular pore size of the various soft lenses has not yet been determined.

The permeability of a specific metabolite, such as oxygen or sodium, may be important in the clinical use of the lens in the treatment of certain corneal pathological conditions. In addition, the lens permeability will undoubtably influence the drug-uptake and -release characteristics of the lens.

These studies have established some basic permeability characteristics of the currently available soft contact lenses and may serve as the baseline for future studies of the lens-tear-cornea interrelationships.

This study was supported in part by USPHS grants EY-00446 and EY-00428 from the National Eye Institute and a Fight for Sight Award for Dr. Morrison.

REFERENCES

1. Morrison, D. R., and Edelhauser, H. R.: Permeability of hydrophilic contact lenses, Invest. Opthal. 11:58-63, 1972.
2. Edelhauser, H. F., Hoffert, J. R., and From, P. O.: In vitro ion and water movement in corneas of rainbow trout, Invest. Ophthal. 4:290, 1965.
3. Green, K.: Dependence of corneal thickness on epithelial ion transport and stromal sodium, Amer. J. Physiol. 217:1169-1177, 1969.
4. Rogers, C. E.: Permeability and chemical resistance of polymers. In Baer, E.: Engineering design of plastics, New York, 1964, Reinhold Publishing Corp., pp. 609-688.
5. Fatt, I., and Helen, R. S.: Oxygen tension under an oxygen-permeable contact lens, Amer. J. Optom. 48:545, 1971.
6. Seiderman, M., Stone, W., and Culp, G. W.: Diffusion-permeability of labeled compounds of various transparent synthetic polymers in relation to the rabbit cornea, J. Macromol. Science Chem. 3:101-111, 1969.
7. Morrison, D. R., and Capella, J. A.: Dynamics of oxygen utilization under a soft contact lens. See Chapter 4.
8. O'Driscoll, K. F.: Polymeric aspects of soft contact lenses. See Chapter 1.

Chapter 4

Dynamics of oxygen utilization
under a soft contact lens

Dennis R. Morrison, Ph.D., Joseph A. Capella, M.S., and Ida Schaefer, B.S.

Normal corneal physiology is largely dependent on an adequate supply of oxygen.[1] The methylmethacrylate or hard contact lenses restrict the oxygen available to the corneal epithelium.[2] The oxygen permeability of these contact lenses is so low that an adequate blink rate is required to maintain normal corneal hydration.[3] The concern about changes in normal corneal physiology that result from a restricted oxygen supply has been extended to the new hydrophilic and silicone soft contact lenses. The oxygen permeability of soft contact lenses have therefore been the subject of many recent investigations.[4-6] These experiments have shown that, although there are large differences in the maximum oxygen permeability of various soft contact lenses,[4] all of the lenses tested are capable of transmitting more than enough oxygen to fulfill the cornea's requirements. In addition to the oxygen that will diffuse through these lenses, the lenses flex during blinking, producing some tear exchange under the soft lens and providing another route for oxygen to get to the corneal epithelium.

The rate of oxygen diffusion through these soft lenses is dependent on the diameter and thickness of a particular lens, as well as the oxygen gradient that exists between the outside atmosphere and the concentration of oxygen under the lens. Fatt and St. Helen[5] have extended oxygen diffusion data for some typical hydrophilic soft lenses to predictions of the oxygen transmissibility through a given thickness lens based on either the oxygen concentration under the lens or whether the atmospheric oxygen is restricted by eyelid closure. They include graphic data that predict the difference in lens thickness required to maintain a given oxygen transmission through the lens when the eyelids are open compared with when they are closed.

These various reports are based on the measured oxygen diffusion rates for the lenses in vitro. They reflect the theoretical capacity of the lens to transmit oxygen, not the actual transmission in vivo.

Polse and Mandell[7] have shown that the corneal epithelium requires a minimum oxygen tension to maintain normal corneal hydration. If the oxygen tension falls below the critical amount, the corneal epithelium swells and becomes edematous. The previous diffusion studies do not reflect the actual rate of oxygen transmission through and around the lenses under true physiological conditions. Corneal oxygen consumption and other unknown factors may influence the dynamics of the oxygen supplied by these lenses. It remained to be determined whether the normal patient wear of hydrophilic contact lenses restricts the oxygen supply to the corneal epithelium.

This study describes the atmospheric oxygen level required to maintain normal corneal hydration during normal soft contact lens wear, and the dynamics of corneal hydration that occur when the atmospheric tension is reduced below the critical range.

MATERIALS AND METHODS

Thirty-one separate experiments were performed on 10 normal subjects selected from a large group of well-adjusted hydrophilic soft contact lens patients of the Shaler Richardson Eye Clinic at the University of Florida, Gainesville, Florida.

Each subject wore a specially designed, goggle type of mask that sealed both eyes from the normal atmosphere. A carefully controlled atmosphere of specific oxygen content, humidity, and temperature was circulated through the bilateral eye chamber within the mask. The corneal thickness, under a hydrophilic soft contact lens, was measured before, after, and at 30-minute intervals throughout each 3-hour experiment. The corneal swelling rate was determined at each level of available oxygen then contrasted with the constant corneal thickness observed when the available oxygen was adequate.

Apparatus. A constant temperature bath, surrounding two mixing chambers, maintained the temperature of the controlled atmosphere at $37 \pm 0.2°$ C. (Fig. 4-1). Analyzed gas mixtures, containing exact amounts of oxygen between 1% and 21%, were humidified then added to the recirculating air in the second chamber. The second chamber was connected by aircraft type of oxygen hoses to the goggle mask worn by the patient. The controlled atmosphere was circulated by an in-line

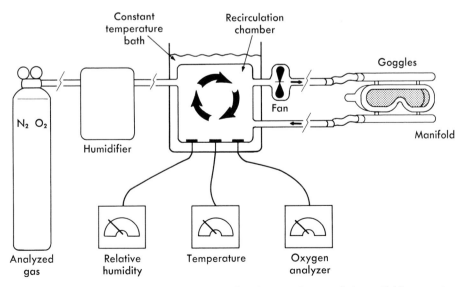

Fig. 4-1. Diagram of closed system for control and recirculation of air available to patients wearing goggles over soft contact lenses.

fan from the recirculation chamber (Fig. 4-1) through the mask and back to the recirculation chamber. The addition rate of analyzed gas was adjusted to maintain the exact oxygen content of the recirculating air. A Biomarine, Model 255, oxygen analyzer was used to monitor the oxygen content of the air returning from the mask. The relative humidity, monitored with a LKB hygrometer, was maintained at 50%. The temperature of the recirculated air was kept constant and the addition of analyzed gas provided a slight positive pressure that prevented atmospheric leakage into the closed recirculation system. This method allowed circulation of the experimental air mixture around both eyes without causing any interference with normal blinking or evaporation from the surface of the hydrophilic lenses.

Corneal thickness measurements. A Haag-Streit pachometer, with the Mishima modification,[8] was used to measure the thickness of corneas and hydrophilic contact lenses. The mean of 10 thickness measurements was used as the representative thickness of the cornea and/or the soft contact lens before, during, and after each 3-hour experiment. The total thickness of the corneal and soft lens image was found to be identical to the sum of both measurements recorded separately.

Corneal thickness was recorded before insertion of the hydrophilic lenses. The thickness of the lens and the cornea was measured through the goggles under normal atmospheric conditions, at 30-minute intervals during exposure to the experimental atmosphere, and immediately after removal of the goggles.

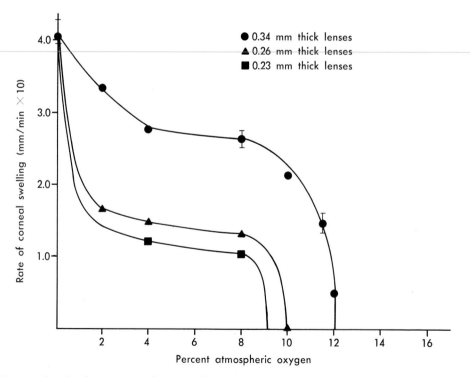

Fig. 4-2. Graph of corneal swelling *rate* dependence on the available oxygen concentration for several different thicknesses of Griffin Naturalens. *Brackets,* Standard deviation of mean rates for three or more subjects.

DYNAMICS OF OXYGEN UTILIZATION UNDER A SOFT CONTACT LENS

The rate of corneal thickening was determined by linear regression of the mean thickness observed at each time interval during the experiment, A BMDOSC–Linear Regression Program, from the Health Sciences Computing Facility of the University of California at Los Angeles, was used on the IBM 360-65 computer to determine the rate and statistical parameters of the corneal thickening.

Statistical analysis of the pachometer measurement showed that very accurate rates of corneal swelling were determined by linear regression of the means of only 10 thickness measurements.

Ostensibly we wished to use the experimental data to predict the oxygen tension that would be required to prevent corneal swelling under any particular thickness lens. Curvilinear regression analysis of these data, using the corneal swelling rate as the dependent variable and the corresponding oxygen content of the controlled atmospheric mixture as the independent variable, was carried out on the IBM 360-65 computer with a BMDO5R–Polynomial Regression Fitting Program also from the Health Sciences Computing Facility of UCLA. A sixth-degree polynomial expression, Y = corneal swelling rate = $a + b(\%O_2) + c(\%O_2)^2 + \ldots g(\%O_2)^6$, was used to exactly fit ($p = 0.002$) the observed data (Fig. 4-2). The

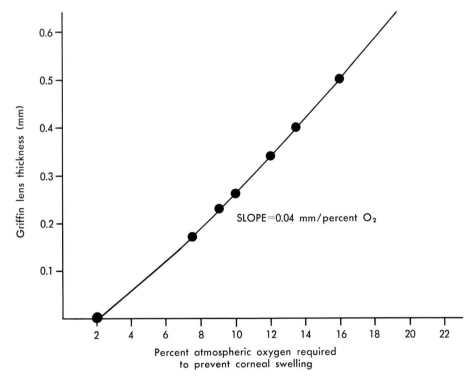

Fig. 4-3. Graph of linear relationship between lens thickness and atmospheric oxygen required to prevent corneal swelling under lens of that thickness. Part of these data was taken from the X-intercepts in Fig. 4-2 and the rest are computer-predicted values. An increase in lens thickness of 0.04 mm. requires a corresponding increase of 1% more oxygen to maintain corneal physiology.

oxygen tension required to prevent corneal swelling, with no lens and under three different thickness experimental lenses, was compared with the oxygen tension requirement predicted by the polynomial expression for several other lens thicknesses (Fig. 4-3).

A variation of the polynomial regression program was also used to fit the graphic model of the effect of oxygen restriction that resulted from the presence of the soft contact lens. The exponential decay model was subtracted from the observed data to allow prediction of the expression that represented the oxygen-restricting effect of the hydrophilic lens. The expression that described the lens effect for one particular lens was then used to predict the oxygen restriction effect imposed by another thickness lens. The predicted effect was then verified by comparison with the experimental data observed for that lens.

Lenses. Naturalenses of 14.0 mm. diameter and thickness ranging from 0.20 to 0.45 mm. were supplied by Griffin Laboratories, Buffalo, New York. Soflenses of the C series, ranging from 0.20 to 0.25 mm. thick were supplied by Bausch & Lomb Company, Rochester, New York.

RESULTS

Corneal hydration and swelling were found to occur in normal patients, without contact lenses, when the atmospheric oxygen was reduced below 2% ($P_{O_2} = 14.2$ mm. Hg). Corneal swelling was not observed at oxygen levels of greater than 2%. The magnitude and rate of swelling that occurred at oxygen levels of less than 2% was comparable to the previous findings of Polse and Mandell[7] for normal patients.

The swelling rate was found to be a very accurate index of the physiological changes that result from induced oxygen deprivation of the corneal epithelium. Subtle changes in the swelling rate were statistically more significant and reproducible than the percent change in thickness that occurred during the experiments. The soft lenses did not change in thickness during the 3-hour experiments in the controlled atmosphere.

The maximum rate of corneal swelling in a pure nitrogen atmosphere was $4.15 \pm 0.10 \times 10^{-4}$ mm./min. Regression analysis of the corneal swelling that occurred during the 3-hour period gave accurate rates of swelling with only 5% standard deviation. Even rates as low as 0.5×10^{-4} mm./min. were statistically significant ($p = 0.05$) when compared to the normal corneal thickness measurements observed during the same time interval.

The mean rate of swelling was plotted against the atmospheric oxygen content maintained inside the mask (Fig. 4-2). The corneal swelling rate was inversely proportional to the oxygen concentration in the atmosphere that the eyes were exposed to, however, the relationship was not linear. Fig. 4-2 shows that the swelling rate dropped dramatically when the mask atmosphere was changed from zero up to 4% oxygen. Minimal change in the swelling rate occurred at atmospheric oxygen levels between 4% and 8%. A comparison of the curves for different thickness lenses (Fig. 4-2) illustrates that the rates of swelling that occur between 4% and 8% atmospheric oxygen (plateau regions of curves) are directly proportional to the thickness of the hydrophilic contact lenses. At oxygen levels above 8% the swelling rate decreased rapidly with increasing concentrations of oxygen. Ten percent oxygen was sufficient to maintain normal corneal hydration under a 0.26 mm.

thick Griffin lens, whereas 12% oxygen was required to maintain normal hydration when a 0.34 mm. thick lens was worn.

Computerized curvilinear regression provided sixth-order polynomial expressions that accurately described the relationships between the rate of corneal swelling and the atmospheric oxygen level that determined that swelling rate. Comparisons between the polynomial regression coefficients for the expressions describing the results for different thickness soft lenses gave the basis for developing a general polynomial expression for other thickness lenses. The computer-predicted rates of swelling, at particular oxygen levels and for a particular thickness lens, were spot-checked by additional experiments. The predicted rates were found to be well within the standard deviation of the measured corneal swelling rates.

The percent oxygen required to prevent corneal swelling under different thickness lenses was determined from the observed data for three different thickness lenses. Comparison of these data with the predicted oxygen requirements for other thickness lenses indicated that linear regression analysis showed that each 0.04 mm. increase in lens thickness required an increase of 1% more oxygen in the mask atmosphere to supply corneal requirements (Fig. 4-3).

The swelling rates were determined at various oxygen tensions equivalent to those that exist when the eyelids are closed (P_{O_2} = 55 mm. Hg = 7.8% O_2 at STP).

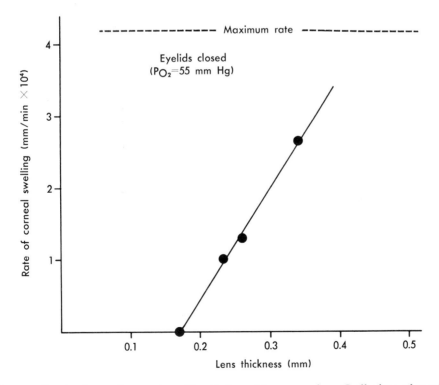

Fig. 4-4. Graph of rate of corneal swelling that would occur under a Griffin lens of specified thickness whenever eyelids remain closed. No corneal swelling should occur under lenses thinner than 0.17 mm.

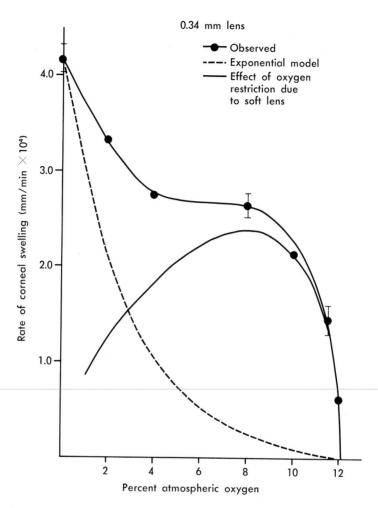

Fig. 4-5. Graphic comparison of observed rate of corneal swelling and exponential decrease in rate of swelling (as predicted by the model) that occur at different atmospheric oxygen levels. *Plain solid curve,* For a 0.34 mm. thick Griffin lens, the differences between the observed and theoretical curves describes the effect of oxygen restriction resulting from the presence of the lens.

Fig. 4-4 shows that the cornea will swell at a significant rate if the eyelids are closed over typical thickness Griffin lenses (0.4 to 0.5 mm. thick). If corneal swelling under a hydrophilic contact lens is to be avoided, a lens of only 0.17 mm. thick or less should be worn when the eyelids are closed.

The model interpretation (Fig. 4-5) indicated that the maximum oxygen-restricting effect of these lenses was quite critical at oxygen levels below 8%. The magnitude of this restricting effect was directly proportional to the thickness of the lenses. The lens restriction rapidly disappeared at oxygen levels above 8%, thus the corneal swelling rate correspondingly dropped to zero.

Preliminary experiments indicate that the Bausch & Lomb Soflenses will also produce corneal swelling under closed eyelids. Soflenses of 0.21 mm. thick were found to cause corneal swelling rates equivalent to the swelling that occurred under a Griffin lens that was approximately 30% thicker (0.27 mm.) when the oxygen level was 7.8% (equivalent to P_{O_2} under closed eyelids). The entire profile of this relationship between the thickness of the Soflens and the corneal swelling rates, however, had not been completed at the time of this report.

Another investigation occurred during patient selection. A small percentage of normal patients who have soft contact lens demonstrated a substantial rate of corneal swelling during a 3- to 6-hour period at normal atmospheric oxygen levels. When these patients were followed by slit lamp inspection, clinically observable corneal edema was not detectable during this period. However, pachometer measurement of corneal swelling was consistantly detectable within 1 to 3 hours of lens wearing. None of these subjects were used in this study. The lenses worn by these patients were of usual diameter and thickness (0.35 to 0.45 mm. thick) and should not have caused oxygen deprivation of the cornea. Normal atmospheric oxygen levels apparently did not prevent this swelling in these few subjects. It appeared that other, unknown, factors may have been responsible for this corneal swelling.

DISCUSSION

The *rate* of corneal hydration and swelling, as well as the degree of corneal hydration[7] is dependent on the oxygen available to the corneal epithelium. The rate of swelling was found to be a most sensitive parameter for evaluation of the effects of oxygen restriction on normal corneal physiology. Although normal corneas do not swell in atmospheres containing 2% oxygen or more, a cornea under a typical hydrophilic contact lens will swell at atmospheric oxygen levels less than 12% to 16%. In contrast corneas under a methylmethacrylate corneal lens require approximately 95% atmospheric oxygen to maintain corneal physiology in lieu of blinking.[9]

Previous reports[4,10] have indicated that hydrophilic contact lenses are capable of transmitting more than enough oxygen to meet the cornea's requirements. This present study demonstrates that the presence of a hydrophilic contact lens does alter the oxygen available to the corneal epithelium. The hydrophilic lenses are not transmitting oxygen at their maximum capacity during normal patient wear. This condition seldom produces any troublesome consequence whenever the eyelids are open; however, the cornea will invariably swell when the eyelids are closed over the lens.

The simplest model that delineates how corneal physiology and hydration vary with the available oxygen would be described by a decreasing first-order exponential function (Y = swelling rate = Ae^{-kx}). This model would dictate the rate of corneal hydration and swelling, Y, would decrease exponentially from some maximum, A, as the oxygen concentration was available to the cornea, x, is increased. When the oxygen concentration is great enough, the rate of corneal swelling will drop to zero and the corneal thickness would remain constant.

Although it has been reported that some corneal swelling occurs overnight[10] because of the reduced oxygen supply (P_{O_2} = 55 mm. Hg under closed eyelids), our results indicate that a 2% oxygen atmosphere is sufficient to prevent measurable rates of corneal swelling during a 3-hour period. When these corneas are covered by hydrophilic contact lenses, however, a considerably higher concentration of oxygen is required to prevent corneal swelling. In effect, the range of the independent variable (O_2 concentration) of the exponential model has been extended to a much larger oxygen concentration (necessary to prevent corneal swelling). If we graphically compare the effective exponential model to the observed rates of corneal swelling (Fig. 4-5), it is apparent that the difference between the theoretical and observed swelling rates (at a particular oxygen concentration) represents the physiological effect of corneal oxygen restriction rendered by the presence of the lens, that is, the effective oxygen deprivation of the cornea.

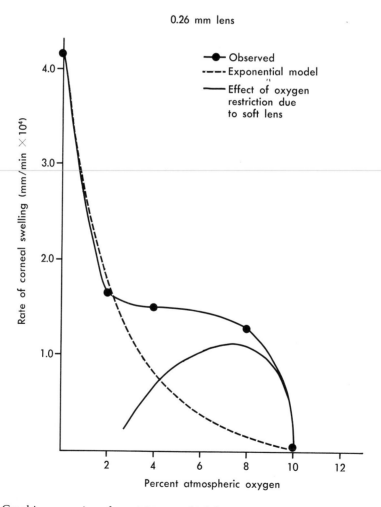

Fig. 4-6. Graphic comparison for a 0.26 mm. thick lens similar to that in Fig. 4-5. Note that maximum effect of lens-induced oxygen restriction also occurs at approximately 8% atmospheric oxygen.

DYNAMICS OF OXYGEN UTILIZATION UNDER A SOFT CONTACT LENS

The maximum effect on corneal swelling caused by the lens-induced oxygen liability occurs at approximately 8% atmospheric oxygen for a 0.34 mm. thick Griffin lens (Fig. 4-5). For a thinner lens (0.26 mm.) the maximum effect of the lens restriction of oxygen occurs at approximately the same oxygen concentration (7.5% O_2) as shown in Fig. 4-6. The magnitude of the maximum lens influence on the corneal oxygen supply is proportional to the thickness of the lens. The lens thickness also determines the independent variable (x) intercept, that is, the oxygen concentration at which there will be zero corneal swelling.

This model implies that the oxygen diffusion through the hydrophilic lens is minimal at low atmospheric oxygen levels, even though the corneal consumption rate may be greater than the diffusion rate through the lens. The cornea may be, in effect starving for oxygen under the lens at these low concentrations. There is apparently not enough partial pressure gradient across the lens to force enough oxygen through to meet the cornea's needs. This results in an obvious oxygen liability until the atmospheric oxygen reaches a level greater than 6% to 8%. At oxygen concentrations above 6% to 8%, the P_{O_2} gradient across the lens becomes so large that the oxygen diffusion increases rapidly with increasing concentrations of atmospheric oxygen. As the oxygen diffusion approaches a rate that will meet the cornea's requirements, the observed swelling rate drops to zero.

Ostensibly the rate of oxygen transmission through a lens, under a particular P_{O_2} gradient, is inversely proportional to the thickness of that lens. The critical atmospheric oxygen level that will maintain normal corneal hydration is therefore a function of the thickness and diffusion dynamics of a particular hydrophilic lens under the P_{O_2} gradient that exists across that lens.

The oxygen restriction imposed by these lenses appears to be a function of the concentration of oxygen available at the anterior surface of the lens and the operational diffusion rate that exists under these conditions. It is clear that the physiological response to this oxygen deprivation, that is, corneal swelling, was critically dependent on the thickness of the hydrophilic lens. Neither the tightness of fit nor the diameter of the lens appeared to play a major role. The lens thickness was so critical that the observed swelling at subnormal oxygen levels must have been a function of the limited oxygen diffusion through the lens. The oxygen supplied in the tears that are pumped around and under the soft lens was not nearly as important as previously reported for hard corneal lenses.[2,3] If the hydrophilic lens is reasonably thin enough, corneal swelling should not occur even during normal sleeping periods.

Normal patient use of Griffin lenses up to 0.7 mm. thick should not result in corneal swelling at normal atmospheric oxygen levels. The 24-hour use of hydrophilic lenses is often indicated in the treatment of certain corneal diseases, (such as bullous keratopathy).[12] Such treatment may require a lens of less than 0.17 mm. thick to avoid physiological complications that may result from lens restriction of the corneal oxygen supply.

Other hydrophilic contact lenses are currently under study. The preliminary results indicate that any of the hydrophilic lenses may result in corneal swelling whenever the eyelids are kept closed over too thick a lens. The magnitude of this problem also appears to be a function of the oxygen diffusion capability of the lens[10] and the average thickness, rather than the diameter of the various lenses.

Occasional observations of corneal swelling under a hydrophilic contact lens during normal wearing have been noted. Until now, these occurrences have been attributed to the lens restriction of the corneal oxygen supply. This study clearly shows that oxygen deprivation is probably not the cause of the observed swelling in these cases. Indeed, it indicates that there may be other, unknown, factors that involve the presence of a contact lens and its subsequent effects on corneal physiology. The hydrophilic contact lenses do not deprive the cornea of its oxygen supply under normal conditions. Since they do not seriously interfere with the oxygen supply, they may become important tools in the study of the unknown, more subtle, effects of contact lens wear.

SUMMARY

Corneal swelling of patients wearing hydrophilic soft contact lenses was measured at various oxygen tensions below normal atmospheric levels. The critical concentration of oxygen required to maintain normal corneal hydration was determined for various lenses. The *rate* of corneal hydration and swelling was found to be dependent on the oxygen tension available to the eye and the thickness of the hydrophilic lens. Mathematical functions were used to describe the relationship between the rate of corneal swelling and the available atmospheric oxygen for different thickness lenses. The critical oxygen tension for a wide range of lens thicknesses was predicted. The oxygen restriction, and hence the rate of corneal swelling, is critically dependent on the thickness of the hydrophilic lens. It is clear that the oxygen diffusion dynamics through the lens plays the major role in regulating the oxygen that is supplied to the cornea under a hydrophilic lens. A simple model is proposed that indicates that the lens-induced oxygen restriction is most severe at oxygen concentrations below 6% to 8%.

Corneal swelling will probably occur if the eyelids are closed for long periods of time over the hydrophilic lenses that are presently available. If overnight swelling is to be avoided, the hydrophilic lens most permeable to oxygen should be no thicker than 0.17 mm. The use of these lenses during waking hours, under normal wearing conditions, should not interfere with the oxygen requirements of the corneal epithelium.

This study was supported in part by USPHS grants EY-00446 and EY-00266 from the National Eye Institute and a Fight for Sight Award for Dr. Morrison.

REFERENCES

1. Langham, M.: Utilization of oxygen by the component layers of the living cornea, J. Physiol. 117:461-470, 1952.
2. Dixon, J. M.: Ocular changes due to contact lenses, Amer. J. Ophthal. 58:424-443, 1964.
3. Fatt, I.: Oxygen tension under a contact lens during blinking, Amer. J. Optom. 46:654-661, 1969.
4. Morrison, D. R., and Edelhauser, H. F.: Permeability of hydrophilic contact lenses, Invest. Opthal. 11:58-66, 1972.
5. Fatt, I., and St. Helen, R.: Oxygen tension under an oxygen-permeable contact lens, Amer. J. Optom. 48(7):545-555, 1971.

6. Seiderman, M., Stone, W., and Culp, G. W.: Diffusion permeability of labeled compounds of various transparent synthetic polymers in relation to the rabbit cornea, J. Macromol. Science Chem. 3:101-111, 1969.

7. Polse, K. A., and Mandell, R. B.: Critical oxygen tension at the corneal surface, Arch. Ophthal. 84:505-508, 1970.

8. Ginsberg, S. P., Capella, J. A., and Kaufman, H. E.: Normal patterns of corneal thinning after penetrating keratoplasty using refrigerated and cryopreserved donor material, Amer. J. Opthal. (In press.)

9. Polse, K. A., and Mandell, R. B.: Hyperbaric oxygen effect on corneal edema caused by contact lens, Amer. J. Optom. 48:197-200, 1971.

10. Morrison, D. R., and Edelhauser, H. F.: Corneal metabolite and ion permeability of hydrophilic contact lenses. (In preparation.)

11. Mandell, R. B., and Fatt, I.: Thinning of human cornea upon awakening, Nature 208:292-293, 1965.

12. Gasset, A. R., and Kaufman, H. E.: Bandage lenses in the treatment of bullous keratopathy, Amer. J. Ophthal. 72:376-380, 1971.

SUMMARY AND DISCUSSION OF PART II
Significance of hydrophilic contact lens effects on corneal physiology
Dennis R. Morrison, Ph.D.

Hydrophilic soft contact lenses are quite different from conventional corneal lenses in both physical properties and their effects on corneal physiology. Although hydrophilic lenses do not actually contain holes, they do have a molecular porosity that permits water, oxygen, and small molecular weight substances to easily permeate the lenses.

Essential corneal metabolites such as oxygen, sodium, chloride, and calcium have little trouble diffusing through the lens to the cornea underneath. Even metabolic by-products (such as lactate) will permeate through the lens quite readily. Substances with a molecular weight of less than 500 demonstrate substantial and predictable diffusion through these lenses. The permeability characteristics of a particular lens may be affected by the lens thickness, state of hydration, and size and ionic character of the diffusing substance. The hydrogel lenses are adequately permeable to essential nutrients, tear ions, and metabolic by-products of normal corneal physiology. Under normal wearing conditions they would not be expected to interfere with corneal homeostasis.

Under certain conditions, however, the permeability characteristics of these lenses may provide several advantages and/or minor difficulties. Prolonged use of the lenses at reduced oxygen tensions will cause corneal swelling if the lens is too thick. Sleeping, while wearing even the most oxygen-permeable lens, will result in corneal swelling if the lens is thicker than 0.17 mm.

Many aircraft personnel are exposed to reduced oxygen levels in aircraft cabins that are pressurized to an equivalent of 8,000 feet above sea level. Patients who work or live in high mountainous areas should also be given special attention. If such a patient encounters mild oxygen deprivation, corneal swelling, and consequently hazy vision, from wearing too thick a lens for the existing conditions, he should be fitted with a thinner lens.

The physical characteristics of the hydrogel lenses will undoubtedly affect their therapeutic use. The uptake and release of drugs by these lenses is already under investigation. The elution of specific metabolites may become important in the clinical use of the lens in the treatment of certain corneal pathological conditions. The predictable physical behavior of the hydrogel lenses will undoubtably play a major role in their future therapeutic applications.

The semipermeable nature of soft contact lenses will be important in determining the acceptable handling and sterilization procedures for patient use. These features may also be pertinent to future studies of the lens-tear-cornea interrelationships.

In general, the hydrophilic contact lenses do not seriously interfere with tear-cornea exchanges and normal corneal physiology. They do not cause oxygen deprivation of the corneal epithelium under normal wearing conditions as do conventional corneal contact lenses. Special wearing conditions and certain therapeutic applications will require additional consideration of the physical properties of the lenses. The permeability of a particular lens, which is a function of its thickness, is one of the most easily regulated parameters available to the clinician.

SUMMARY AND DISCUSSION OF PART II

Discussion

First question by Dr. Gasset: Was there a fixation device involved in these technique measurements similar to what Dr. Mandell has used?

Dr. Morrison: Yes. There was a fixation device. We used a Haag-Streit pachometer, modified by Dr. Mishima with a fixation device for the patient.

Second question: Dr. Mandell has pointed out with his experiments that when you measure corneal thickness relative to oxygen deprivation, it occurs over the total cornea. Is this so?

Dr. Morrison: In our experiments, we considered the mean of 10 central corneal thickness for each data point shown. Obviously when the total cornea thickens, the central cornea also thickens. Even if our measurements are less sensitive, I think they approximate his measurements, and we have clearly determined that the rate of corneal thickening is perhaps a much more sensitive parameter than determining the percent of corneal thickening that may occur.

We can determine rates of thickening very quickly within the first hour or two of an experimental run with the patient under these conditions. It takes longer to produce any clinical signs of edema. And just looking at the percent changes does tend to be a little difficult to interpret as Dr. Mishima has previously pointed out. We are dealing here with a small amount of percent change, when we look at the total corneal thickness, because of thickening of the epithelium alone.

Third question: Aren't there reports that in an eyes-open condition (no blinking), rabbits don't seem to get enough oxygen through either the Griffin or Bausch & Lomb lens?

Dr. Morrison: In our experiments, we had a blinking situation, as normal as possible, with our patients merely wearing a goggle with controlled atmospheric oxygen, temperature, and humidity. In addition, there is undoubtedly a difference in oxygen sensitivity between rabbit and human corneas. I think our experiments with normal patients are certainly significant.

Fourth question: Do we understand that essentially there is enough oxygen available to the cornea under the soft lenses under normal wearing conditions, provided that the lens is not too thick?

Dr. Morrison: If we will look at this extrapolation between the rate of thickening and the actual oxygen concentration required, we would see that, indeed, for a Griffin lens a range specified from 0.25 to 0.30 would only require about 10% or 11% oxygen available.

We can go up to actually as high as an 0.7 mm. lens, which is much thicker than is available currently, before we get to the point where eyes that are open under normal conditions (21% oxygen) would ever incur any thickening. And it turns out that the Bausch & Lomb lens is in approximately the same range.

There is a difference in oxygen transmission. Even though the Bausch & Lomb lens transmits a little less per square centimeter, it is a little thinner than normal by comparison to the Griffin lens and has a little smaller diameter. Our preliminary experience has shown it to be comparable. So there is no problem with the currently available lenses.

It brings up the main point that if we do find edema in some of the patients fitted with these lenses, why? We are beginning to get to the point where we can think it is perhaps not all dependent on oxygen as was previously referenced by the experience with hard lenses.

Dr. Mishima has pointed out higher tear osmolarity can cause changes in corneal physiology. There are undoubtedly some other factors we have not been able to evaluate that have been relatively clouded by the oxygen problem. And now, as we eliminate the oxygen problem with these soft lenses, we will be able to evaluate these more subtle factors that can cause corneal edema under these lenses.

Fifth question: Dr. Friedberg, can the changes in corneal curvature with the use of contact lenses be beneficial by reducing myopia, and do you place any credence in orthokeratology?

Dr. Friedberg: My feeling is that any change that we make in corneal curvature is purely of a haphazard nature. I don't attempt to create any corneal curvature. I look for something that would not create it.

And so far as orthokeratology is concerned, I look at it with suspicion until a lot more work is done and we do know what we are doing besides changing the corneal curvature.

Sixth question: Professor Nakajima, you have stated seven cases of some impairment in vision out of some 37,000 cases. Did any of these result in blindness from contact lens themselves?

Dr. Nakajima: I am very grateful to my colleague, Dr. Gasset, who asked this. Dr. Hamano's survey is directed to around 300 ophthalmologists and asks how many cases of eye trouble that were caused by contact lenses they have seen during a certain period. And they collected 18,000 replies. All have some trouble, and the majority of the cases disappeared in 1 day.

Probably, guessing from my experience, the total population of contact lens wearers from which those patients had been extracted may be half a million or a few hundred thousand. All seven cases had a slight scar formation, but nothing serious.

As far as I know, in Japan, I know of two cases who lost eyes because of hard contact lens wear. And one case was fitted by a layman. We are going to make a nationwide survey to get more information about eye trouble caused by contact lens wear as well as by spectacles. The government is going to give us a small amount of money.

Dr. Kaufman: Could I just comment on that? Arthur Keany, as you probably know, has published a very nice paper where he has accumulated at least 40 cases where eyes were lost from wearing of spectacles. Nothing in the world is absolutely safe.

Seventh question: The question was asked in connection with fitting of soft contact lenses. "What is the equilibrium time for each of the three terms?" Dr. Bailey, I presume here the inquirer is speaking of the two hydrophilic lenses and the silicone lens. At least those are the only three we have spent any time on.

Dr. Bailey: I think with the hydrophilic materials, a few minutes—and here I would say 4 or 5 minutes—perhaps is sufficient. Normally, however, we wait approximately a half hour because it fits into our office schedule well and I think often gives us a little more firm base, that is, before we depend on overrefracting.

Eighth question: Do refractive changes occur with time?

Dr. Bailey: I am not sure how much time is being spoken of here, whether this is in connection with a so-called myopic control or whether they mean just over a matter of weeks. I think, in general, because vision sometimes is quite variable, we have noticed no changes.

PART III
Correction of refractive error

Chapter 5

The Bausch & Lomb Soflens: Basic concepts and fitting techniques

Neal J. Bailey, O.D., Ph.D.

DEVELOPMENT OF CONTACT LENSES

Some evidence is available to show that contact lenses were dreamed about by Leonardo da Vinci in 1508 and later in 1637 by René Descartes. But it remained for the British astronomer, Sir John Herschel, to describe the mathematics of these devices. Sir John not only discussed the first hard contact lens but went a step further and speculated on the possibility of filling a glass contact lens with transparent gelatin to correct for corneal irregularities. This might very well have been the first "soft-lined" contact lens.

Unfortunately, none of these men are known to have made a wearable hard or soft contact lens. In 1887, however, a hard scleral contact lens was made and worn for 20 years, not as a visual device, but as a protective cover for the eye of a patient whose lid had been destroyed by cancer.

But the glass scleral contact lenses that were made from 1887 until 1938 were fitted by a tedious method of trial and error from a fitting set that might contain more than 1,000 lenses. In addition, glass contact lenses were heavy and adjustments on them by the fitter were impossible. Their life in the eye was short since glass is vigorously attacked by the lacrimal fluid. Hence, in 6 months or so this same tedious process often had to be repeated because the lens became too rough to wear or to see through. Glass could, however, point to one advantage: tears wet it easily.

Hard contact lenses

When, in 1938, polymethylmethacrylate (PMMA) appeared on the scene, it brightened markedly the future of contact lenses. This material is readily fabricated by lathe cutting and by a variety of casting and molding techniques. Adjustments can be made on a lens after its original fabrication and its light weight, optical clarity, and relative chemical and physical stability are highly desirable qualities. A PMMA lens may have an indefinite life on the eye.

Two of its characteristics have made it a less than perfect material, however: (1) PMMA does not wet readily and (2) gases, especially oxygen and carbon dioxide, do not pass through it readily. And, of course, the physical stability on which some of its optical effectiveness depends means that this lens, just like the glass contact lens, may produce harmful physical pressure effects upon the cornea.

Soft contact lenses

In 1960, a paper by Dr. Otto Wichterle[1] and Dr. Drahoslav Lim of the Institute of Macromolecular Chemistry in Prague, Czechoslovakia, announced the development of a new hydrophilic plastic material, hydroxyethylmethacrylate (HEMA). This hydrophilic polymer was fashioned into a contact lens by a spin-casting technique. Prior to its introduction into the United States in 1964, the resulting soft contact lenses had been fitted successfully on several thousand patients in Czechoslovakia.

In Europe (except Czechoslovakia) and in England, HEMA lenses of both cast and lathe-cut construction were used prior to and after 1964, but the success of these lenses was so limited that they had been largely discontinued in Europe and England by the time they reached the United States. The apparent popularity and success of these lenses in Czechoslovakia can be understood only by realizing that in Czechoslovakia at that time there were no hard contact lenses. Contact lens wearers wore the HEMA lens or no contact lens. In some parts of Europe and in England, hard contact lens technology rivaled that in the United States, and consequently the HEMA lens, in its very underdeveloped stage, found itself in rough competitive company.

In 1964 this material and the spin-casting process were brought to the United States under a license from the Czechoslovakian government that was granted to the National Patent Development Corporation of New York City. A sublicense by the National Patent Development Corporation was granted to the Bausch & Lomb Company, which then started the necessary safety studies in the Department of Ophthalmology at the University of Rochester in October 1966. During 1967 a clinical evaluation program of somewhat limited nature was started, also confined primarily to the Rochester, New York, area.

Ironically, in late 1968, Bausch & Lomb placed ads in a number of eye care journals for publication in their December 1968 issues. These ads announced that the Soflens soon would be available to all interested eye care practitioners. But, in the middle of December 1968, a ruling by the Food & Drug Administration declared that all contact lenses would be classified as drugs rather than as devices. The long history of the safe use of a hard (PMMA) contact lens allowed it to be accepted immediately. However, in order for any contact lens made of a new material to be used on the public, it became necessary to follow the procedures for new drug approval already outlined by the F.D.A. From December 1968 until March 18, 1971, when the F.D.A. agreed to release the Soflens for general distribution to practitioners, the HEMA lens was used only by investigators selected and accepted by Bausch & Lomb and the F.D.A.

SOFT LENS MATERIAL AND MANUFACTURE

The material from which the Bausch & Lomb Soflens is made is closely allied to polymethylmethacrylate and is named hydroxyethylmethacrylate, or HEMA. It absorbs 41.7% water by weight if the water is pure, and 38.6% if it is a normal saline solution. The refractive index changes from 1.53 in the dry state to 1.43 when fully hydrated in normal saline.

When HEMA is dry, it is much more brittle than PMMA. But when fully hydrated, a lens made of the material is so flexible that it cannot be removed from the eye even with a suction cup unless air is allowed to get under it. It recovers its original shape almost regardless of any deformation it may undergo. In addition, it is biologically inert and compatible with human tissue. Bacteria and fungi are claimed to be incapable of penetrating the surface of the hydroxy-ethylmethacrylate lenses.

If the lens should dry out, at first it becomes rather sticky and may stick to the lids and be rolled out of the eye with blinking. In an automobile with the top down, for example, these lenses sometimes dry sufficiently so that the wearer must be very careful that he does not open his eyes too wide.

The lens is spin cast; that is, the monomer-polymer cross-linkage agent mixture is poured onto a spinning female mold where it is polymerized. Only a female mold is used and Bausch & Lomb refers to the front or convex curve of the Soflens as the *base curve*. Since no male mold is used, the ocular surface of the Soflens is free to assume a controlled shape that depends on the speed of rotation, the viscosity of the material, and the rate at which polymerization occurs. A paraboloid probably best describes this ocular surface.

Polymerization is completed on the mold, but hydration is only partial when the lens comes off. After removal from the mold, the lens is completely hydrated in 0.9% saline solution (normal saline), and its power is measured in the completely hydrated state. Incidentally, in the practitioner's office, no parameter of this wet, ultrathin, and very flexible lens can be measured with an accuracy approaching that possible with a hard contact lens.

FITTING SOFT LENSES

A Soflens might be fitted from a trial set, but a fitting set is preferred for at least two reasons:

1. The shape of this lens may be changed markedly when it is placed on a given cornea. Hence, the performance of a given lens can differ radically on two different eyes.
2. Since the parameters of these lenses cannot be evaluated precisely by the practitioner in his office, both he and his patient can be assured that the lens selected does perform as it was intended even before the patient leaves the practitioner's office. After the practitioner is assured that the lens does perform satisfactorily, he will order a new lens to fill his fitting set.

Since the lens is thin and extremely flexible, there is a radical difference in the mathematics of this contact lens as compared to that of a hard contact lens. First, the lacrimal lens layer is clinically without refractive power. Secondly, the refractive power of the lens itself changes rather noticeably as it bends to adhere to the cornea.

Lens power

Our first consideration, that is, the lack of power in the lacrimal layer, allows a somewhat simpler initial approach to the fitting of the Soflens since no lacrimal lens power allowance need be made for a steep or a flat base curve. Unfortunately, this same factor precludes the use of the Soflens on any eye that requires refractive aid from a cooperative lacrimal lens. An eye with more than 1 to 1.5 diopters of refractive astigmatism is rarely a good candidate for a Soflens.

The second problem, that is, the power change, occurs because the shape or the "bend" of the lens on any given cornea depends on the shape of this cornea rather than on the initial shape of the Soflens. And when the bend of a given lens changes, its back vertex power changes: if the bend of the lens is increased, its back vertex power increases in minus refractive power; if the bend decreases, the back vertex power decreases in minus refractive power.

Lens dimensions

During most of the time that the investigational work was being done for the F.D.A. approval, the only Soflens available had a functional curve on its front surface of 45.00 diopters (keratometer power), which is equivalent to a radius of curvature of 7.5 mm. If this lens with a given marked power, such as −4.00 diopters, were placed on a cornea that had a keratometer reading of 45 diopters, its back vertex power effect on this eye would be −4.00 diopters. A 45.00 diopter cornea requires zero compensation in the back vertex power of the lens selected. However, if the cornea upon which this were placed had a keratometer reading of 46.00 diopters, the back vertex power of the minus lens would be greater than −4.00 diopters and a Soflens with less minus refractive power would be required on the eye in question. And if the cornea had a keratometer reading of 44.00 diopters, the back vertex power of the lens would be less than −4.00 diopters so that a Soflens with more minus refractive power should be used on that eye. Fortunately, the additional plus or minus refractive power that is required in any eye rarely exceeds about 0.50 diopter.

At present, three series of Soflenses are available in the 72-lens fitting set. Each series has its own front (convex) curve. And each lens in a given series of lenses, whether this lens has a back vertex refractive power of −0.25 diopter or −9.50 diopters, has the same front (convex) curve throughout this range of powers. As is obvious, this means that a lens of a given series and power will have a different ocular (concave) curvature from that of another given lens of the same series but of different power. As the minus refractive power increases in a given series, the ocular surface curve becomes steeper. However, because all of the molds, regardless of the lens power, have the same sagittal depth, all Soflenses of a given series have the same diameter and the same sagittal depth. Only the relatively small optical zone curve will steepen as the minus power increases since the aspherical concave curve flattens more rapidly toward the periphery in a high minus lens than in a low minus lens.

One further point is that the zero compensation cornea for all lens series is the cornea that has an average corneal curvature of 45.00 diopters or 7.5 mm. radius; that is, for a cornea of 45 diopters, the marked power of the Soflens should be its effective back vertex power for this eye. This point will be further clarified in connection with the use of the power selection procedure chart later.

One of these lens series was used throughout much of the investigational period: Series C. This design produces a monocurve lens with a front (convex) curve of 7.5 mm. radius (45.00 diopters). Its chord diameter is 13.3 mm. and the optical zone is 6.0 to 6.5 mm. In center thickness it varies from 0.09 to 0.36 mm., and its edge is almost knifelike. The Series C lens was originally available from −1.50 through −9.00 diopters. Today, relatively few C lenses are used and the available power range has been restricted markedly. This lens performs about equally well on corneas of 40.50 to 49.00 diopters in average curvature. Patients with tight lids and small apertures often are pleased with this lens because of its thin, tapered edge. Initially, the C series lens had to be used for myopia of above −6.50 diopters because such powers were not available in any other series. And again, because of its very thin edge, this lens still may be preferred for contact sports.

Also in the Soflens fitting set are F series and N series lenses. The F series is intended for corneas that are flatter than 44.50 diopters and the N series for corneas of 44.50 diopters and steeper. These are bicurve lenses with the same type of aspherical curve on the ocular side as the C lens but with a front chamfer curve of 0.5 mm. width on the edge of the front (convex) surface. The chord diameter is 12.3 on both series, and each series maintains a center thickness of 0.17 mm. regardless of the lens power.

N and F lenses have somewhat thicker edges and are not quite as comfortable initially as is the C lens. In a very short time, however, the lid sensation diminishes to complete comfort in most cases. The thicker edge does seem to provide better centering.

In practice, the N series, the F series, and the C series lens often are tried on the same cornea. Whichever lens provides the best centering and the best vision may be the lens chosen for the patient.

Before November 1, 1971, minus lenses only were available. In the N series, powers between 0.25 diopter and 9.50 diopters could be obtained; for the F series, 0.25 diopter through 6.00 diopters were available; and, in the C series, 3.00-diopter through 8.50-diopter lenses could be obtained.

A series of lenses currently is being tested for use with keratoconus cases, and a series of lenticular, high plus lenses is being tried for aphakia. Also, in the testing stage are Soflenses with one toric surface so that residual astigmatism may one day present less of a problem to the soft lens wearer than is the case today.

Fitting the Soflens is not difficult, since, for a given eye, only a few choices are possible. The Power selection procedure chart (Fig. 5-1), which accompanies the Soflens fitting set, may help the reader understand how to procede. We shall take an example and follow it through the prescribed steps.

We shall assume that the patient's right eye has a corneal curvature of 43 diopters along the horizontal meridian and 44 diopters along the vertical meridian. The assumed refractive error is −6.50 −50 cylinder axis 180. Look at the chart and note in the upper left *"Step one."* It points out that the spherical equivalent of the refractive power is calculated by adding one half of the cylinder power to the sphere power. In our example the spherical equivalent is −6.75 diopters, that is, −6.50 diopters plus one half of the half diopter cylinder. *Step two* says to con-

1. **Calculate the sphere equivalent of the refractive power: add half the cylinder power algebraically to the sphere power. Note.**

2. **Convert the sphere equivalent for vertex measuring distance by using the Vertex Power Conversion Chart. Note.**

3. **Calculate the average corneal radius: add the two K readings, divide by two. With this number, refer to the Corneal Radius Power Change Chart to determine the corneal power compensation. Note.**

4. **Add 1 + 2 + 3 to determine the SOFLENS Power.**

VERTEX POWER CONVERSION
for refractive distances from 9mm to 14 mm

Power at Measuring Distance	Vertex Compensation
−1.50 to −4.00	0 D.
−4.25 to −5.25	+0.25 D.
−5.50 to −7.25	+0 50 D.
−7.50 to −8.75	+0.75 D.
−9.00 to −10.50	+1.00 D.
+9.00 to +10.75	+1.00 D.
+11.00 to +12.35	+1.25 D.
+12.50 to +13.75	+1.50 D.
+14.00 to +14.75	+1.75 D.
+15.00 to +15.75	+2.00 D.

CORNEAL RADIUS POWER CHANGE

Corneal Radius: Millimeters	Diopters	Corneal Power Compensation
6.50	52.00	+1.00 D.
6.75	50.00	+ .75 D.
7.00	48.25	+ .50 D.
7.25	46.50	+ .25 D.
7.50	45.00	.00 D.
7.75	43.50	− .25 D.
8.00	42.25	− .50 D.
8.25	40.87	− .75 D.
8.50	39.75	−1.00 D.

Fig. 5-1. Soflens power selection procedure (From Bausch & Lomb, Inc., 1969.)

vert the spherical equivalent for the vertex distance by using the vertex power conversion chart. Note the vertex power conversion table in the upper right corner. For powers of −5.50 to −7.25, a compensation of +50 sphere is added to the −6.75 so that the lens power now becomes a −6.25 sphere. For *Step three,* calculate the average corneal radius. In our example the average corneal radius is 43.50 diopters since one meridian is 43.00 diopters and the other is 44.00 diopters. If we look at the lower right corner we find 43.50 diopters on the corneal radius power change table. This line tells us to add −0.25-diopter sphere to the −6.25 diopters calculated in Step two, since the Soflens will lose −0.25 diopter because it is bent less than the 45.00-diopter cornea, which represents its zero compensation point.

After these steps have been taken together, the practitioner would select a −6.50 sphere for this eye. And, since this cornea has an averaged corneal curvature of 43.50 diopters (7.75 mm. radius), the −6.50 sphere selected would be an F series lens.

In preparing to place the lens on the eye, the lens is removed from its vial, and normal saline is squirted on the lens in sufficient amounts so that the lens is well wetted. The lens is then rubbed between the thumb and forefinger in much the same manner as would be the case when using a wetting solution on a hard lens. It is then flushed again with the saline solution. When the lens is considered to be clean, it is placed on the tip of the index finger of the preferred hand. After turning the eye up as high as he can, the patient pulls down the lower lid and presses the lens against the sclera of the eye inferior to the cornea. The eye is then closed and the patient looks straight ahead through the closed eye while he rubs the lid very gently with his finger. Rubbing the cornea through the closed lid serves two functions: first, it helps to center the lens; second, it rubs out any air bubbles that may have remained under the lens.

After a minute or two, the practitioner should assure himself that the lens has positioned itself centered on the cornea or no more than 2 mm. low on the cornea. When the patient is instructed to blink, the lens moves 0.5 to 1 mm. vertically but should recenter itself immediately.

At this stage of the examination, even if visual acuity is poorer than 20/30 and lens centering is less than ideal, the patient may be allowed to wear the lens for 30 minutes, after which time the position and performance of the lens is rechecked and a spherical refraction is done. If the addition of spherical power alone (or no addition of power) allows the patient to obtain a best acuity of 20/30 or better in each eye, he is considered a potentially good Soflens wearer.

If on the other hand, visual acuity cannot be brought to 20/30 or better, the practitioner should change the lens from the F series to an N series lens and even to a C series lens, if necessary, to achieve optimum centering. After the best of the three series of lenses has been determined, the patient is tested for refraction again. Should visual acuity with full correction still be less than 20/30 in each eye, the patient is regarded as a potentially poor Soflens wearer.

When the patient is to remove the lens, he turns his eye up as high as he can. His second finger pulls down the lower lid while the first finger reaches up and contacts the lens, which is on the cornea. The first finger pulls the lens down onto the sclera and by swinging the thumb over toward and against the sclera, the lens is grasped between the thumb and the first finger and pinched off the eye. This "pinching" procedure is necessary because the lens is so firmly adherent to the eye that air must be allowed to get under it before it can be freed from the eye. The lens is so flexible and has such a thin edge that the lids will not grasp and eject it as they will a hard contact lens.

When the lens has been removed from the eye, it is cleaned again by squirting it liberally with normal saline solution and rubbing the lens between the fingers. If this lens is not to be taken out of the office by the patient, it is replaced in its original marked vial and placed aside for asepsis before it is replaced in the practitioner's fitting set.

Should one decide that the Soflens can provide an acceptable visual device, a continuous reel super-8 movie is used to teach the patient the care and handling of his lenses at this visit or at a subsequent visit.

Patient care kits

In addition to the Soflenses, a patient care kit also is provided for each patient. This kit contains the following:

    1. Soflens case

2. Asepticizer
3. 200 Salt tablets
4. Small plastic bottle in which the normal saline solution is mixed and stored
5. Instruction booklet

The case provided for this lens has a small hemisphere on each cap and the lens is placed on this convex hemisphere. The case is kept filled with normal saline solution, and each end of the case is screwed on in much the same way as with any hard contact lens case. At least once daily the case should be rinsed under running water and refilled with fresh saline solution.

Each day the contact lens case and the lenses inside of the case are made aseptic in the rather simple asepticizer, which looks like a baby bottle warmer. About 2 ounces of water are placed in the asepticizer well. The lens case is filled with saline solution, and the Soflenses are snapped into a clip in the top of the cap of this device and placed over the water. A small switch on the bottom of the asepticizer is depressed and an indicator light comes on, showing that the unit is in operation. The unit runs through a cycle of about 20 minutes, during which time the water inside the little bottle warmer device is brought to a boil and continues to boil until the water is boiled away. When the water is gone, the temperature of the device rises sufficiently so that the unit is automatically turned off by the thermostatic switch. In the morning the lenses are at room temperature and can be removed from the clip on the cap of the asepticizer and are ready for insertion.

The wearing schedule is extremely flexible. It is generally safe to start with a "3 hours on–1 hour off" schedule throughout the day for the first 2 days. For the next 2 days, "4 hours on–1 hour off" throughout the day is acceptable. On the fifth and sixth days, "6 hours on–1 hour off" should be safe. Our patient returns to the office on the seventh day, and if there are no adverse effects apparent, the lens can be worn "8 hours on–1 hour off" for 3 days. After that, 10 to 14 hours wear daily is acceptable. The patient is cautioned against wearing the lens for more than 30 minutes if steamy or foggy vision should occur. Sometimes the foggy or steamy vision may be the result only of a dirty front lens surface. Blinking may clear the vision, and the patient can extend his wearing time. Also, in common with the hard contact lens, a break of 30 minutes to 1 hour during the middle of the day will be helpful.

If the patient should accidently place the lens in plain water instead of normal saline solution, hydration will be increased and the lens will be tight and uncomfortable on the eye. On the other hand, should the saline concentration be increased, for example, if the patient should err when he makes up his saline solution, the lens would seem to be loose on the eye and also uncomfortable. In both of these instances, so long as the patient knows that the problem is one of salinity difference, he may elect to leave the lens on the eye, and in about 5 minutes the salinity of the Soflens will be approximately equal to that of the tears and comfort again will be apparent. A hypotonic lens may be especially difficult to remove. Flushing the eye liberally with normal saline solution can be very helpful.

Care of the Soflens is not difficult. A normal saline solution is prepared daily by the patient in the small plastic bottle provided in the care kit. One salt tablet is dropped into the bottle and the bottle is filled with distilled water to the horizontal line. Distilled water of the type normally used in steam irons is adequate. After about 10 minutes the solution is ready for use.

Advantages of the Soflens

1. Insertion and removal techniques are easily learned.
2. Lens dislocation onto the sclera rarely occurs, and if it should, no damage to the sclera or cornea could take place.
3. Comfort is excellent in most cases.
4. Corneal staining occurs rarely.
5. Spectacle blur is very uncommon and if it is apparent, rarely lasts longer than 10 to 15 minutes.
6. Full-time wear on the first day is possible.
7. Ejection or loss of the lens from the eye is not common even in contact sports.
8. Foreign bodies cannot get under the lens.
9. Contact lens care is simple since only one available solution is required.
10. Cosmetically, the lens is excellent.

Disadvantages of the Soflens

1. Erratic, often poor, visual acuity at far and near distance.
2. Lens durability, especially in regard to torn edges, is not good.
3. Daily sterilization by boiling the lenses can be a nuisance. This procedure may also account for a gradual loss of comfort and a decrease in vision.
4. The possibility that the lens may soak up water-soluble chemicals, which could damage the eye, still remains as a most serious potential problem.

Three of the disadvantages might be amplified. First, patients usually claim that vision with the Soflens is not as good as that with spectacles or with a hard contact lens.

At least three known factors can account for this "poor" vision complaint:

1. All soft contact lenses are sufficiently flexible so that the lacrimal lens provides very little help for an astigmatic eye; in addition these lenses change shape almost constantly as a result of lid and eye movements. And the constantly changing shape produces constantly changing visual acuity.
2. The Soflens has a relatively small optical zone, often not larger than 6 mm. If this lens centers poorly or moves excessively on the eye, the non-optical section may cover a sufficient pupillary area to produce poor vision.
3. Spectacle blur does not occur as it does with most hard contact lens wearers, hence Soflens patients can make a valid comparison between their vision with contact lenses and their vision with spectacles. The hard contact lens wearer commonly compares his good or poor vision with hard contact lenses against the rather poor "spectacle blur" type of vision common to the hard lens wearer. Naturally, his hard contact lens vision wins out most of the time even though it may not be a passable 20/20 on the Snellen chart.

In regard to the second and third disadvantages, that is, lens durability and daily sterilization of the lens, it might be well to point out that since bacteria and other foreign microorganisms are believed not to invade this lens material (with a few possible exceptions), it is probable that a sterile (or near sterile) lens may not be so critical if a simple, suitable, and safe Soflens cleaning system could be devised. A clean Soflens should be no more prone to produce conditions favorable to bacterial invasion of a normal eye than is the case with a clean hard contact lens. And few of us today would argue for the absolute necessity of sterilization of a hard contact lens except on the pathological eye. Much lens deterioration (such as, edge tears) and nearly all of the progressively occurring discomfort and reduced vision appear to be related to cleaning, storage, and sterilization problems. Harsh rubbing with normal saline alone in an effort to clean the lens is highly ineffective and undoubtedly this procedure damages the edges and the surfaces of the Soflens. The elevated temperature necessary to heat asepsis coagulates proteins on the lens surface, and this gradual buildup of foreign materials on the lens produces discomfort and poor vision.

Only the fourth disadvantage appears to be without a real solution aside from patient education.

THERAPEUTIC USES
Keratoconus

The Soflens has so far proved a rather poor substitute for the hard contact lens in keratoconus or other highly irregular corneas. As a general rule, even the addition of noticeable amounts of sphere or cylinder over the Soflens may provide too little improvement in visual acuity to make their use in place of hard contact lenses feasible. Without question, however, this is an area that should be diligently explored. Corneal deterioration undoubtedly occurs with or without the use of any type of contact lens, but few practitioners with long experience in this field can deny that hard corneal or scleral lenses rarely are the gentle, helpful devices that these pathological corneas require. A soft contact lens that can smooth out the irregular cornea would represent a giant step forward.

Aphakia

Aphakia has, in general, been a more favored area, perhaps because the lenticular high plus power Soflens is thicker and therefore firmer. This Soflens has a chord diameter of 13.3 mm. and a front lenticular bowl of 7.7 mm. in its hydrated state. Some patients admit that vision with this lens can be as good as vision with a hard contact lens, but most of them insist that this good vision may not always be present with the Soflens. Without question, however, the aphake who is uncomfortable with hard contact lenses will accept the Soflens. This is a promising area.

A Soflens design that employs at least one toric surface is being tested. If the Soflens does not rotate around the eye's anteroposterior axis as some clinicians claim, such a lens design could produce decided improvements in visual performance.

Distribution

In September 1970, Bausch & Lomb claimed that approximately 1,300 patients were wearing this lens. Two thirds of them were females and 51% of the 1,300 patients formerly wore hard contact lenses. The refractive error distribution was normal (for myopes only) except for the fact that refractive and corneal astigmatism were each less than 2.00 diopters.

It was pointed out that visual acuity in more than 80% of these patients was 20/20 or better and that acuity appeared to improve as the lenses were worn. No data were given as to the number of patients who had tried the Soflens and failed; hence we cannot judge the adequacy of performance of this lens except to point out that at least 80% of the patients who accept the Soflens get 20/20 or better acuity.

Patients wear the Soflens daily about as long as is expected for hard contact lens wearers or, often, even for longer periods. Comfort is not usually a real deterrent to Soflens wear although comfort sometimes decreases as the weeks of wear accumulate. There is little question, however, that poor visual acuity rather than discomfort causes most Soflens failures.

The Soflens already undoubtedly plays an important role for at least three types of patients:

1. Unsuccessful hard lens wearers.
2. Those who wish to wear contact lenses only occasionally, including actors and actresses or even the housewife and public speaker.
3. Athletes, especially for contact sports but not for swimming.

Soft contact lenses seem certain to stay, in some form. It probably is far too early to talk about them in terms of the "lens of the future," but this type of lens will provide a very useful addition to the visual devices available to eye care practitioners of today and tomorrow. More than 80 years have passed since the first successful hard contact lens was put on a human eye. Perhaps time is the essential ingredient for maturity of the Soflens also.

REFERENCE

Wichterle, O., and Lim, D.: Hydrophilic gels for biological use, Nature **185:**117-118, 1960.

Chapter 6

The Bausch & Lomb Soflens

Chester J. Black, M.D.

LENS MATERIAL AND COMPOSITION

The material of the Bausch & Lomb Soflens is really not the same as that of the Czechoslovakian lens. The difference is a result of stringent quality controls in both compounding the material and the method of processing. This is responsible for a more stable lens. This lens is more difficult to tear and, to my knowledge, I have heard no one complain that it spontaneously split.

The reason for deciding to fabricate the lens so that it is 38% water by volume when it is soaked in saline, was that this resulted in the most stable state of the material and lens.

The lens does not pass the estimated amount of oxygen to the epithelium of the cornea by way of the tears on tests measuring the oxygen deprivation of the underlying epithelium. This is corroborated clinically by complaints suggesting edema in some instances during the adaptation period. This edema is usually transient and in most instances does not recur.

BACTERIAL CONTAMINATION

As far as bacterial contamination is concerned, the problem is no greater than that of the hard lens, except one must use the unconventional technique of boiling instead of ophthalmic preservatives. Neither are lenses actually placed sterile on the eye. Obviously this is not customarily expected, for one would have to use operating room techniques sterile gloves, and so on. One is, however, concerned with the control of an overgrowth of bacterial pathogens. *Pseudomonas* is probably the most common and serious offender followed by *Aspergillus niger*, which has been observed as a contaminant on some hydrogel lenses (I have never observed such contamination of a Bausch & Lomb Soflens).

In addition with the Bausch & Lomb Soflens, as with most hydrogel lenses, saline solution is needed. This presents a problem as far as supply is concerned. Distilled water is used to make the saline with the use of salt tablets without iodine and a minimal amount of other contaminents. The patient inadvertently may substitute another kind of water on occasion. This may or may not irritate the eye. It may cause a discoloration of the lens, particularly if iron is present in the water.

Saline itself will not support the growth of *Staphylococcus aureus, Aspergillus niger, Escherichia coli, Candida albicans, Bacillus globigii,* and is bacteriostatic for all except *Staphylococcus aureus,* against which it is lethal. However five strains of

Pseudomonas aeruginosa continued to grow. If organic constituents are instilled in the saline as contaminants, this will of course alter the results, as other organisms may be able to survive.

The Bausch & Lomb Soflens can stand autoclaving up to about 230° F. (111° C.). It was found that the asepticizer was lethal to all the above mentioned organisms. I am told that there are some sporeformers to which this process is not lethal.

LENS CHARACTERISTICS AND FITTING PROCEDURES

Since the lens is so flexible, the back surface of the lens takes on more or less the shape of the front surface of the cornea, and the only lens parameter one needs to know is the power.

Corneal measurements

The part of the cornea one measures with the keratomer is only the central part of the two principal meridians. Since the lens covers both it and the peripheral part of the cornea, which is unmeasurable by conventional methods, one has to resort to some degree of trial lens fitting.

One can have two corneas each with a central area of the same radius, as measured by the keratometer. One of these corneas can have a peripheral area that is flatter than the other. Thus two series of lenses of the same power are available, a steep series N and a flat series F.

Lens power and visual acuity

The power of the lenses, as labeled on the container bottle, is determined for a cornea of about 44.50 diopters. If these lenses are placed on corneas of different radii, the power will be different from that marked on the bottle. To compensate for this difference, a power selection procedure chart is available. One notes that the steeper corneas would need less minus refractive power than that calculated for a 44.50-diopter cornea and that the flatter corneas need more minus power.

Vertex distance is important and one must take this into consideration on powers over −4.00 diopters. Less power is needed than that found in spectacles. The keratometer findings are not used for determining the central posterior curve of the lens, but for determining the correct power of the lens.

The new concept of fitting the Bausch & Lomb Soflens is that one needs to know only the power of the lens. This is calculated by compensating for the vertex distance as well as the change in radius from that of a 44.50-diopter cornea.

Corneas with over 1.00 diopter of astigmatism, as read by a keratometer, or again 1.00 diopter, as found on refraction, are rarely good candidates for the Bausch & Lomb Soflens as one usually finds an appreciable residual astigmatism present.

The fitting of a Bausch & Lomb Soflens can be very difficult or very simple. The difficulty arises from the fact that as many as three to six lenses can be used to obtain a visual acuity of one line less than that obtained with the best spectacle correction. The lens tends to take a longer period of time to bed down than the hard lens, causing the patient to complain of a watery vision. It usually takes some patients 6 to 8 weeks before the best visual acuity is obtained.

CORRECTION OF REFRACTIVE ERROR

When the Bausch & Lomb Soflens is first placed on the eye, the front surface of the lens tends to have waves. As one watches the front surface of the lens with a Placido disc, one sees these waves tend to disappear in about a half hour or so. Yet, if the patient has a wet eye (subclinical tearing), there will be some residual waves. It is possible to use the keratometer to measure the front power of the lens on the eye. One can, with the appropriate tables, calculate what it should read. Keratometer readings tend to be unreliable, particularly on the initial visit. This could very well be attributable to the need for the lens to bed down. The use of the keratometer, though, can be of some help in fitting. If one finds after wearing the lens a half hour that the reflected images of the circles of the keratometer are wavy, one probably has an improper lens on the eye. It may be too flat or too steep or one may have a wet watery situation. If the keratomer readings show little astigmatism and the images of the circles are not wavy but visual acuity is poor, then the power may be off. The lens series is probably right.

Actual calculation of what the front surface of the lens should be and what one finds can be similar, especially when one is fitting a spherical cornea. When fitting astigmatic corneas, since one is using the spherical equivalent to ascertain power and an average of the two principal keratometer corneal readings, greater differences do occur. Calculating both the flattest and steepest meridians, using their respective powers, does seem to bring about a closer relationship. All this is predicted on the premise that one is not measuring a wave of the front surface of the lens.

The variation of the powers of the two principal meridians can be observed when the patient blinks by viewing the front surface of the lens with the keratometer. The power may change on blinking. This is ascertained by a separation of the mires of the keratometer. These mires should quickly become approximated to their original position after the blink is completed. If there is a prolonged period of time before the return of mires to their original approximated position, then, of course, the patient will experience blurred vision. If the mires have to be readjusted after a blink to another power, then one has variable vision. This is usually caused by a poor return of the lens to its original position on the cornea upon blinking or, as some might say, by poor return to center.

The parameters of the corneas are responsible for the centering of the lens. An eccentric apex of the cornea would normally result, to a degree, in a decentralization of the lens on that cornea. A lens too steep for a particular cornea would result in a decentralization of the lens with the usual waves on the front surface of the lens, as seen by viewing the images of the circles of the keratometer. A lens too flat for a particular cornea would usually result in a decentered lens with an exaggerated residual astigmatism of the front surface of the lens. The lens hardly moves when the patient blinks as viewed by the observers naked eye. With the use of the slit lamp 0.25 to 0.5 mm. of motion downward may be seen. This is tolerated provided that the lens rapidly returns to its original position.

On the initial visit one does not always get all of these fitting parameters precisely as one would wish, but the patient acquires more of them as time passes.

Retinoscopy and manifest refraction can be very tedious and misleading unless waves and unusual astigmatism are not prevented. In addition, the lens must center promptly on blinking. It can also be complicated by a subclinical tearing (wet) eye.

Fitting procedure

After a keratometer reading is taken and the spectacle correction is ascertained, the first lens fitting is as calculated by the use of the power selection procedure card. After the lenses have been on the eye for a half hour, note if they are centered, preferably by the use of the slit lamp. If the lenses are greatly decentered, try another lens of the same power but the other series. If the lens is fairly well centered, note if the eye is very moist by observing whether there is an unusual amount of tears at the lower lid margin. If so, wait another 15 minutes until this is minimal or disappears. Check the motion of the lens to see if it returns rapidly to its original position after a blink. Some sluggishness is acceptable at this time, but it must return to its original position. Check the front surface of the lens with the keratometer. If the images of the circles of the mires are wavy, the lens is probably incorrect or the eye is wetter than normal. If it is the latter, then wait another 15 minutes or so. Whenever the images of the circles of the keratometer are wavy or there is an unusual amount of astigmatism, as read by the keratometer, try another series of the same power first.

Whether the two keratometer readings of the principal meridian of the cornea are the same or about 0.75 diopter apart will, of course, depend on the original astigmatism of the cornea provided that one is not measuring waves. Visual acuity will usually be good when the keratometer readings of the two principal meridians are the same or 0.75 diopter apart. One is more prone to find this on the second or third visit than on the initial one. Now the visual acuity is checked. If the visual acuity is poorer than expected, try a manifest refraction or retinoscopy. Usually a power change using the same series is all that is needed. Rarely, a power change of the opposite series is needed.

The patient has by this time seen the movie on the handling and care of the lens. In my office, a patient must remove the lens three times and place it on his eye three times before he can take it home. Precautions and particularly a method of cleaning the lenses by rubbing the convex surface in the palm of the hand using saline as a cleaning media, are again demonstrated. The lens surface may collect some debri that cannot be removed as it may be cooked on the lens by the asepticizer. These lenses have to be replaced. Lenses are never soaked in a wetting solution or soaking solution, but some can be used to clean a lens when one cannot clean them with a saline solution. The same procedure is used as with the saline, except one should rinse off the solution with water and saline and then make the lens aseptic. Patients are cautioned that baby water and spring water are not distilled waters. Rarely do patients buy saline. A bottle in which the patient can mix and boil the saline will soon be available.

The wearing schedule prescribed is as suggested by the instruction insert found in the package.

FOLLOW-UP EXAMS

In 2 weeks the patient is seen again. The cornea is checked with the slip lamp in the usual manner. The centering and motion of the lens are checked. With the use of the keratometer the power of the front surface is ascertained. A waviness of the images of the circles is noted. A minor amount may be tolerated, particularly if it disappears on blinking several times, as it may be caused by loose debris on the lens surface. If the keratometer readings of the two principle meridians are within 0.75 diopter, depending again on the original astigmatism of the cornea, it is acceptable. One will usually get good visual acuity. Observe if any power change occurs on blinking and if it does, how fast it returns to its original reading. The visual acuity will probably be less watery than it was at the time of the initial visit. The visual acuity will improve more so in a month.

A manifest refraction with spheres only will usually suffice for determining any necessary power changes. Check the near point and question the patient about his reading ability for evidence of any overcorrection of minus power. If any power changes are necessary, they are done at this visit. After a new lens is provided, it is again checked after 10 or 15 minutes for the visual acuity and, with the slit lamp for centering and motion, use the keratometer for the usual similarity of power of the two meridians as well as the presence or absence of waves by the use of the images of the reflected circles.

Only two more visits, a month apart, are really needed. Visual acuity is difficult to obtain initially for some. It takes work by trial fitting. A full complement of lenses at your disposal is very important for this reason.

COMPLICATIONS OF THE BAUSCH & LOMB SOFLENS

Symptoms of scratchiness, which occur when the lens is inserted, are usually caused by foreign material under the lens. In most cases, removing the lens and rinsing it with saline will remove any debris and alleviate the symptoms. Patients do not complain of foreign bodies getting under the lens while they are wearing them.

Conjunctival injection with tearing is caused usually by a contaminant the lens has absorbed such as soap from a patient's hand. Tearing without conjunctival injection when the lenses are first put on the eye, or after 2 hours or so, can occur on unusually sensitive eyes. Initially, for 4 or more days proparacaine hydrochloride (Ophthaine) instilled in the eye once a day, or as needed, for this period of time may eliminate the problem.

Corneal stippling may occur when a patient attempts to remove a lens that is not there. Localized conjunctival injection at the position of approximately 6 o'clock because a patient tries to remove a lens not present, has been observed. Rarely, an abrasion can be found.

Edema may occur during the adaptation period. Edema is usually controlled by limiting the wearing time and more slowly increasing the wearing time than originally suggested. Rarely, an abrasion can be found.

Approximately 42% of my patients have never had to have the lenses replaced because of loss or tearing.

The original asepticizers were made of pot metal and corroded. These have been replaced by stainless steel. Now no such problem is anticipated. The original carrying case leaked and was replaced by a new design.

I have seen one patient who has ulcers that recur on wearing the lenses.

THERAPEUTIC USES

In general, Soflens wear for bullous keratopathy cases rarely results in improvement of visual acuity and this only with the adjunct use of 5% sodium chloride solution. Most of the bullous keratopathies were secondary to endothelial dystrophies and primary or secondary to complications of cataract surgery. All essentially were painful. The pain is usually dramatically relieved by the use of the lens as a protective shield, as similarly accomplished by the old hard scleral lenses. The use, of course, of this lens is much simpler. No moldings of the eye or keratometer readings are necessary. These were worn day and night, cleaned once a day to once a week depending on the severity of the pain. Half percent chloramphenicol (Chloromycetin) drops twice a day were used with no preservatives added as a prophylaxis to control bacterial growth.

The few recurrent ulcers were not improved by the use of the lens in my hands but were aggravated. Although, I must admit, they were not subjected to debridement before the lens was used.

Exposed noninfected ulcers do well. The lenses are worn day and night. The lenses are cleaned and made aseptic once per day. A tendency toward neovascularization at 6 o'clock position does occur but is minimal. These cases really have not been followed long enough (5 to 10 years) to note what the long-term effects will be.

Moderate to mild keratitis sicca patients do well with the lenses when they are soaked in a hypotonic solution. One fills the mixing bottle to the top, instead of to the mark, with distilled water. The usual one tablet is dissolved in the bottle. The lenses are usually taken off at night.

Better visual acuity can be obtained more easily in some instances with the use of acetylcysteine 10% or 20% four times or so a day, as one does not have the problem of ascertaining the proper parameters of the lens to be used.

If the keratitis sicca is severe the edges of the lens may dry out.

Patients with a trichiasis do well with the lens. It can be removed at night, and if any residual astigmatism occurs, it can be corrected with spectacles.

Keratoconus patients with minor cones can be fitted with the lens. If irregular residual astigmatism occurs, it can be corrected by a hard contact lens fitted on top of the Soflens. This is done for patients who cannot tolerate the hard lens. Residual regular astigmatism may be corrected by spectacles in lieu of a hard contact lens.

If a pinhole effect is needed because of corneal scars or multiple holes of the iris, a hard cosmetic lens can be made to fit over the Soflens. This again is only done when the patient cannot tolerate the hard lens.

Many keratoconus patients cannot be fitted with the Soflens as the lenses are not steep enough. The lens tends to produce a pleat or fold interiorly that projects off the eye onto the margin of the lower lid. On blinking, the lens tends to pop out.

ADVANTAGES OF THE SOFLENS

The iatrogenic aspects of the hard lens have, to a great extent, been alleviated by the Bausch & Lomb Soflens. Little or no problems occur on overwearing the lenses. No abrasions are usually found. The eyes are white and usually free of conjunctival injection.

Initially the patient experiences a very minor foreign body effect. This may not be so with successful hard lens patients.

There is no need for any adjustment equipment, but this advantage is offset to some degree by the need of using the trial method of obtaining the proper lens.

Chapter 7

Some considerations and basic fitting of the Soflens

Maurice G. Poster, O.D.

In consideration of the value of new contact lens materials and designs it becomes important to develop a model from which we can evaluate any new modality that is available or which we hope will be available. The following I consider to be a realistic model with the information available today, notwithstanding new scientific research, which undoubtedly will be pursued in the future. The model is a change in the physical dimensions of the surface of the cornea in order to satisfy the visual requirements achieved with a material so closely compatible to the cornea and its surrounding tissue that we can consider it to be a part of the cornea. Within this context a few of the requirements needed to achieve this model are the following:

1. Physical comfort
2. Continuous wear
3. Best obtainable visual acuity commensurate with the patient's visual status
4. No physiological involvement with the eye or the supporting tissue
5. Maintenance of a normal biological environment
6. Material stability and longevity

Using the model and the few requirements listed, have we approached our needs? Contrary to some, we have approached and possibly arrived for a very small number of patients. There are reports of patients who wear the PMMA contact lenses continuously for months and years and, according to these reports, meet the requirements of the aforementioned model. Similarly, there are reports of a few cases that seem to meet all these requirements with hydrophilic contact lenses.

The conclusions we can draw are that the parameters of comfort, acuity, physiology, tissue tolerance, compatibility, and other requirements seem to have been met in these few cases. This by no means indicates that the material or its design is universal in its application. To the contrary, it points up the need for a multitude of materials and designs, and for the improvement of what we have, to increase the practitioner's ability to approach the model with each patient. Great strides have been made in recent years in the development of new materials, which have expanded our horizons.

There is no question of the need for further research in these areas. We must also be aware of the complexity of the problem. The following is only an abbreviated list of what must be considered in developing a new material and in evaluating it:

Stability	Tear resistance
Material matrix	Optical properties
Absorptive properties	Hardness
Adsorptive properties	Resiliency
Surface chemistry	Diffusion
Chemical inertness	Permeability
Chemical reactivity	Service life
Rigidity	Toxicity

With all this in mind let us look at what we are gaining and what we may be giving up with the use of this new modality:

Advantages
Initial comfort
Ease of adaptation
Little to no spectacle blur
Ease of fit
Reduced dust problem
Minimal corneal physical change
Minimal dislodging
Almost no recentering
Part-time wearers
Use in highly sensitive corneas
Reduced amount of flare
Transition lens, when refitting patient with hard lenses

Disadvantages
Visual
Acuity (Snellen chart)
Fluctuation of vision
Limitations imposed by refractive error or corneal topography
Tearing
Splitting
Cleaning
Duplication
Verification
Aseptic techniques
Evaluation of fit
Fragility
Inspection

Things to consider
Environment
Humidity
Temperature
Pollution
Contamination

Hydration variations
Scratches
Service life
Stability
    Aging
    Chemical reactivity
    Surface chemistry
Permeability
Corneal physiology
Long-term effects
Total package (lens, solutions, case, aseptics)

Obviously, even the limitations imposed by the manufacturer relative to patients who may be fitted with this lens tells us that it is not a panacea.

The practitioner must in the last analysis make the professional judgment as to which material and design will best suit each patient's needs. Undoubtedly, even with this added modality we still have patients for whom we cannot prescribe a contact lens. I do feel this new material has enlarged our armamentarium, but we are only at the threshold of greater things to come.

Assuming examination and questioning of the patient reveals no contraindications and we have a healthy eye, what criteria can we use to determine when to use this new modality in place of the time-tested PMMA lens. An initial refractive screening can be made on the basis of the manufacturer's recommendations:

1. 2.00 diopters (D.) or less of corneal astigmatism

2. 1.50 diopters or less of refractive astigmatism

My experience has shown that these guidelines are too broad and the use of the spectacle astigmatic correction is the principle key.

Let us consider the following situations:

1. *Corneal astigmatism with appropriate spectacle astigmatic correction.* Since the spectacle correction contains the astigmatic element and is correcting most, if not all, of the corneal astigmatism, a Soflens placed on this cornea would take an astigmatic shape. The degree of uncorrected astigmatism on the front surface would impair the visual acuity. My limits are 1.00 D. or less of spectacle astigmatism to evaluate these patients with lenses.

2. *Virtually no corneal astigmatism with a spectacle astigmatic correction.* As the spectacle astigmatic correction is neutralizing the astigmatism produced within the eye, a different situation now exists than in situation no. 1. A Soflens on this eye would take the shape of the cornea, which has virtually no astigmatism. The resultant front surface of the lens therefore would be spherical for all practical purposes. The astigmatism created within the eye is uncorrected and we would have a residual astigmatic error left, causing visual problems. My limits are less than 0.75 D. to evaluate the lens on the patient.

3. *Corneal astigmatism with no spectacle astigmatism.* In the situation of corneal astigmatism with no spectacle astigmatism the Soflens will assume the approximate toric surface of the cornea and will neutralize most of the astigmatism produced within the eye. Although the manufacturer uses 2.00 D. of corneal astigmatism as the upper limit there are cases that could benefit visually with a greater amount. This type of case generally does well visually with the Soflens.

4. *Spherical cornea with a spherical spectacle correction.* This is the best possible situation for visual success with these lenses.

The four categories mentioned are guidelines when predicting. Surely a lens should be evaluated while being worn in any situation.

The fitting parameters of the Soflens are limited. Basically there are the F and N series, with the ability of resorting to the C series when physical comfort is not achieved with the other two series. The F series has a front curve of 7.70 mm., the N series 7.25 mm., and the C series 7.50 mm. The inside curve is aspheric and its curvature is dependent on the power of the lens. This as well accounts for variations in optical zone sizes.

If we calculate the lens needed for the patient, we find the optic zone radius is steeper than the cornea, and as we increase it in power, the radius becomes much steeper than the cornea of the given eye.

The method for determination of the initial lens necessary for the patient depends on the ametropia and the radii of curvature of the cornea. Since the power of the lens as marked holds true only for corneas having a 7.50 mm. radius, a cornea that is steeper requires plus power added to it and a flatter cornea requires minus power. A rule of thumb is that 1 mm. of change in corneal radius requires 1 diopter of change in prescription.

The radii of the cornea determines the series to be used. After averaging the corneal radii in diopters, a cornea of 44.75 D. or flatter requires an F series. A cornea of 45.00 D. or steeper requires an N series.

Thus, an eye with a cornea of 39.50 D. (8.54 mm.) requiring a −4.00 D. spectacle lens will need an F series of approximately −5.00 D. The reliability of this method is only fair and surely requires modification through evaluation of the fit and prescription. In general, a prescription change of over 0.75 D. (as an overrefraction with the lens in place) seems only accurate to ±0.50 D.

Evaluation of the fit and prescription should be done at least one-half hour after insertion of the lens because of changes in hydration, pH, and other factors. The fit is assessed by determining the positioning of the lens on the cornea. A well-fitting lens will have little movement in the primary position. This should be approximately a half millimeter. Horizontal versions of the eye should not change the positioning of the lens appreciably. In superior and inferior gaze the lens lag may be as much as 2 mm. The downward gaze, as in reading, should be carefully checked to ensure, not only positioning, but reading acuity.

There is only a limited ability to alter the fit. One can try for better centration, if he is using an F series, by changing to an N series. Conversely, an N series can be loosened by using an F series. As diameter, central thickness, and all other parameters are fixed in these lenses there is no ability to alter the lens except by changing the series, or the prescription. In the latter case the lens will be flatter by adding plus power and tighter by adding minus power, but acuity will be sacrificed.

There is no doubt that increasing the number of parameters will increase its potential use.

Chapter 8

Soft and hard contact lenses:
A comparison

Harold I. Moss, O.D.

My clinical experience is with the Griffin Naturalens and the Bausch & Lomb Soflens. We must remember, in any discussion of this nature, that when discussing soft lenses we are referring to a completely new modality—a visual aid that is in its infancy. If we were to compare soft lenses, at the present stage of development, with hard corneal lenses, at the same stage of development, we would be hard pressed, I believe, to ever place a hard corneal lens on a patient's eye. The stage of development must be kept uppermost in one's mind when discussing a comparison between soft and hard lenses.

Lens construction must first be considered when drawing a comparison. Hard lenses, as currently prescribed, have many variables. They may be listed as follows: base curve, secondary curve, tertiary curve, blend curves, visual zone diameter, overall diameter, thickness, and color. We may alter these variables according to the corneal topography and the external factors involved in corneal lens prescribing. Most laboratories are fairly capable of making these lenses to exact specifications, and after the lens is received from the laboratory, we can verify these specifications.

Lens verification of the soft lenses, however, leaves a great deal to be desired. The only accurate procedure to check a soft lens, at the present time, is to place it on the eye and determine if the performance is what was desired.

Regarding the Soflens, we are, at present, limited to two series of lenses. They are referred to as the N (7.2 mm.) series and the F (7.7 mm.) series. The numerical figures refer to the outside curves of the lenses—the outside curve being the base curve of the Soflens in the dry state. The inside curve of the lens is varied to encompass the power. We readily understand, therefore, that if the power is changed, the fit of the lens is automatically changed. The lenses have a standard thickness of 0.17 mm. and a standard overall diameter of 12.2 or 12.3 mm. Also incorporated is a standard outside chamfer.

The Griffin Naturalens, on the other hand, more approaches our thinking insofar as the hard lens is concerned. It has variable base curves as we understand them. The base curves vary from 7.2 to 8.7 mm. in 0.3 mm. steps. The lenses have an optical zone of approximately 8 mm. All lenses have an edge bevel. The Soflens has an optical zone of about 6 mm. and an aspherical periphery on the inside of the lens. The Griffin lens has variable diameters, from 13 to 15 mm. in 0.5 mm. steps. The Naturalens has a single inside radius. All the lenses have a lenticular cut to control edge thickness. All lenses should, therefore, have approximately the same peripheral thickness.

The next point in this comparison is the prescribing procedure. When prescribing the hard lens, we prescribe or we follow that particular routine that resolves our patients' problems and leads us to conclude that the lens construction arrived at will provide the best clinical results for that patient. The Soflens, as just stated, is rather limited in its application because there are only two series available to us. As Dr. Poster pointed out, "It either works or it doesn't work."

The Naturalens, on the other hand, can be varied considerably. The prescriber may combine any of the specifications outlined. The prescriber can do anything he desires within the parameters that are available.

The next consideration is the degree of difficulty in prescribing. Because of the flexibility of the lens, one need not be as exacting with the curvatures prescribed as with the hard lens. You are all aware of the fact that the soft lenses change curvature on the cornea and tend to assume the same curvature on its inside as the outside corneal curve.

I feel safe to state, therefore, that it is easier to prescribe a soft lens than it is a hard lens. It should not, however, be considered easy. The prescriber must fully understand the limitations of the lens being prescribed. Soft lenses are, in fact, complicated to prescribe if one considers all of the factors mentioned in other chapters. Lens stability must be achieved, but the proper amount of lens movement must be retained. Lens centration is of paramount importance. All these factors must be considered if we are going to achieve a good clinical result without interfering with corneal integrity.

The Naturalens can best be described as a semiscleral lens. The periphery of the lens should always rest on the sclera. It should be prescribed approximately 2 mm. larger than the visible iris diameter. The Soflens is basically a corneal lens, but in a great number of cases, with small corneas, it is also a semiscleral lens. The Soflens diameter is 12.2 mm. We often encounter 10.5 and 11 mm. corneas for which we are attempting to prescribe this lens. The lens now rests in the limbal area or possibly beyond it. In these situations the lens cannot be classified as corneal. Extreme care must be exercised in these cases.

In any discussion of soft lenses I prefer to talk about visual efficiency rather than visual acuity. If good visual efficiency can be achieved, we have prescribed for that particular patient a lens that will provide the kind of vision required to perform their visual tasks properly and efficiently. It is difficult to talk about soft lenses in terms of visual acuity only. I feel that visual efficiency is a much more encompassing term.

Patient adaptation to soft lenses has already been discussed. Adaptation is infinitely easier with soft lenses. If we were to take a beginning contact lens patient and place on one eye a Naturalens and on the other eye a Soflens, the immediate patient reaction, in the average situation, is greater comfort with the Naturalens. Reference here is to the immediate patient reaction and not to the eventual comfort attained with the Soflens, which, in most instances, is excellent. Both soft lenses are considerably more comfortable, for the average wearer, than is the hard lens of any construction.

Flare, glare, and photophobia are practically nonexistent with the Naturalens.

Wearers of the Soflens are not, however, completely free of this problem. If the patient has a rather large pupil, he will complain about flare almost to the same degree as the hard lens wearer. The symptoms are magnified at dusk and at night. When good lens centration is achieved with the Soflens, the flare factor is minimized.

Sporting activities. I do not like to compare the soft lenses used in sporting activities with hard lenses because I never did consider hard corneal lenses the lens construction of choice for contact sports. In all my years in practice I did not knowingly prescribe hard lenses for contact sports. I prescribed the minimum-clearance haptic (sceral) lens. The haptic lens was and still is an excellent sport lens. It in no way, however, compares with efficiency achieved with either of the soft lenses.

Length of wearing time. I have always limited my hard lens patients to a maximum of 10 hours wear at any one wearing time. This procedure has just about eliminated the overwear syndrome. It has, as well, reduced the afterblur (spectacle blur) time. In like manner I limit my soft lens wearers to a maximum of 10 hours at any one wearing time. The lenses are cleaned upon removal, stored in their proper solution and rinsed prior to reinsertion. I have not experienced any adverse patient reaction to these instructions. Little or no objective or subjective symptomatology has resulted by following this procedure.

Our instructions to the patient are given many times over. The patient, in addition, is admonished to use his common sense. If any symptoms occur such as a red or irritated eye, the patient is instructed to call the office at once. One of the problems encountered in my early experiences was that an eye could become somewhat congested and the lens wearer may not be aware of it. They only became aware of the increased redness because someone told them about it. When calling, the inquiry usually was concerned with the fact that they did not feel anything wrong—should they continue to wear the lens despite the congestion. This, of course, was only a minor problem, but the prescriber should be aware that it may occur.

A soft lens wearer may vary his schedule considerably. He may wear the lenses 2 hours one day, 10 hours the next, skip a day, and go back to 10 hours the fourth day. We all know that this is relatively impossible with hard lenses. The soft lens wearer may alternate between lenses and spectacles as desired. We all know that this change is very difficult for the average hard lens wearer.

Care of the lenses. Care of all lenses, soft and hard, is exceedingly important. We must follow proper hygienic procedures with all forms of lenses. We must admit, however, that the care of soft lenses is much more exacting than the care of hard lenses. We can have surface contamination on a hard lens and clean it off by rubbing with a cleaning solution. We are fully aware that this is much more difficult with the soft lens. There has not, however, been any patient objection to the hydrogen peroxide procedure for the Naturalens or the boiling procedure for the Soflens.

Lens durability. I have been keeping a log on causes of replacement for soft lenses as opposed to hard lenses. Lens replacement is a factor and most patients ask about this prior to getting their lenses. My data tend to confirm the fact that the replacement ratio of soft lenses, for whatever reason, tends to be very much the same as the loss ratio of hard lenses combined with the replacement of lenses for scratches and chips.

The need for insurance exists for the soft lenses. The lenses however are not generally replaced for the same reasons as are hard lenses; soft lenses are rarely lost. The need for replacement is that the lenses become coated, tear, or are chipped. The primary reason for the replacement of hard lenses is loss.

Percentage of people for whom the lenses may be prescribed. For the past several years, in the practice of a good clinican, 85% success is about the maximum one could expect to achieve in the prescribing of hard contact lenses. Approximately 65% of these cases were total successes, which is determined by good wearing time, good visual efficiency, and a minimum degree of interference with the corneal integrity. The totally unsuccessful and the partially successful cases stemmed, in the main, from the sensitivity factor.

I agree with Drs. Poster and Bailey in their conclusion that, at the present time, only about 20% success may be achieved with the Soflens. This percentage is taken from patients at random and not after screening the patients for suitability. I use the same successful criteria as I did above with the hard lenses. The primary reason for this fact is the limitation of lenses available for prescription and the standardization of the overall diameter of the lens. To achieve better success, Bausch & Lomb will have to increase the numbers of base curves available and will have to permit variation in diameter. We may reasonably conclude that Bausch & Lomb will supply more parameters for us to prescribe. Another reason for failure is the resultant decrease in visual efficiency in some situations.

My success with the Naturalens has been infinitely greater. The success ratio in my practice approaches 85%. The failures are not attributable to the inability of the patient to wear the lens but rather to our inability to achieve adequate visual efficiency. Included in my study are cases of corneal astigmatism of 3.00 D. and more. As with the Soflens I did no prior screening. With the Naturalens, I can mask some corneal astigmatism, and I have found it better not to attempt to predict the outcome but rather to put lenses on and then make a clinical judgment.

Under other headings I have discussed patient symptomatology and corneal integrity, and other chapters explore these subjects in great detail.

Publicity relating to soft lenses has, in the main, been very negative. If you think back 6 or 8 years, you may remember the headlines in newspapers and magazines stating "Contact lenses cause blindness." They could not have been referring to soft lenses. The fact is that most of what appeared in print then were totally distorted statements. The same appears to be true today regarding the soft lenses. Lecturers have been misquoted or quoted out of context. Poorly designed pharmacological and bacteriological studies have been quoted as gospel. Contact lenses have been and still are an emotional and highly readable topic. References to them get into the public press far more often than they should. I feel it essential that the professional organizations involved correct the misinformation that has so sorely confused the public.

The therapeutic use of the Griffin lens has been covered completely by other chapters. The hard lens cannot be used at all for this purpose.

Time does not permit a comparison of lenses as to laboratory fabrication and the difficulty encountered by some wearers of soft lenses in areas of low humidity.

Chapter 9

The Griffin Naturalens:
A preliminary report

Michael A. Friedberg, O.D.

This is, indeed, a preliminary report involving 375 patients who were fit over a 2-year period with the Griffin Naturalens, a product of the Griffin Laboratories, Buffalo, New York. It is significant to note that the following data involve all of the patients that were fit, regardless of their degree of success, the duration of their wearing time, or the type or amount of visual acuity obtained.

It must be noted that the lenses used in 1969, and those used in 1971, were not necessarily of the same soft lens design. Technological improvements in manufacturing did unquestionably influence results.

PROCEDURE

In the beginning, patients were fit with the soft lens after routine visual analysis, corneal topography measurements, and biomicroscopy examination. With these data, which of course included a complete refraction, lenses were selected from a 12-lens trial set.

"Best fit" has different meanings to different practitioners. To me, it represents a lens that does not disturb corneal integrity, that provides satisfactory visual efficiency and visual acuity, and offers the patient comfort in wearing for an 8-hour period when at least that amount of time is desired or required by the wearer.

Obviously, "satisfactory" visual efficiency and visual acuity lends itself to patient and professional interpretation. The same holds true for patient comfort. This latter fact has been borne out repeatedly by former satisfied "comfortable" all-day conventional (hard) lens wearers who, when they wear soft lenses, are ecstatic with the additional or improved comfort.

The patients involved in this report include, in varying degrees, all types of refractive errors (such as myopia, hyperopia, astigmatism). Included are persons who had not worn contact lenses before and those who had successfully or unsuccessfully worn hard lenses.

These data include those patients who for any number of reasons reverted to spectacles or hard lenses. No specific effort for the basis of securing statistics or research data was made that would have patients continue wearing soft lenses beyond the point of their own desire.

A detailed indoctrination was part of the office routine before the patient was accepted for soft lens fitting. This included a discussion of (1) the nature of the lens material; (2) the visual problems that might be encountered; (3) splitting of

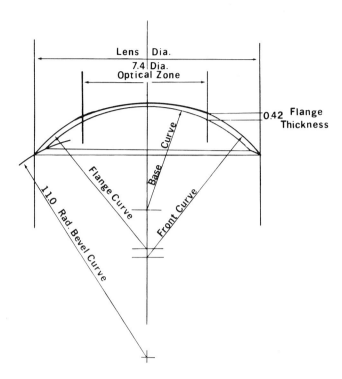

Fig. 9-1. Sketch of Griffin lens in a hydrated form. Standards for minus lenses. (Courtesy Griffin Laboratories, Buffalo, N. Y.)

the material, formation of calcium or other deposits, and change of parameters, all of which lessen lens longevity; (4) the possibility of prescription changes; and (5) the costs involved.

The presentation was made factually and not negatively. This position is mentioned so that the conclusions drawn must be weighted by the routineness of patient selection and indoctrination in earlier cases, in contrast to a later selective sampling of patients.

The Griffin Bionite lens is lathe cut in a dehydrated form and then maintained in a hydrated state (Fig. 9-1).

At present, the laboratory is attempting to standardize all lenses. The purpose of this standardization is twofold. First, repeatability in manufacture simply means that one can get a lens the same as he originally ordered in the case of replacement, and second, in fitting the lens, if there isn't repeatability in manufacturing, then one will have to maintain a large bulky inventory of trial lenses.

In Fig. 9-1 note that the inside curve of the lens is one curve. It is a spherical curve. The outside curve is the prescription curve with a lenticular cut creating an optical zone (7.4 mm.).

You will notice that the flange begins at the end of the optical zone and continues down to the edge of the lens. The flange thickness is approximately 0.42 mm. thick at the juncture.

THE GRIFFIN NATURALENS: A PRELIMINARY REPORT

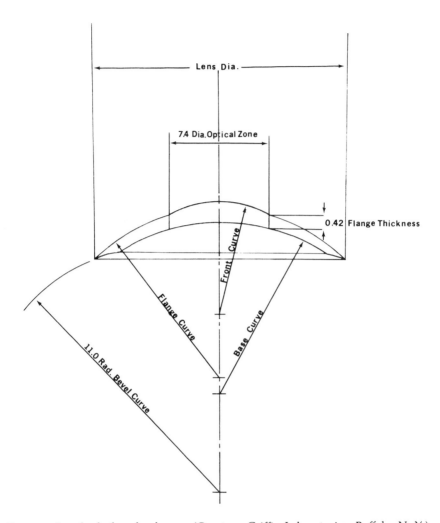

Fig. 9-2. Standards for plus lenses. (Courtesy Griffin Laboratories, Buffalo, N. Y.)

In Fig. 9-2, the important thing to understand is that this diagram is for plus lenses. The only difference should be the center thickness, except in very high powers. Fig. 9-3 shows more or less a rounded edge, approximately 0.21 mm. thick with an 11 mm. radius of curvature and a bevel 0.5 mm. wide. The edge is the same for plus and minus lenses. This standardization of lens edges and flanges accomplishes a very important factor, in that the same type of peripheral flexing in the peripheral area of the lens is obtained.

Fitting procedure

The basic steps for fitting the Griffin lens are as follows:
1. Refraction
2. Keratometer readings

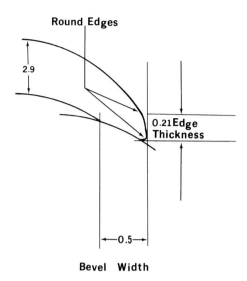

Fig. 9-3. Sketch of Griffin lens edge (plus and minus lenses). (Courtesy Griffin Laboratories, Buffalo, N. Y.)

3. Trial lens testing

4. Overrefraction

Since most of these fitting steps have been reviewed in several other chapters, I will elaborate only slightly on "keratometer readings." Keratometer readings, K, tell us something about the topography of the cornea and monitor any changes caused by contact lens wear. In this way, they help in patient selection and follow-up.

The criterion of a good fit is stable positioning with a slight lag on the blink. It must not be so steep as to cause a fluctuation of vision or so loose as to create rubbing or discomfort. Lenses that are fit improperly, because of technique or fabrication, may create injection, discomfort, edema, or visual problems.

RESULTS

The number of patients with the Griffin Naturalens, broken down to their present wearing time, are as follows:

Wearing lenses 8 or more hours	276
Social wearers	64
Discontinued wearing lenses	35
Total	375

One should keep in mind that many of the patients selected early in the program did have measurable corneal astigmatism in excess amounts. It was intended at that time to mask this astigmatism as much as possible. In most cases this effort failed but resulted at times in satisfactory visual acuity.

Some of the patients, more of the earlier ones than those selected later, changed from all-day wearers to social wearers.

Previous conventional methylmethacrylate lens failures comprised a substantial number of cases fitted, as follows:

No previous contact lens experience	238
Previous hard contact lens failure	137
Total	375

Some of these people had long discarded their hard contact lenses but maintained the desire to find a substitute for eyeglasses. Others still wore their conventional lenses periodically but with much less than complete satisfaction.

Following are the reasons that wearers discontinued use of the lenses:

Poor vision	24
Moved to other area	6
Other	5
Total	35

This analysis clearly shows that the patients who discontinued wearing the the soft contact lens did so in most instances because of inadequate vision. Good visual performance does not necessarily correlate with good visual acuity.

An individual, for example, who demonstrates 20/20 visual acuity may not be able to perform specific visual tasks with uncorrected astigmatism or with fluctuating vision.

There were some patients who for personal reasons moved from the area and were unable to complete or continue with the fitting procedure. And others, for such reasons as scleral injection or general discomfort, became discouraged and discontinued wear.

Patients' lenses were replaced for a myriad of reasons: poor vision, splitting or tearing, deposit formation, irritation, and discomfort. I must emphasize that the very high percentage of replacements were indirectly related to the quality of fabrication especially in the early stages of production.

DISCUSSION

It was a hindrance in the beginning days of soft lens fitting to be limited by a trial set of only 12 lenses. As the inventory of available lenses increased, the degree of success increased. One can assume then that those patients who received the Naturalens in 1969 had less probability of attaining longer periods of comfortable wear, or comfortable wear at all, than those fit later.

All contact lens practitioners agree that there are many reasons why patients have discontinued wearing their conventional contact lenses, but this report does not reflect a breakdown in the reasons for the failures in conventional lens wear. If these data were analyzed, the information on successful wearers might be more meaningful when compared with a similar breakdown analysis of those recorded as failures.

Many patients are searching for the panacea in contact lenses. The placing of any material, hard or soft, between an eyelid and an eyeball will indeed have some sensation. To some it is of no significance, whereas to others it is significant.

The procedures for asepsis and the care and handling of contact lenses are more detailed and more time consuming than those needed with spectacles and sometimes provide reason for the discontinuance of contact lens wear. As minor as this reason is to some, it is significant to others and must be considered.

Poor vision in a patient who has been properly selected is usually caused by poor optics. The quality of the optics in the Griffin Naturalens can be determined by the target image in a lensometer or Nikon Vertometer. When properly fabricated, the image should be very good.

The edge of the soft contact lens must be well formed and the geometrical design so constructed as to cause no scleral indentation or excessive pressure on the limbus. The stability of the parameters may be related to the manufacturing procedure, climate, or tonicity or lenses and solutions used. Earlier lenses were less stable and required exchange.

Deposits that sometimes form on lenses are attributed to calcium from the tears, possibly abetted by poor surface quality. These deposits may interfere with vision or cause discomfort and injection. The lenses were replaced when this condition occurred.

Splitting and nicking of soft contact lenses is primarily caused by poor patient handling and care. Fabrication and material, too, could be a factor.

SUMMARY AND CONCLUSION

Approximately 85% of the patients that were fit with the Griffin Naturalens continue to wear their lenses 8 hours a day to all day. This high degree of success can be attributed to repeated changes of lenses. As experience in fitting increased, less lens changes were required or desired.

Good patient selection is paramount for good visual performance with soft lenses. Thorough patient indoctrination that includes a discussion of the lens material, the limitations as well as the advantages, is vital to successful practice.

Special office management techniques for soft contact lens practice have evolved. It includes a close liaison between the practitioner and his aides with the patient, especially when exchanges of lenses are necessary.

A comprehensive inventory of lenses is desirable for ease of fitting. This new material is not completely predictable and until greater repeatability in fabrication is attained, fitting from inventory is the preferred technique.

Soft contact lenses afford excellent comfort, ease of adaptation, a minimum of spectacle blur, relatively low incidence of corneal insult, ability to be worn sporadically, and stability for use in sport activity.

CORNEAL CURVATURE CHANGES

Along with corneal integrity, corneal curvature changes are of great concern to all practitioners. Constant corneal compression over a period of years with its resultant refractive changes making spectacles ineffective is most distressing to both patient and practitioner. The design of the lens, upper lid structure, corneal composition, response, and duration of wear contribute to spectacle blur. Even with sophisticated handling of these entities, I doubt that any office has not encountered corneal curvature changes, regular or irregular.

In a negative sense we may appreciate this phenomena. During the adaptive stage the patient compares his contact lens vision with his new spectacle vision and rushes back to his contact lenses. Small degrees of uncorrected residual astigmatism with contact lenses are not noticeable when compared to this new blurred spectacle vision. But even if experience has proved that these changes may not be detrimental, other avenues where this does not occur would be most welcome.

The hydrophilic lens creates little if any spectacle blur. When the lens is fitted properly, it ensures immediate interchange between soft lenses and spectacles. We must infer therefore, that compression of corneal tissue and/or corneal edema is minimal as compared to methylmethacrylate lenses.

Whatever mechanisms come into play in adaptation to contact lenses, the hydrophilic material is far superior to hard methylmethacrylate. The initial comfort, little lid irritation, slight tearing, and minimal interference in corneal metabolism set the stage for long, comfortable, safe wear.

Clinical experience demonstrates that most patients quickly adapt physically, physiologically, and psychologically to the soft lenses. Other hydrophilic materials may vary but in most cases are superior to conventional lenses in achieving maximum wear rapidly.

Caution, however, should be exercised that ease of adaptation should not be the deciding factor in selecting a type of lens. We must not be diverted from professionally analyzing all other criteria that are in the best interests of the patient. We must not be deceived by short-term success if there are other recognizable problems.

Chapter 10

Fitting flexible contact lenses in Mexico

Victor Chiquiar Arias, O.D.

For 10 years we have been hearing or reading conflicting reports about flexible contact lenses at the meetings or in the professional literature. On one hand, we hear that flexible contact lenses are a panacea: the ideal contact lens that anyone can fit on everyone for everything. On the other hand, we hear the lenses condemned as being complicated, useless, and potentially dangerous. Those of us who have been fitting contact lenses for almost a quarter of a century cannot fail to see the similitude of this stage of development of the flexible contact lens with the similar stage experienced with stable contact lenses in the early 1950s. It seems to be that innovations in the health care field—and contact lenses are no exception—tend to conform to a three-stage pattern as follows:

First stage—optimistic. This is where the inventors or first researchers present overenthusiastic reports, which virtually place their discovery as a panacea with few or no complications. In this case it is the "ideal" lens that *anyone* can fit on *every*one for *every*thing.

Second stage—pessimistic. As soon as clinicians begin to use the new discovery with their everyday patients and specifically with their difficult ones, they begin to report problems and complications. In part, because of the overenthusiastic initial reports, the clinicians feel frustrated at their lack of success and bitterly condemn the new device as worthless, pointing out its deficiencies, inconveniences, and complications to the exclusion of any advantages.

Third stage—realistic. With the passage of time, the development and improvement of materials, and refinement of fitting techniques, a more scientific and sober tone comes forth in the technical papers and reports. Finally we are able to assess the true value and uses of the new device, with its indications and contraindications, its advantages and limitations.

I believe that in stable contact lenses, after 25 years of development, refinement, and extensive use, we are in the third, realistic, stage. It is my impression that in flexible contact lenses we are in the emotional controversy of the first and second stages. In an effort to find out for myself what the true "stage of the art" in flexible contact lenses was, I accepted Dr. Gasset's invitation, and in March 1970 came to the University of Florida. I was impressed with the seriousness of the work done here and the potential of the new device. Therefore, after adequate instruction, I decided to obtain the necessary lenses and equipment to begin fitting my patients in Mexico with flexible contact lenses. The lenses I have been fitting are Griffin Bionite lenses, and I have used them on refractive cases only.

94

I have also been called as a consultant for the fitting of these lenses on pathological corneas, by a number of ophthalmologists.

I have fitted almost 100 cases between April 1970 and January 1972. This paper is based on the results of the first 64 patients fitted up to November 1971. They were chosen from unsuccessful or undesirable candidates for stable contact lenses for some of the following reasons:

1. Hypersensitivity
2. Frequent epithelial edema
3. Excessive fragility of the epithelium leading to frequent staining or recurcurrent ruptures
4. Recurrent or slow-healing ulcers

Most of the patients had simple ametropias ranging from −1.25 to −15.75 diopters (D.) and from +3.00 to +17.50 diopters. Included in the group were 10 cases of aphakia with edema and 8 cases of keratoconus with recurrent ruptures and/or slow-healing ulcers.

This is a summary of my observations:

1. In 58 cases, physical tolerance was excellent from the first moment.
2. In 50 cases, insertion and removal were learned without difficulty. Elderly patients had problems in mastering the removal. Ladies had to have their fingernails cut short (3 had corneal abrasions and conjunctival wounds caused by their fingernails).
3. With the exception of the 8 keratoconus cases and 6 cases of corneal astigmatism above 2 diopters, as well as 2 cases with tight lids, the vision obtained was almost as good as with stable contact lenses or spectacles.
4. The majority of patients started wearing their lenses from 8 to 12 hours the first day without problems.
5. Photophobia was not seen.
6. Excessive tearing was not present except in 6 cases, where it may have been related to the solutions used.
7. All 64 patients were instructed to use the chemical sterilization method of hydrogen peroxide–sodium bicarbonate–sodium chloride solution.
8. In 16 cases, stinging or burning of more or less intensity after the third day of use was reported. The burning sensation began upon insertion and lasted several hours. This problem was solved by changing the length of time lenses were kept in the various sterilization chemicals.

Later, 20 patients were instructed to change this method for the use of two new solutions, Flexsol and Hexaphen.* All the 20 patients welcomed the simplified techniques. Of the 10 patients using Flexsol, 7 reported stinging or burning sensation of variable degrees, and also a lowering of the quality of vision, which, as one reported, "is like seeing through a dirty window." The other 3 patients reported no stinging or lowering of vision. Of the 10 patients using Hexaphen, 8 reported a drying of the lens, which would tend to adhere to the upper lid, with consequent discomfort and variations in vision.

---

*Flexsol (Burton, Parsons & Co., Washington, D. C.) and Hexaphen (Barnes-Hind, Sunnyvale, Calif.) are investigational drugs.

9. Twenty patients reported diminished vision in poorly lighted places and at night.
10. Twenty-four reported difficulties in seeing at close distances such as reading. Perhaps lid position and pressure have a role in this problem.

There were no serious lens-related complications. The general aspects of the patients' eyes were good. Three of them developed conjunctivitis while wearing their lenses. It was not ascertained whether this complication was directly related to the use of the lenses.

On the other hand, the patients with a history of frequent breakages of the epithelium did very well. No breakage was seen while they wore their flexible lenses. The cases with slow healing or recurrent ulcers also did very well with the ulcers healing while the lenses were worn.

Among these two above-mentioned categories were the patients with keratoconus (see Chapter 21). Here I will only state that although their vision was considerably less than with stable contact lenses, the integrity of their epithelium was preserved. With respect to the pathological cases fitted with the Griffin lens by ophthalmologists in Mexico, the results were in general satisfactory. There were dramatic improvements in cases of bullous keratopathy and Stevens-Johnson syndrome.

SUMMARY AND CONCLUSION

Summarizing, I will weigh the advantages against the disadvantages of flexible contact lenses as seen in my 2-year experience.

Advantages
1. Comfort. The majority of patients experienced very little physical sensation.
2. Practically, there is no adaptation period. Patients begin using lenses almost all the waking hours.
3. Epithelial edema is present in only few cases.
4. No cases of epithelial rupture were seen, while the patients wore their lenses.
5. No photophobia or excessive tearing was observed.
6. Vision for distance was good, where corneal astigmatism was less than 2.00 diopters.

Disadvantages
1. The serious problem of sterilization, which although improved and somewhat simplified, requires more time and operations than handling of stable lenses. Therefore, we are always in doubt as to whether the patient will follow the instructions. If not, there is a potential danger to the patient's eyes.
2. When corneal astigmatism exceeds 2.00 D. or in cases with tight lids, the vision is less than with stable contact lenses or spectacles.
3. Some patients report diminished vision at night or in places with poor light. Others report insufficient vision for reading.
4. A number of patients report variations in vision related to changes in the temperature and humidity of the environment.
5. Breakage of the lenses is still a serious problem although it has greatly diminished.

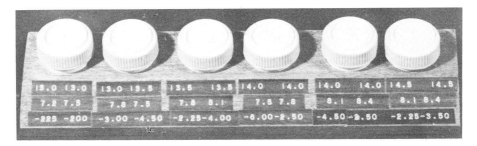

Fig. 10-1. Minimum trial set of soft lenses, suggested by Kaufman and Gasset.

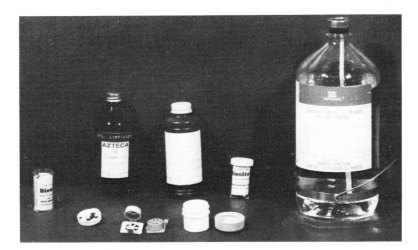

Fig. 10-2. Equipment and material for chemical sterilization.

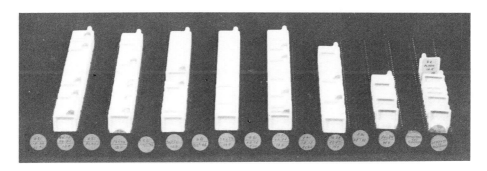

Fig. 10-3. Small inventory of hydrophilic contact lenses.

6. For some patients, especially females, the handling of the lenses, particularly "bending" them for removal, offers problems and dangers in view of the long fingernails of women.

CONCLUSIONS

In this age of superspecialization, let us keep in mind the following points:
1. The patient comes to us because he has a visual problem.
2. Our goal is to preserve and improve human vision.
3. We are in the field of vision, *not* contact lenses, flexible lenses, and so on.
4. We should be conversant with *all* types of optical devices and techniques for improving vision, whether they are scleral lenses, corneal lenses, flexible lenses, spectacles, subnormal vision aids, orthoptics, or pleoptics.
5. We should choose the device or devices that best suit the individual needs of each particular patient and fit them properly.
6. Then and only then, can we say that we are performing our duty of preserving and improving human vision.

Figs. 10-1 to 10-3 demonstrate some of the materials necessary for fitting and sterilization.

Chapter 11

Cosmetic fitting of the Griffin Naturalens

James V. Aquavella, M.D.

The use of hydrophilic polymers for cosmetic contact lenses has been accompanied by an extraordinary degree of interest from the general public. Despite the ministrations of the news media, business community, and Food and Drug Administration, the hydrophilic lens has managed to survive a rather stormy postnatal period.

Although improvements in the manufacturing and fitting of methylmethacrylate lenses have occurred over a period of more than 20 years, the use of flexible materials is new. Some of the present hydrophilic lenses are good, and improvements are appearing almost daily. Many of the problems that were considered almost insurmountable a few months ago have already been solved. One can reasonably expect continued progress in the future.

The individual practitioner should try to keep in mind the inherent differences between standard methylmethacrylate lenses and the hydrophilics. Thus, many of the techniques employed with hydrophilic lenses will vary considerably from those employed in the fitting of hard contact lenses. A second important consideration is the fact that each specific hydrophilic polymer is a distinct chemical entity and will demonstrate specific physical and chemical properties. These properties may have a direct bearing on the performance of the resulting contact lens. The practitioner is urged to follow the individual recommendations of the manufacturers carefully during the period of initial experience with any one or all of the existing polymers.

GRIFFIN LENS COMPOSITION AND CHARACTERISTICS

This chapter deals with methods employed in fitting over 300 cosmetic cases with the Griffin Naturalens. This lens is composed of the Bionite polymer, which is a composite-graft copolymer resulting from the polymerization of 2-hydroxyethylmethacrylate (HEMA) in the presence of ethylene glycol dimethacrylate (EGDM) and polyvinylpyrrolidone (PVP).[1] The resultant polymer, when molded for use as a cosmetic contact lens, possesses certain unique properties that have a direct relationship to the performance of the lens. Paramount among these properties are flexibility, permeability, and architectural configuration. Thus, although flexible, the lens has sufficient rigidity so that when placed on the corneal surface there is no disruption of the underlying corneal tear film.

The fluid permeability of the finished lens is such that almost 60% of the weight of the lens is represented by water. Recent reports may have tended to overemphasize the importance of oxygen permeability in relation to the function of hydrophilic contact lenses, but the Bionite polymer does possess a significant degree of oxygen permeability.[2] This particular polymer has a very high degree of stability (despite its great water content). Thus, a number of varying architectural configurations are possible, and the lens is available in a wide variety of diameters, curvatures, thicknesses, and refractive power.

The lenses are manufactured in six standard base curves ranging from 7.2 to 8.7 mm. in steps of three tenths of a millimeter, as follows:

7.2 mm.
7.5 mm.
7.8 mm.
8.1 mm.
8.4 mm.
8.7 mm.

The actual curvature is measured by means of an optical gauger consisting of a series of plastic gauges each ground to a specific curvature. When a lens is placed on one of the gauges, an air bubble is visible in the interface if the curvature of the lens in question is steeper than that of the underlying gauge.

If the lens curvature is flatter than that of the gauge, the edge of the lens is seen to extend. If the curvatures of the gauge and the lens are identical, there is a flush fit.

Lens diameter is easily measured with a standard contact lens reticle or even with more sophisticated projection devices. Lenses are available in diameters ranging from 13.0 to 15.5 mm. in increments of 0.5 mm., as follows:

13.0 mm.
13.5 mm.
14.0 mm.
14.5 mm.
15.0 mm.
15.5 mm.

Lens power may be ascertained with a standard lensometer, or more easily with a projection vertometer. Lenses are currently available in powers ranging −20 to +30 diopters. Other powers may be specially ordered.

The average thickness of cosmetic lenses is from 0.33 to 0.45 mm. Aphakic lenses are slightly thicker. Bandage lenses for use in pathological corneas are generally thinner.

FITTING PROCEDURE

Although the specific procedure employed in fitting a patient with the Griffin hydrophilic lens is simple, experience and attention to detail are extremely important. The fitting procedure is based on three steps: manifest refraction, trial lens selection, and overrefraction. In most cases, the manifest refraction is sufficient as a starting point, and here we deviate considerably from methylmethacrylate lens fitting. Keratometer readings are of limited value and at the early stages of the fitting experience they may even prove misleading.[3]

COSMETIC FITTING OF THE GRIFFIN NATURALENS

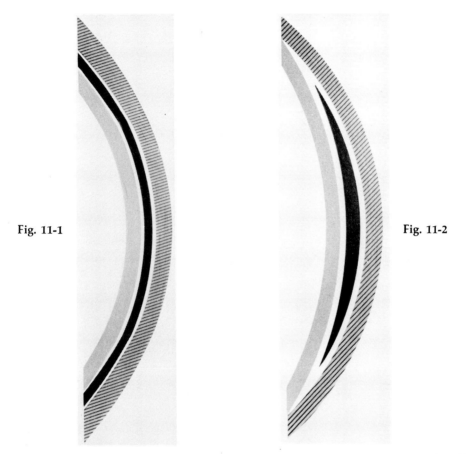

Fig. 11-1   Fig. 11-2

Fig. 11-1. Diagram of the flat-fit situation with virtual contact between anterior surface of central cornea and posterior surface of lens.

Fig. 11-2. Diagram of the steep-fit situation with its expanded interface area.

A relatively elaborate trial lens set is supplied with the Naturalenses and is extremely useful in certain select cases. However, the overwhelming majority of cosmetic cases can be successfully fitted by employing one or two lenses.

An excellent starting point is a 14 mm. lens of a relatively flat curvature 8.4 or 8.1 mm. A second choice would be a lens of slightly greater diameter (14.5 mm.), which may prove to be more versatile. A properly fitted lens is self-centering, although a certain amount of motion is desirable with blinking and ocular rotations. The importance of centering cannot be overemphasized. This attribute is paramount to the success of the Bionite polymer.

A good guiding principle is to fit flat so that virtual contact exists between the posterior surface of the lens and the central corneal area (Fig. 11-1).

If the lens is too steep there will be apical clearance and the subjective acuity will vary with blinking (Fig. 11-2). In addition, the convexity of the expanded

Table 11-1. Sagittal relationship of various base curves and diameters

Flat							
13.0	8.7	14.0	8.4	15.0	8.7	15.0	8.1
13.0	8.4	13.0	7.5	14.0	7.8	15.5	8.4
13.5	8.7	14.5	8.7	14.5	8.1	14.0	7.2
13.0	8.1	13.5	7.8	15.0	8.4	14.5	7.5
13.5	8.4	14.0	8.1	15.5	8.7	15.0	7.8
14.0	8.7	13.0	7.2	13.5	7.2	15.5	8.1
13.0	7.8	14.5	8.4	14.0	7.5	15.0	7.5
13.5	8.1	13.5	7.5	14.5	7.8	15.5	7.8
						Steep	

interface tear film layer will produce a plus lens effect and the subsequent over-refraction will require more minus power than is indicated by the manifest spectacle refraction.

The relationship between the base curve and the diameter of an individual lens is fixed and results in a specific chord diameter. This relationship is important to a proper understanding of the fitting process (Table 11-1).

Thus if we desire to change from a 14.0 mm. diameter lens to one slightly wider (14.5) we must also make a corresponding increase of one step in the base curve to maintain the same fitting relationship between lens and cornea.

When the lens is first inserted, the patient may experience a few seconds of mild discomfort and there may be some excessive lacrimation. This should subside within a minute or two and the patient should be completely comfortable with hardly any sensation that the lens is in place. If the lens seems to demonstrate excessive motility even after a minute or two, a larger diameter is often indicated to provide for greater adherence. A slightly steeper lens may also be selected at this point. If immediately after insertion of the lens an air bubble is noted in the interface, the lens selected is probably too steep and a lens with a flatter radius of curvature should be selected.

After the proper trial lens has been allowed to settle for 15 minutes, simple overrefraction determines the final power of the lens. At this stage, the quality of the retinoscopic image may be used as a guide. If there is no distortion with blinking, the fit is generally a good one. Some practitioners prefer to judge the quality of the reflex with the keratometer; a modified keratoscope can also be of value at this juncture. The Naturalens is primarily recommended for those individuals having 1.5 diopters of astigmatism or less.[4] However, with careful fitting, even patients with moderate to high amounts of astigmatic error may occasionally achieve good acuity. This often depends on the relationship between corneal and lenticular astigmatism.

Patient handling is not difficult to instruct. Female patients with long fingernails must be warned to exercise caution so that they will not lacerate the lens. Insertion is easily learned. The danger of corneal abrasion is almost nonexistent. Because Naturalenses have a relatively wide diameter and excellent centering properties, they are difficult to dislodge accidentally. Removal is accomplished by shifting the lens to either the lateral or inferior sclera where a pinching maneuver allows for air to pass under the lens.

LENS HYGIENE

As far as lens hygiene is concerned, the Griffin lenses may be boiled, or asepsis may be accomplished by a simple peroxide cycle.[5] In addition several ancillary systems are currently under investigation. One includes storage in a solution called Flexsol (Burton, Parsons & Co., Washington, D. C.) and then rinsing the lens with a modified saline solution for insertion. A second system employs a slightly larger lens case and the single solution Hexaphen (Barnes-Hind, Sunnyvale, Calif.) is used for lens storage. Regardless of the system employed patients should be instructed to mechanically clean the lens between thumb and index finger. It is important to realize that bacterial contamination is primarily a surface phenomena.

One reason that lens hygiene is perhaps more important than with the methylmethacrylate medium is the extreme comfort of patients wearing the Griffin lens. Patients with epithelial damage (inflammatory or traumatic) may elect to wear their lens because there is no discomfort, and thus a potentially serious problem may be masked. Instruction should stress not using the lenses if the eyes are red or irritated.

Because the Naturalens is so flexible, it can on occasion turn inside out. This is readily ascertained by means of the simple taco test, named after the popular Mexican sandwich. When the lens has its proper side out and it is bent between the thumb and forefinger, the edges of the lens are easily approximated. If the lens is inside out, when it is bent, the edges will flare and not come together easily. If a reversed lens should be inserted on the cornea, minor discomfort and inconstant acuity may result, but there are no harmful effects on the eye.

TIGHT LENS SYNDROME

It has been mentioned that fitting a steep lens may cause variable acuity because of the compression of the lens by the upper lid with blinking, and the subsequent collapse of the underlying interface area. Clinically a steep lens may produce the so-called tight lens syndrome, consisting of variable acuity, mild discomfort, and circumcorneal injection. This diagnosis is characteristic and can often be made on the telephone. When a patient is fitted with a flatter lens, the symptoms immediately subside. It is extremely important to understand this phenomenon. When you first see a patient with a tight lens syndrome, you will be certain that you are dealing with an infection. Many of these patients have a culture made, and several nonpathogenic bacteria, which normally inhabit the conjunctival fornices, have recently been accused of possessing virulent qualities. More important, some individuals have been concerned that there was a relationship between the hydrophilic lens and the "virulence" of these bacteria.

If the lens is removed from a patient suffering with a tight lens syndrome, fluorescein staining will undoubtedly reveal some areas of staining. There may be peripheral epithelial edema.

The Griffin Naturalens should be instantly comfortable, and in all our routine cosmetic cases, there has been no necessity of adaptation to the lens. The patients should have white and quiet eyes and they should be able to wear their lenses all waking hours from the first day without discomfort. In addition, patients do not demonstrate a spectacle blur in switching from the lenses to spectacles and vice versa. The incidence of epithelial edema has been extremely low and has always been controlled by adjusting the fit. If the patient reports the necessity of restricting wear or delayed blurred vision, we don't consider the fit to be a good one and the patient is recalled for a reevaluation.

Should such reevaluation be necessary, one of the first steps is to recheck the actual parameters of the patient's lenses. If they are not as exactly prescribed, the lenses should be exchanged. If the parameters are exact, perhaps a slightly flatter lens may be the answer. On occasion as especially thin lens must be specially ordered.

THERAPEUTIC USES

There are certain types of cases where specialized fitting techniques may be necessary. These are aphakia, keratoconus, Fuchs' dystrophy, postoperative keratoplasty, and high astigmatism. In all these cases a valuable technique has been to take a keratometer reading from the front surface of the properly fitted Griffin lens. Invariably a single clear astigmatic axis can be found, and the patient can in many cases be given good visual acuity by wearing the residual correction in spectacle form over the hydrophilic contact lens. These techniques are discussed at length in Chapter 24.

DISCUSSION

Certainly there are variations of the techniques described that may prove successful in others' hands, but these are the techniques that we have found beneficial. In well over 300 cosmetic contact lens cases, we have seen no overwear phenomena. I have seen overwear with Griffin lenses once or twice, and they have always been aphakic patients who have been allowed to wear their lenses for more than 24 hours at a stretch. In aphakic patients who have worn their lenses all day and removed them before retiring, we have not observed overwear.

The monocular aphake may be fitted in the early postoperative period. A lens of approximately +14.00 diopters will enable the patient to benefit from peripheral fusion. The residual refractive error (especially the astigmatic portion) may be supplied in a spectacle form. This is readily accomplished since most of these individuals wear bifocal correction.

In keratoconus the resultant acuity may be excellent even in advanced cases. Usually a rather thick lens (0.45 to 0.55 mm.) of approximately 8.1 mm. radius of curvature and 14.0 mm. diameter may be used to eliminate most of the irregular astigmatism. Supplemental correction of residual astigmatic error can be supplied in spectacle form.

Postoperative corneal grafts are among the most difficult patients to fit with these lenses. High astigmatism may be corrected in some cases with smaller steeper lenses. However, real success with these patients will have to await the advent of toric lenses.

A certain percentage of patients with bullous keratopathy or Fuchs' dystrophy may be improved visually by fitting a relatively flat lens and supplying the astigmatic correction with spectacles. In these cases the addition of hypertonic saline drops may be necessary to maintain clarity. We have tried removing the epithelium and allowing reepithelialization to occur under the lens (as advocated by Gasset[6]), and this method has proved successful on occasion.

SUMMARY

Over 300 cosmetic cases have been successfully fitted with the Griffin Naturalens. The success of this medium as a cosmetic device seems to be related to the specific physical and chemical properties of the Bionite polymer. A standard fitting technique is presented that differs considerably from the procedures usually advocated for methylmethacrylate lens fitting. The main advantages of this material are ease of fitting and patient comfort. The main disadvantages are currently the difficulty in fitting individuals with high astigmatism and the lack of a single, simplified, inexpensive method to maintain lens hygiene. Advances in this field are being made at a rapid rate; however, even in its present form this lens system is capable of delivering excellent acuity, as well as comfort, to a significant percentage of all contact lens candidates.

REFERENCES

1. Aquavella, J. V., Jackson, G. K., and Guy, L. F.: Therapeutic effects of Bionite lenses: mechanism of action, Ann. Ophthal. 3(12):1341-1350, 1971.
2. Morrison, D. R., and Edelhauser, H. R.: Permeability of hydrophilic contact lenses, Invest. Ophthal. (In press.)
3. Aquavella, J. V., Jackson, G. K., and Guy, L. F.: Bionite hydrophilic contact lenses used as cosmetic devices, Amer. Ophthal. 72(3):527-531, 1971.
4. Kaufman, H. E., and Gasset, A. R.: The new soft hydrophilic contact lens, Highlights Ophthal. 12(3):177-190, 1969.
5. Kaufman, H. E., Uotila, M. H., Gasset, A. R., Wood, T. O., and Ellison, E. D.: The medical uses of soft contact lenses, Trans. Amer. Acad. Ophthal. Otolaryng. 75:361-373, 1971.
6. Gasset, A. R., and Kaufman, H. E.: Bandage lenses in the treatment of bullous keratopathy, Amer. Ophthal. 72:376-380, 1971.

Chapter 12

The Griffin Naturalens:
Basic concepts and
fitting techniques

Antonio R. Gasset, M.D.

Heretofore hydrophilic lenses have been available only to a selected group of investigators. A nationwide evaluation for safety and efficiency has already been conducted in the two main lenses, the Basuch & Lomb Soflens and the Griffin Naturalens. The approval by the Food and Drug Administration of the first type of soft lens (the Soflens), and the imminent approval of the Naturalens marked the beginning of the era of the soft lens.

It is of the utmost importance to the practitioner to realize that hard lens concepts cannot be used in the fitting of soft lenses. In addition, it is essential to realize that the fitting of the Naturalens is not only different from convention acrylic (hard) lens but also from other types of soft lenses.

The Griffin lens is not a panacea; knowledge and skill is required in fitting to obtain maximum vision and comfort. I emphasize that, in contrast to hard lenses, soft lenses can significantly impair vision if lenses are not properly fitted.

THE LENS

Griffin Naturalens is a new contact lens manufactured from a hydrophilic plastic called Bionite. It is semisoft, or it might be better described as being semirigid; yet it has a very high water content of approximately 55% water by weight. The refractive index is approximately 1.40.

Both the inside and front surface are spherical. The inside aspect of the edge has a bevel that is 0.5 mm. wide on larger lenses and 0.3 mm. wide on smaller lenses. The front surface always has a lenticular cut to reduce the edge thickness.

Base curve

There are four base curves to cover the entire range of normal corneas from relatively flat to relatively steep corneas. The radii of curvature in millimeters are as follows: 8.4, 8.1, 7.8, and 7.5.

Diameter

There are five diameters to cover variations in corneal size. The lens diameters are 13.0, 13.5, 14.0, 14.5, and 15.0 mm. with an 0.5 mm. increment of change in diameter.

Thickness

The center thickness of a minus lens is usually 0.30 to 0.40 mm. in the hydrated state. Lenses could be obtained from the manufacturer thinner or thicker on request.

For plus lenses, the lenticular form is used, which provides a center thickness from 0.40 to 0.60 mm. depending on the power. The front lenticular zone is usually 9.0 mm. in diameter.

Optical considerations

The index of the material in the hydrated state is approximately 1.40. The index change from tears to plastic at the lens-tear interface is much less than we are used to with hard contact lenses (1.49 to 1.33). Therefore, the tear layer has less refracting power, or rather it requires a greater difference in curvature to create a significant amount of refracting power in the tear layer. This difference almost always induces a small amount of minus refracting power in the tear layer amounting to an approximately −0.25 or −0.50 diopter. Therefore, the refracting power of the Griffin Naturalens will be the same as the spherical refracting power of the patient's spectacles (stated in minus cylinder) corrected by the vertex distance change and this small amount of minus power in the tear layer. However, this minus power correction can vary by 0.75 diopter and is not precisely predictable.

Adherence and form of the lens

Although the concept of adherence has been used in fitting regular hard acrylic contact lenses for many years, it is usually referred to in different terms. Lenses are spoken of as being "loose" or "tight," and this usually refers to movement or the appearance of tear exchange under the lens with fluorescein (that is, the "fluorescein pattern").

In the case of these new lenses, there is very little adherence to the cornea. The lens glides easily on the cornea at the touch of the finger. Yet it is not so loose that ordinary lid pressure from blinking causes it to move. It clearly has a substantial tear layer under it from the ease with which it slides. The lens also weighs much more than a hard acrylic contact lens.

Because there is so little adherence and because the lens needs more adherence as a result of its mass, the lens is almost impossible to fit when it is smaller than the diameter of the cornea. We have been able to produce sufficient adherence with larger diameters. The lens is most stable when it is fitted so that the overall diameter is 1 to 2 mm. larger than the cornea.

The inside curve is almost always flatter than the curve of the cornea in its central region. It therefore rests on the cornea in two places, the central region and a circular peripheral region, while vaulting a section in the region of the limbus.

LENS MEASUREMENTS

Semirigid hydrophilic contact lenses are supplied by Griffin Laboratories fully hydrated in normal saline as a finished lens. Each finished lens should be carefully inspected, and the following variables must be checked:

Base curve
Refracting power
Diameter
Physical quality
Optical quality

Base curve

The inside curve is measured with reasonable degree of accuracy by a system known as "optical gauging." This method has been used in the optical industry for a great number of years. In this case, we have adapted it to the specific requirements of measuring a semirigid wet material against a hard acrylic surface. The gauges are clear acrylic spheres and the increment of change between its surface is marked on the base of the stand.

If the lens is steeper than the sphere, an air bubble will be trapped under the lens at or near the center of the sphere. If a lens is flatter than the surface, the edge will not align the sphere uniformly and will show a convoluted shape.

The lens must be fully hydrated in normal saline; the gauging surface must be absolutely clean and wet with normal saline. Finally the procedure should be repeated two or three times.

Refracting power

The refracting power is measured in the conventional way with a lensometer or vertometer that is properly adapted to measure the posterior verted focal length of a regular methylmethacrylate contact lens. A lensometer with special conical choke for contact lenses should be used.

The lens must be blotted with a lint-free tissue to remove excess water. After it is mounted in the instrument with the curved surface toward the light source, the lensometer is set in the vertical position to avoid gravity from distorting the lens. After 30 seconds, the image will clear and the power can be read to +0.50 diopter.

Lens diameter

The diameter can be measured in two ways, either by a measuring lens magnifier or magnifying reticle, similar to the one used for checking the diameter of hard lenses, or by use of base curve gauges.

Physical quality

The quality of the edges and anterior and posterior surfaces of the lenses may be ascertained by observation at arm's length with the naked eye or by using a hand magnifier or slit lamp biomicroscope. Of particular importance is the evaluation of the edges of the lenses. Small chips or scratches can produce more irritation than do large easily detected cracks.

To facilitate lens inspection, a special instrument was designed (Fig. 12-1). The lenses are placed in the plastic plot form and rotated in all directions. This simple instrument has proved to be most useful.

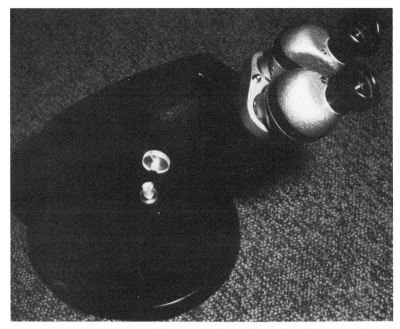

Fig. 12-1. Special instrument designed to evaluate lens edges for chips or scratches.

Optical quality

The optics can best be evaluated by the images of the mires of the lensometer. Clear images indicate good optical quality.

FITTING PROCEDURES

Griffin Naturalenses are fitted in a somewhat empirical manner. Lens selection is determined by a mixture of science and art. Careful corneal measurements are combined with the trial lens procedure in determining the lens dimensions that will give the best vision and optical performance.

There are several steps that should be followed to arrive at the final lens. The following special examinations must be performed:
1. Keratometry
2. Corneal diameter
3. Lens power determination
4. Additional tests for evaluation of optical performance
   a. Retinoscopy
   b. Keratometry
   c. Biomicroscopy

Keratometry

The patient's keratometer (K) reading and corneal diameter provide the starting point for the trial lens testing. In our experience a single careful reading with the keratometer has been adequate.

The selection of the base curve of the trial lens can be made by use of the following tabular material for the relationship between the patient's corneal curvature found by keratometry and the suggested lens radius of curvature.

For a corneal curvature, in diopters, of:	Select a test lens with a respective millimeter radius and diameter of:	
40.00 to 42.00	8.4	14.5
42.00 to 43.50	8.1	14.0
43.50 to 45.00	7.8	13.0
45.00 to 48.00	7.5	13.5

The following points must be emphasized:

1. Steeper lens curvature increases adherence and may also cause apical clearance and variable vision.

2. Flatter lens reduces adherence and may cause movement and lag.

3. A larger diameter lens always increases adherence and may cause apical clearance.

4. A smaller diameter lens always decreases adherence and may cause movement and lag.

Determination of the power of the lens

The power that is prescribed can be determined by using the spectacle refraction and vertex distance and refining the refraction through a trial lens procedure.

The selection of the trial lens is made as follows:

1. Take the spectacle refraction in minus cylinder form; ignore the cylinder.

2. Correct for the change in effectivity attributable to the vertex distance when necessary.

3. Add +0.25 diopter to correct for the minus power in the tear layer.

Usually the selected lens does not require any change in power. However, in some patients overrefraction revealed a difference of 0.50 or 0.75 diopter. In our experience the only accurate way to arrive at the correct power is to refract over a test lens.

EVALUATION OF OPTICAL PERFORMANCE
Retinoscopy

The retinoscope is used to evaluate the quality of the reflex and the amount of residual astigmatism. A properly fitted lens will give a reflex that will be essentially the same as the eye without a lens in regards to its quality. A steep lens with significant apical clearance will show an irregular reflex similar to that seen in irregular astigmatism.

Keratometry

The measurement of the front surface of the lens on the eye should be performed routinely. The quality of the image should be as good as the quality of the reflected image from the cornea itself. Moreover, the amount of astigmatism on the front surface of the lens should be measured.

Biomicroscopy

Biomicroscopy must be done routinely after the patient is first fitted and in each follow-up visit. The following points should be checked:
1. Relationship between the lens edge and the sclera
2. Appearance of lens surface
3. Evaluation of the cornea
4. Evaluation of the conjunctiva
5. Lens centering
6. Lid pressure

A properly fitted hydrophilic soft contact lens results in stable visual acuity and maximum comfort. However, such results can only be achieved by the proper selection of the lens diameter.

EXAMPLE

Refraction
O.D. $-2.75 +0.25$ cyl. axis 175
O.S. -2.50 sphere

Keratometer readings
O.D. 41.50/41.75 cyl. axis 175
O.S. 41.25/41.75 cyl. axis 180

Corneal diameter
12.5 mm.

Base curve is the most important single factor. For selection of the trial lens, the K readings provide the starting point; the base curve selection is done as follows:

Eye		K reading range (diopters)	Base curve (mm.)
O.D.	41.50	40.00 to 42.00	8.4
O.S.	41.25	42.00 to 43.50	7.8
		43.50 to 45.00	7.5
		46.00 to 47.00	7.2

Diameter. Selection of the lens diameter is made after the corneal diameter is carefully measured. The following table will give the relationship between corneal and suggested lens diameter:

True corneal diameter	Corneal diameter range (mm.)	Lens diameter (mm.)
	11.0 to 11.5	13.0
	11.5 to 12.0	13.5
12.3 ⟶	12.0 to 12.5 ⟶	14.0

Corneal diameter measurement to 0.5 mm. accuracy is difficult and time consuming. However, at least in our hands the following "rule of thumb" has worked in most cases: A steep cornea, a small cornea; a flat cornea, a large cornea. Therefore in most cases the following normogram, in millimeters, can be applied:

For a corneal curvature of:	Select a lens diameter of:
8.4	14.5
8.1	14.0
7.8	13.5
7.5	13.0
7.2	13.0

Power. The power is calculated by use of the spectacle refraction as follows:

1. If spectacle refraction is in minus cylinder form, ignore the cylinder.
2. Correct for the change in effectivity attributable to the vertex distance when necessary.
3. Add +0.25 diopter to correct for the minus power in the tear layer.

Therefore, the power should be O.D. −2.75 and O.S. −2.75.
Trial lens selection:

Corneal curvature	Lens diameter	Power (sphere)
O.D. 8.1 mm.	14.0 mm.	−2.75
O.S. 8.1 mm.	14.0 mm.	−2.75

Trial lens evaluation

A comparison of trial lens testing for hard versus soft lenses reveals both similarities and differences. Trial lens testing is easier with soft lenses than with present-day hard lenses because of comfort and almost total lack of tearing. However, the purpose for the testing is somewhat different and it takes some experience to appreciate this point. The main purpose of testing is to find the proper dimensions, mainly base curve and diameter, which will give the best and most stable visual acuity.

Visual acuity evaluation

Most reliable results are obtained if a few minutes are allowed from the time the lens first goes on the eye to the time visual acuity is tested.

Rule. Never rely on the results of a given lens until the lens has been on the eye for 10 minutes.

Let us consider the following possibilities in this case:

1. Visual acuity is stable and comparable to best spectacle correction. Prescribe a lens 8.1/14.0/−2.75.
2. Visual acuity can be corrected with refraction over trial contact lens (such as −0.50) to the best spectacle correction. Prescribe a lens 8.1/14.0/−3.25 ([−2.75] + [−50] = −3.25) thickness 0.44 mm.

Variable visual acuity. Occasionally the patient has the readings of 20/20 but then blurs to 20/40 and 20/60, not improved with overrefraction. In this case there are two possibilities. First and by far the most common cause is that the lens is *too steep*, and second the lens is *too flat*. If the lens is too steep, visual acuity improves immediately after blinking; if too flat, vision will blur immediately after blinking. This can be explained on the basis that a steep lens will create a significant amount of apical clearance, which will be abolished immediately after blinking; on the contrary, if the lens is too flat, it will not make contact at the periphery and will decenter immediately after blinking. Neither of these lenses will provide good visual acuity.

A lens that is too flat can easily be identified. It will move up and down on each blink or be displaced in the opposite direction to ocular movement (upward-downward, and so on). A lens that is too steep cannot be easily recognized unless it is extremely steep (7.5 for an 8.1 mm. lens). We have found that after some experience the eye can be used essentially in the same way we use the optical gauging and an indication of a too-steep lens can be obtained. Additional tests as retinoscopy and keratometry will help in the evaluation. In the former a reflex similar to irregular astigmatism is usually seen. In the latter the keratometer mires will change with each blink.

Lets consider our example patient again. Suppose we have determined that the lenses were too steep, what can be done?

Either diameter or base curve can be changed. It is advisable to change only one parameter at a time. In deciding which parameter or dimension to change first, visual acuity and trial lens–to–corneal diameter relationship must be considered. First, if the patient's eye is blurred to 20/40 and cannot read 20/20 after a blink, usually the base curve has to be changed. For example, in this case we could make the lens an 8.4/14.0. Second, if vision is 20/20 but blurs to 20/40, it probably can be corrected with an 8.1/13.5 lens; however, we must always keep in mind that a smaller lens is less comfortable than a larger lens. Third, more than one combination might be necessary.

If the trial lens in this case were too flat, the lens should be made larger. Rarely does the base curve have to be changed to a steeper curve than the one predicted.

Comfort

There is usually no complaints about comfort. However, if the lens is too flat, it will move excessively and the patient would be aware of the lens. Usually a larger lens is more comfortable. Let us assume that in our example the same visual performance and stability could be obtained with an 8.1/14.0 and an 8.1/14.5. Most patients would prefer larger lens. However, we do not advise fitting larger lenses if they are not necessary.

EXAMPLE

Refraction
     O.D.   −2.25 sphere   20/15
     O.D.   −1.75 sphere   20/15

Keratometer readings
     O.D.   41.00/42.75   cyl. axis 90
     O.S.   41.25/42.75   cyl. axis 90

Corneal diameter
     12.0 mm. for each eye

CORRECTION OF REFRACTIVE ERROR

QUESTIONS
1. *Give the lens dimensions that will give the best and most stable visual acuity.*
O.D. (8.4) (14.0) (−2.50)
O.S. (8.4) (14.0) (−2.00)
Total astigmatism of the eye is composed of both corneal and lenticular astigmatism. In patients such as the one presented in this example the corneal astigmatism is neutralized completely by the lenticular astigmatism of the opposite axis.

Therefore, if this patient is fitted with hard acrylic lenses, the corneal astigmatism will be neutralized by the hard lens and the lenticular astigmatism becomes manifest. On the contrary, if the patient is fitted with a Griffin soft lens most of the corneal astigmatism will be preserved and neutralized by the lenticular astigmatism of the opposite axis.

It is evident from this example that in cases such as this Griffin lenses will result in better vision than will the hard acrylic lenses.
2. *How common is this type of residual astigmatism?*
The frequency of occurrence is generally believed to be between 30% to 50%.
3. *How would astigmatism affect visual acuity with these two types of lenses?*
The hard acrylic contact lenses will neutralize at least nine tenths of the corneal astigmatism bringing out the lenticular astigmatism. This may very well be why hard acrylic contact lenses seldom give perfect vision in low refractive errors.
The Griffin soft lenses are available in different thicknesses. In this type of case a thin lens will correct far less than one fifth of the corneal astigmatisms as demonstrated by K readings with and without the lens. Most likely thickness is the reason for the high success rate of these lenses in low refractive cases.

EXAMPLE

Refraction
O.D. −2.25 +1.25 cyl. axis 180 20/15
O.S. −2.25 +1.00 cyl. axis 180 20/15

Keratometer readings
O.D. 46.50/46.50 cyl. axis 180
O.S. 46.00/46.25 cyl. axis 180

QUESTIONS
1. *Give the lens dimensions that will give the best and most stable visual acuity.*
O.D. (7.5) (13.0) (−1.25)
O.S. (7.5) (13.0) (−1.25)
Normal thickness
2. *How will visual acuity compare with hard spherical contact lenses?*
Neither hard nor soft contact lenses will give satisfactory vision.
3. *How can vision be improved?*
Front cylinder hard lenses will improve vision to 20/20. This type of lens is not yet available for soft lenses. Glasses with a cylindrical correction could give satisfactory results for both types of lenses.

EXAMPLE

Refraction
O.D. −2.50 +2.00 cyl. axis 90
O.S. −3.00 +2.50 cyl. axis 90

Keratometer readings
O.D. 42.00/44.25 cyl. axis 90
O.S. 42.50/45.00 cyl. axis 90

QUESTIONS

1. *Give the lens dimensions that will give the best visual acuity?*
   O.D.   (8.1) (14.0) (−1.00)
   O.S.   (8.1) (14.0) (−0.75)

2. *What is the greatest degree of corneal astigmatism that can successfully be fitted with Griffin soft lenses?*
   There is none.

3. *Has any work been done with toric or bitoric Griffin soft plastic contact lenses?*
   Only a small amount of testing has been done using toric inside surfaces on corneas with three or more diopters of astigmatism. Calculations have shown that only inside toric lens would be required for astigmatism up to 5.00 diopters. This lens will orient and eliminate the corneal astigmatism.

4. *What percentage of the population has corneal astigmatism in excess of 2.00 diopters?*
   Less than 5% have that excess.

This study was supported in part by USPHS grants EY-52868 (Gasset) and EY-00446 from the National Eye Institute.

Chapter 13

The soft contact lens in Japan

Akira Nakajima, M.D., and Hisao Magatani, M.D.

In the department of ophthalmology at Juntendo University, research on soft contact lenses began in 1956. With support from a government grant, we tested literally all available materials (such as polyvinyl-alcohol derivatives, combinations of plastics, agar, gelatin, cyanogum) in our search for a substance that would produce a contact lens with a more hydrophilic surface and oxygen permeability.

In early 1963 we noted the Czech reports on soft contact lenses, and in September 1963, conferred with Professor Wichterle on this new modality. Some practitioners have noted that the first Czech soft lenses were comfortable with good central, but rather poor peripheral, vision. In all, our experience with the Czech lens indicated it was a bit inferior to hard contact lenses in optical quality and we were especially concerned with the possibility of soft lens contamination.[1,2]

It was not until 1969 that we were exposed to the progress of soft contact lenses in the United States. At that time, we were extremely impressed by the scale of research going on and the improvements already made in the original lenses. Although soft contact lenses have become rather well known during the last 3 years, we believe that a few more years will be needed until we digest or determine the best materials and techniques for their manufacture, fitting, and care.

PROBLEMS IN CONTACT LENS FITTING

Contact lens fitting is essentially a technique of adjusting the following lens variables until the most suitable combination is found for the individual patient:

Refractive power

Base curve

Size

Bevel and edge shape

But with soft lenses, we add two new variables:

Softness of material

Oxygen and water permeability

Soft lenses are hydrophilic in varying degrees, and the full importance of this property has not been determined. The factor lens-material softness, is also important. Here we set up a simple apparatus (Fig. 13-1) to determine the softness by using two thickness gauges and measuring the difference in reading caused by the tip of the gauge being pushed into the soft material by force. The correlation between softness thus measured, refractive index of the material in water, and water content of a soft material is shown in Fig. 13-2. Here is one example of a two-component cross-linked two-dimensional copolymer system, and this

THE SOFT CONTACT LENS IN JAPAN

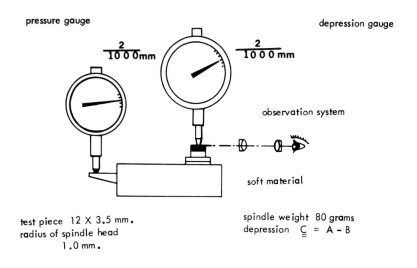

pressure gauge   depression gauge

observation system

soft material

test piece 12 X 3.5 mm.   spindle weight 80 grams
radius of spindle head   depression C = A – B
        1.0 mm.

A : cross section of spindle (mm^2)

W : weight of spindle (gm)

S : stroke of working indicator (mm)

D : depressed depth (mm). diff. of two indicators

K : coefficient of softness

$$D = \frac{K}{AWS}$$

practical data   A :   mm^2

W : 80 gm

S : 0.5 mm

unit of "K"   mm.mm^2. gm. mm

Fig. 13-1. Device for measuring lens material softness.

relationship may apply to any other system of similar nature with the shift of
the line or their inclinations. By showing this, we merely want to say that we
should have a common expression for the measure of material softness.

This measure should be added to the description of the soft contact lens in
addition to the shape that is considered to be most convenient. The interrelationship between shape and softness in lens performance is still empirical, and we
hope this problem will be solved by having some guidelines soon.

Another problem is the aging of hydrophilic soft material. One polymer phys-
icist told me that a polymer of this type will undergo a constant aging process

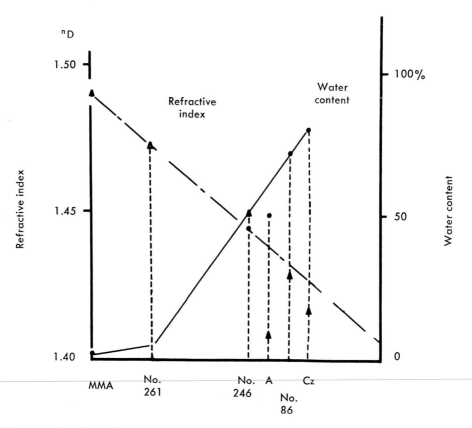

Fig. 13-2. Correlation between softness, refractive index in water (^nD), and water content of material. **MMA,** Methylmethacrylate. **Cz,** Original Czech lens. **A,** p-Hydroxypropyl-methacrylate) (PHP).

in water, caused by thermal agitation of water breaking the cross-linking between molecules. The result of measurement of the strength of soft lens material in relation to the period of storage in water or normal saline of some hydrophilic polymer material is shown in Fig. 13-3. The curve shows constant drop, an indication of the aging of the material. This feature of the material, along with the problem of quality control, may be related to the frequent complaint of breaking or cracking.

Of course, even hard lenses do not last forever. The patient may lose, scratch, or deform the lenses by improper handling. We do not know exactly the distribution of the life of hard contact lenses worn by patients, but we estimate it to be a few years. Soft lenses undergo forced deformation daily when patients insert and remove their lenses, and this practice would seem to shorten the life of these lenses. The possibility of continuous wearing will solve part of the problems related to lens durability. However, the obvious advantages (such as comfort) of the soft lens over the hard lens must be considered in regard to the superior durability of hard lenses.

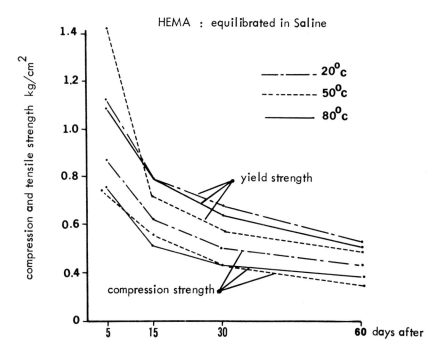

Fig. 13-3. Strength of soft lens material in relation to period of storage in water or normal saline.

Another important concern is soft lens contamination. There are two aspects to this problem. One is not to introduce live pathogenic organisms on or in soft contact lenses into the eye and the other is to ensure that the lenses do not damage (that is, scratch) the healthy cornea, allowing even pathogenic organism to migrate into the conjunctiva and cause corneal infection. Proper lens sterilization will take care of the first aspect, and proper fit the second.

We examined normal flora of the patients wearing contact lenses. Our results[3] (Tables 13-1 to 13-3) shown here, as well as other studies, indicate that the normal conjunctiva of contact lens wearers are comparable to or cleaner than those people not wearing contact lenses. Table 13-4 shows the results of a study done by Dr. Hamano in Osaka[4] from ophthalmologists who have seen eye diseases related to contact lens wear. The exact sample size of contact lens wearers from which these patients were extracted is not clear, but the result shows that around one in 3,000 cases of eye trouble caused by contact lens wear results in permanent loss of vision because of corneal scarring. We feel the safety of the soft lenses should be at least comparable to this.

SELECTION OF CASES

From the beginning, our policy is to try soft contact lenses on patients who really need contact lenses but cannot wear conventional hard lenses. At this

Table 13-1. Number of strains of bacteria cultured from conjunctival sac (in percent)

Number of strains	Kouno*	Hivama†	Juntendo Hospital
0	1.3	7.0	26.4
1	43.8	13.0	66.0
2	39.4	51.0	6.7
3	13.8	22.0	0.6
4	1.9	7.0	0.3
5	0	0	0

*Kouno, G.: On bacterial flora in healthy normal Japanese conjunctival sac, Acta Soc. Ophthal. Jap. **22**:415, 1918.
†Hiyama, H.: Relation between conjunctival bacteria and phlyctane, Acta Soc. Ophthal. Jap. **55**:896, 1951.

Table 13-2. Bacteria demonstrated from conjunctival sac (by culture)

	New patients (150 eyes)	Old patients (150 eyes)	Average percentage (300-eye total)
Staphylococcus albus	66.0%	52.0%	59.0%
Staphylococcus aureus	1.3	2.0	1.7
Corynebacterium	7.3	10.0	8.7
Streptococcus	1.3	2.0	1.7
Pneumococcus	0	0	0
Micrococcus	0.7	0	0.3
Bacillus subtilis	0	0.7	0.3
Citrobacter	2.7	0	1.3
Alcaligenes faecalis	4.7	2.7	3.7
Achromobacter	0.7	1.3	1.0
Cloaca	2.7	1.3	2.0
Bacterium anituratum	0.7	1.3	1.0
Serratia marcescens	1.3	0	1.3
Neisseria	0	0.7	0.3
Klebsiella	0	0.7	0.3
Pseudomonas	0	1.3	0.7
No growth	20.7	32.0	26.4

Juntendo Hospital clinic patients with contact lenses.

moment, we believe that the soft lens is the lens to fill the gap in which hard lenses cannot help. As a guideline, for example, patients with myopia and aphakia, especially in children or the elderly, who cannot wear hard contact lens, or those with bullous keratopathy, corneal ulcers, and xerosis can take soft contact lenses.

The medical indication of contact lenses in children (aphakic infants) is one field where soft lenses can be extremely useful. Fig. 13-6 shows an aphakic baby, a little over 1 year old, wearing soft contact lenses. Hard contact lenses have been

Table 13-3. Bacteria demonstrated from conjunctival sac (by culture)

	Kouno* (1918) (160 eyes)	Hiyama† (1951) (100 eyes)	Cason‡ (1954) (3,208 eyes)	Juntendo (1966) (300 eyes)
Staphylococcus albus	56.9	73.0	68.0	59.0
Staphylococcus aureus	10.6	17.0	7.0	1.7
Corynebacterium	56.2	69.0	33.0	8.7
Streptococcus	22.5	14.0	<1.0	1.7
Pneumococcus	3.1	9.0	<1.0	0
Micrococcus		1.0		0.3
Bacillus subtilis	6.3	2.0	<1.0	0.3
Citrobacter				1.3
Alcaligenes faecalis			<1.0	3.7
Achromobacter				1.0
Cloaca				2.0
Bacterium anituratum				1.0
Serratia marcescens				1.3
Neisseria			<1.0	0.3
Klebsiella			0	0.3
Pseudomonas			<1.0	0.7§
No growth	1.3	7.0	23.0	26.4

*Kouno, G.: On bacterial flora in healthy normal Japanese conjunctival sac, Acta Soc. Ophthal. Jap. **22:**415, 1918.
†Hiyama, H.: Relation between conjunctival bacteria and phlyctane, Acta Soc. Ophthal. Jap. **55:**896, 1951.
‡Cason, L., and Winkler, C. H., Jr.: Bacteriology of the eye; normal flora, Arch. Ophthal. **51:**196, 1954.
§Could not be detected after 2 weeks, without any treatment.

Table 13-4. Eye damage caused by contact lens (data from enquiry to 275 clinics in Japan)*

Total cases treated for condition presumably attributable to contact lens wear	18,490
Healed by itself in a few days	15,937
Needed treatment for 3 days or more without residual symptoms	2,546
With permanent impairment of vision	7

*From Hamano, H., Komatsu, S., Hirayama, K., and Kanai, A.: The damage caused by wearing contact lens studied on questionnaires, J. Jap. Contact Lens Soc. **12:**16-20, 1970.

applied for this purpose for several years, but the more comfortable and convenient (continual wearing) soft lenses are now the best therapy. As soft contact lens therapy develops, we intend to widen their use gradually.

THE SOFT LENSES AS BANDAGES

Soft lenses are also being clinically tested as a bandage and vehicle for applying drugs. Using isotope-labeled compounds, we did some experiments on the

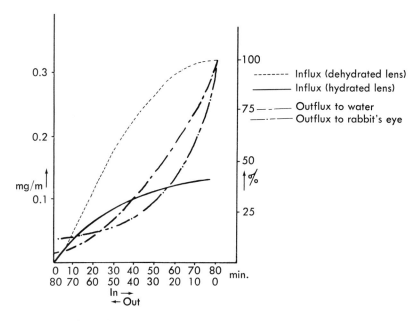

Fig. 13-4. Uptake and release of thimerosal by hydrated and dehydrated soft lenses.

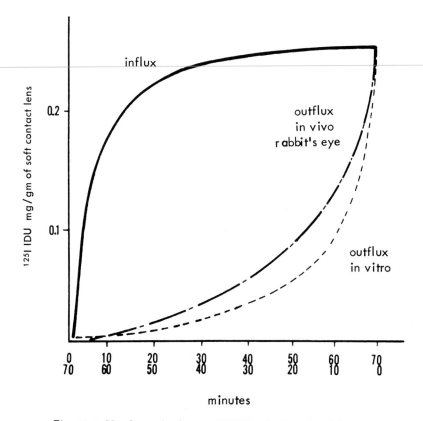

Fig. 13-5. Uptake and release of IDU by hydrated soft lenses.

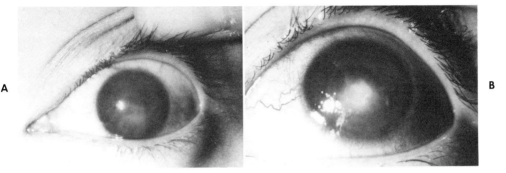

Fig. 13-6. A, Disciform keratitis before soft lens wear (December 13, 1971). **B,** After soft lens wear (January 21, 1972).

uptake and release of various substances to and from these lenses. With thimerosal and iododeoxyuridine (IDU) (Figs. 13-4 and 13-5), inflow and outflow occur fairly quickly and flow comes nearly to an end within 1 hour.

In cases of corneal herpes, we ask the patient to use IDU every hour. One isotopic IDU experiment revealed that IDU instilled directly onto the eye penetrates into the globe and the concentration of IDU in corneal epithelium drops abruptly in 30 minutes. However, the IDU in soft contact lenses decreases slower and takes 1 hour to wear off. This experiment indicates that by using soft contact lenses with IDU, we could feasibly reduce the number of eye drop application in herpes patients. Dr. Kanai tried soft lenses in the following case of disciform keratitis (Fig. 13-6):

> Y. K.: Female, 23 years old
>> First visit: Dec. 4, 1971
>
> Visual acuity
> Right vision: 0.3 (1.0 −4.0 D. axis 90°)
>> Left vision: 0.01 (noncorrigent)
>
> Diagnosis: Dendritic keratitis of the left eye
>
> Treatment: Idoxuridine (IDU) every 2 hours
>> Antibiotic drops every 4 hours
>> Antibiotic drops every 4 hours
>
> Dec. 7, 1971: Ciliary injection, corneal ulcer
>> Treatment: Dexamethasone (Decadron) tablet 1.5 mg.
>> IDU every 2 hours
>> Antibiotic drops every 4 hours
>
> Dec. 11, 1971: Condition of disciform keratitis
>> Treatment: Dexamethasone tablet 1.5 mg.
>> IDU every hour
>> Antibiotic drops every 4 hours

Dec. 18, 1971:
    Treatment: Dexamethasone tablet 0.5 mg.
                 IDU every hour
                 Antibiotic drops every 4 hours

Dec. 22, 1971:
    Treatment: IDU every 2 hours
                 Antibiotic drops evey 4 hours

Dec. 27, 1971: Small corneal ulcer
    Treatment: IDU every 4 hours
                 Antibiotic drops every 4 hours

Dec. 29, 1971: Corneal ulcer ($-$*)
    Treatment: IDU every 6 hours
                 Antibiotic drops every 4 hours

Jan. 8, 1972: Corneal ulcer ($-$), stromal edema ($+$*), Vascularization ($+$)
    Treatment: IDU every 8 hours
                 Antibiotic drops every 4 hours

Jan. 11, 1972: Corneal ulcer ($-$), stromal edema ($+$)
    Treatment: Dexamethasone tablet 1.5 mg.
                 IDU every 4 hours

Jan. 18, 1972:
    Treatment: Dexamethasone tablet 0.5 mg.
                 Stop IDU

Although one has difficulty in evaluating the value of soft lenses from this case alone, they seem to merit further clinical trials. We feel that we are at the dawn of a new soft contact lens age and that future research of these lenses should handle the following problems:

1. Establish methods to measure factors related to the refractive power, base curve, shape, softness, and so on, of soft contact lenses.
2. Establish rules for soft contact lens fitting techniques, taking softness into consideration or as one of the variables that fitters can control.
3. Establish the technique for safe continuous wearing of soft contact lenses. Continuous wear is done by many hard contact lens wearers, but not all hard contact lens wearers can wear them continuously. Continuous wearing may be more important for soft lenses to avoid contamination and breakage of the lens by aging and handling of the material.
4. The possibility of therapeutic application of soft lens, combined with various kinds of drugs, should be further explored.
5. Last but not least important, establish the method of sterilization of the soft lens itself.

At present, we think it is still too early to completely switch from hard to soft lenses.

---

*"$-$" and "$+$" mean 'absence of' and 'presence of', respectively.

REFERENCES

1. Nakajima, A., and Magatani, H.: Contact lens research in Japan. In Girard, L. J., editor: Corneal and scleral contact lenses. Proceedings of the International Congress, St. Louis, 1967, The C. V. Mosby Co., pp. 257-261.
2. Nakajima, A.: Panel one. In King, J. H., Jr., and McTigue, J. W., editors: The Cornea World Congress. London, 1965, Butterworth & Co. (Publishers), Ltd., p. 103.
3. Takahashi, T., and Kanai, A.: Bacterial flora of the conjunctiva of contact lens wearers, J. Jap. Contact Lens Soc. **9:**108-111, 1967.
4. Hamano, H., Komatsu, S., Hirayama, K., and Kanai, A.: The damage caused by wearing contact lens studied on questionnaires, J. Jap. Contact Lens Soc. **12:**16-20, 1970.

Chapter 14

Silicone lens

Chester J. Black, M.D.

LENS HISTORY, COMPOSITION, AND CHARACTERISTICS

Most of us are familiar with the organic macromolecules. The so-called hard lens consisting of methylmethacrylate belongs to this group. The newer materials of the soft lenses are built around the methacrylate molecule and are 2-dihydroxy-ethylmethacrylate, still an organic macromolecule.

A new class of man-made macromolecules are the silicones. These are really semiorganic polymers. Commercially, silicones are made from sand or quartz. Using carbon with the sand or quartz in an electric arc furnace, one obtains a high yield of high-purity elemental silicon, a nonmetal. This is crushed and reacted with methyl chloride to obtain methylchlorosilanes, which are rectified and hydrolyzed to produce polydimethysiloxane. The backbone of the molecular chain itself is made up of two of the earth's most abundant elements oxygen and silica. They are usually called "polyorganosiloxanes." The backbone of this group is made up of alternating atoms of silicon and oxygen. Organic groups are attached usually to the silicon atom. If only methyl groups are attached to the silicon atom, then the material is called a "polydimethylsiloxane." This is the substance in which we are most interested. This is the least organic. It has been known for some time that this polymethyl group is responsible for the lens's being physiologically inert.

The silicones can be resinous fluids or elastomers. The extent of the cross-linkage between the polymer molecules as well as the types of organic molecular groups attached to the silicon atoms will determine which it will be.

For example, if one wishes to extend the thermal properties of the polymer, then one can add a phenyl group. Now this new polymer can withstand both higher and lower temperatures. By substituting a trifluoropropyl group the polydimethylsiloxane is, of course, another polymer and less soluble. These polymers are chemically inert. For the sake of completeness we should mention the fact that there are some that are chemically active. These are intermediates containing silanol groups—a silane with an OH group, which can react with other organics containing hydroxyl groups.

We are interested in the silicone rubbers, the so-called elastomers. They usually contain inorganic fillers, such as silica. They are vulcanized or cross-linked in the presence of a reinforcing agent. One can usually see the silica particles in the lens, using the higher power of the slit lamp.

The silicone polymers are noted for the retention of their ·physical properties or characteristics over a wide range of temperatures. Unfortunately they have a very low surface tension. They have excellent lubricating properties and also are used as releasing agents. One of the most important properties is its chemical inertness; another is its physiological inertness.

We have all heard of this material being used to make implants, functional devices such as heart valves and hydrocephalic shunts. Silicones are used in heart lung machines, artificial kidneys, pacemakers, and so on.

The material from which the Silcon contact lens is made is especially prepared by Dow-Corning and sold exclusively to the manufacturer under a licensing agreement. It is a polysiloxane rubber not unlike that described above. The lens is molded by the conventional male and female dies. High temperatures, pressures, and a curing cycle are needed for vulcanization. As with all molded lenses, the mold determines the quality of the lens produced. The lenses can be made in any diameter, but at the present they are 10.5 mm. in diameter. Anterior and posterior surfaces as well as peripheral curves are molded. The edges are mechanically fabricated. A clean room is necessary as with all molding processes, otherwise bits of foreign material may be molded in the lens. A coating process is necessary to create a hydrophilic surface. One such process (the patent of which is assigned to Dow-Corning) is the use of titanate solution as a dipping solution.

The silicone lens is transparent and has a clear to light straw color. The refractive index is 1.439. The transmission of light for all colors is about equal, and about 91% when the lens is wet as on the eye. The lens has minute birefringent particles because of the silica filler. It is soft wet or dry and takes up to 0.5% to 1% of water by weight.

The silicone lens has the unusual ability to return to its original state on bending and can be broken or split like rubber if one folds it too hard. This property of elasticity is responsible for the good visual acuity one can obtain with it in the thicknesses in which the lens is fabricated. The lenses are made half again as thick as the conventional hard lens. For example a −2.00-diopter silicone lens would have a center thickness of 0.3 mm., whereas the usual thickness of the hard lens would be 0.2 mm. This lens can thus be used to correct refractive astigmatic errors of 2 diopters. The thinner lenses have the problem of a distorted anterior surface when placed on the eye. One can visualize waves and, of course, irregular astigmatism by the use of the placido disk, or by the study of the reflections with the use of an ophthalmometer. The poor recovery of the front surface to its original shape after it has been distorted on blinking is responsible for what is termed "variable vision," when too thin a lens is used. On the other hand, the lens does not center because of its thickness and size. It will usually rest at the 6 o'clock position, sometimes encroaching on the sclera.

Hardness is tested by means of the ability of a blunt rod or ball to indent the material. When the Shore durometer is used (the A scale and ASTM D 676), hardness reads about 80 to 85.

One can use the lensometer to read the lens power, and the radiuscope is used to check the anterior surface and base curve.

The lenses, of course, because of their rigidity must be fitted as the conventional hard lens. They are fitted in most instances on K, the flattest meridian on the cornea as measured by the ophthalmometer.

It is recommended that a special wetting and soaking solution be used, as well as a cleaning solution for this lens. These solutions are supplied by the manufacturer. There is some question about the lens's ability to pick up chlorobutanol.

The edge of the lens can be torn, or the lens itself can be punctured with a hard object.

Hill and Schoessler[1,2] did work on oxygen-deprivation studies of the cornea wearing the Mueller Welt silicone lens and found negligible functional resistance.

Burns, Roberts, and Rich[3] claim "determinations of corneal epithelial glycogen, glucose, adenosine, triphosphate and lactate levels after eight hours, sixteen hours and one week wearing time in rabbits wearing silicone rubber contact lenses showed no significant deviation from normal levels."

It is important to note that resistance to aging, light, and heat is generally excellent for silicone rubber formulation. Tissue in contact with the silicone lens has not shown any changes in either the silicone or the tissue in animals wearing the material for 2 or 3 years.

The lens, of course, is not amenable to modifications.

FITTING PROCEDURE

The fitting procedure is the same as that used when fitting the hard contact lenses. The usual refraction and examination of the eye is done. A keratometer reading and slit lamp examination similar to that done when fitting other contact lenses is also needed.

Contraindications

At present no pathological eyes are being fitted. Eyes with over 2 diopters of corneal astigmatism are poor candidates. Since the lens is highly mobile, it is thought, as occurs with the use of hard contact lenses, that dust particles can get under the lens. Clinically this has not been a major problem. Another environmental condition that would be a contraindication to the use of contact lenses is one in which there is an abundance of noxious chemical vapors.

Other contraindications at present are pathological disorders, poor patient hygiene, poor manual dexterity, and those emotional and psychological problems that are not amenable to wearing contact lenses. Patients who are sensitive to the feel of contact lenses, particularly if the Bausch & Lomb Soflens bothers them, will not accept this type. Thus, since the lens is perhaps at best somewhat less irritating but not much more so than the hard lens, one is prone to avoid using these lenses on the sensitive patient. On the other hand, some patients who gave up the hard contact lens because of their irritating properties found the silicone lens to be more comfortable.

Trial lenses

A trial set of silicone lenses is not necessary except perhaps for the use of ascertaining power when one wishes to fit aphakic cases. Other than this the only other value of a trial set is to familiarize the patient with the feel of the lens.

One should remember that diameters of 10.5 mm. are the largest made. This may be too small in some aphakic cases. The lens tends to position itself at 6 o'clock.

The optic axis of the lens is thus decentered inferiorily and can result in some residual astigmatism.

Lens selection and examination routine

To determine the power of the lens, one expresses the refraction in minus cylinders, and the cylinder is then ignored as in the determination of the power of hard contact lenses. The spherical power only is used. A -0.25 diopter is added to the spherical power to compensate for the tear layer under the lens or for the plus lacrimal lens one may create. One must compensate for the vertex distance as one did when ascertaining power of the hard lens. No overrefraction with the use of a trial lens is necessary for most myopic cases. A trial lens for keratoconus and aphakic cases is helpful.

Usually no difficulty is encountered in fitting patients 0.1 mm. (0.50 diopter) flatter and steeper than their keratometer reading. Personally, I think it is a waste of time to consider such factors as the horizontal diameter of the cornea, palpebral fissures, length or width, and pupil size. If the corneas are small, such as those of a child, the correction of aphakia is usually as good as one can obtain with a hard corneal contact lens. When and if larger diameter silicone lenses are available, then perhaps consideration of these factors will be of some importance.

Lenses are checked as to power and base curve on arrival. The power is usually within a plus or minus 0.12 diopter and the base curve is within the limits of the tolerance of the radiuscope. I prefer the 10.5 mm. size only.

The patient is then and only then given an appointment. On arrival the lenses are placed on the patient's eyes. After 10 minutes to a half hour when the tearing has stopped, examination of the lens on the eye is done. Tearing is usually less than that seen with a hard lens. Visual acuity is checked monocularly with the overhead lights on and then with them off. This is to ascertain whether flares from the edge of the lens will be extensive. Visual acuity with the use of these lenses tends to be surprisingly good, even though the lenses do not center.

Slit lamp examination should reveal a mobile lens whose movement is not unlike that of a hard lens. This movement is to some extent probably responsible for the lack of edema, for if the lens does not move but remains stationary at 6 o'clock, edema could develop under the lens. The usual signs of epithelial disruption and conjunctival irritation are checked, and usually one finds only a faint blush of conjunctival injection. On subsequent visits, if the patient blinks infrequently, conjunctival injection of the area exposed by the palpebral fissure will be found to various degrees.

An overrefraction can be done at this time. The lack of variable vision or the fact that patients do not experience the watery vision as they do with the hydrogel lenses makes an overrefraction not only possible but reliable.

PATIENT INSTRUCTION

Instructions on how to remove and place the lens on the eye is next in order. Patients are required to perform the task at least three times before they are discharged. The lenses are removed in the same manner as the conventional hard contact lenses.

Most important are instructions on the care and handling of the lens. They must never be permitted to dry out, as they will become much more difficult to wet and clean. The special solutions supplied should be used, since experience with some of the other solutions has resulted in dirty lenses or improperly wetted lenses, with subsequent mild eye irritations.

Lenses are worn 4 hours the first day, and a half hour more each successive day. The reason for this wearing schedule is because of my own prejudice. I believe that since the lenses do cause some discomfort it is best to slowly adapt the corneas and lids to the lens. The irritating properties of the lens are probably caused by the area of the junction of the central and peripheral curves of the anterior surface of the lens. The posterior surface is good in this respect as we are not getting abrasions. The 2- to 3-thousandths of the edge thickness is well shaped and rounded.

Follow-up visits and patient instruction

A following visit need not be for 2 weeks. At this time the visual acuity is taken, and the usual manifest over-the-lens-refraction, if indicated, is done.

Slit lamp examination should be done to ascertain any corneal or conjunctival changes. One particularly looks at the 6 o'clock area for evidence of corneal stippling or changes of the adjacent conjunctiva, especially as to injection of the limbal vessels or staining of the area with the use of fluorescein. This rarely occurs. Edema has not been a problem of those cases I have fitted. The surface of the lens is checked as to whether it is clean or dirty and not wetted properly. One must again emphasize the importance of the care and handling of the lens.

Patients then need only be followed at monthly intervals for 3 months.

Irritating symptoms and or blurred vision are usually caused by improper handling and care of the lens.

Insurance should be made available to the patient, since the lens can be torn or the edges chipped. Rough handling can cause damage to the lens, and care in placing the lens in the case is important, since chipping of the edge can occur when the lid is closed.

Patients are told not to sleep with the lenses, since there has been no adequate study on the safety of this habit.

Reproducibility of the lens has been good. Replacement of lost soft lenses has been done with less difficulty than that experienced with hard lenses. As to the wearing schedule of the replaced lenses, I probably have been overcautious, since I treat them as I do the patients with hard lens. If they have been without a lens for 3 or more days, they have to start their wearing time as they did when they received their initial lens. Wearing time is four hours at first and a half hour more each day.

To date no overwearing symptoms of the severity found with the use of hard lenses have been seen. There is some tearing on the initial visit because of the foreign-body sensation. Burning and stinging symptoms are usually caused by improper care and handling. Poor visual acuity with or without discomfort is usually caused by improper care and handling. Poor acuity can also occur when

Table 14-1. Results with silicone lenses

Patients who use lenses							33	
Lenses not delivered							20	
Patients who discontinued lenses							19	
Total							72	
Male patients								
Active							13	
Discontinued							15	
Total							28	
Female patients								
Active							24	
Discontinued							20	
Total							44	

Age group	Preteen	Teens	20s	30s	40s	50s	60s	70s
Males who use lenses	1	3	5	0	0	2	2	0
Females who use lenses	0	5	8	4	1	0	2	0
Males who discontinued lenses	0	6	4	2	0	0	2	1
Females who discontinued lenses	0	8	8	3	2	0	1	2

Occupations of patients

Students	29
Housewives	18
Machine operator	1
Musician	1
Doctors	2
Nurses	2
Clerical workers	3
Banker	1
Marketing specialist	1
Retired	5
Unknown	5

Fitted with plus lenses, aphakic	Total—14
In use	Male—4, female—3
Discontinued	Male—3, female—4
Fitted with minus lenses	Total—58
In use	Male—9, female—17
Discontinued	Male—12, female—20
Two keratoconus patients fitted	In use—1; not delivered—1
Range of K readings	36.50 to 47.00, average 41.00 to 44.00
Lenses torn or nicked	6
Lenses replaced because they became cloudy	4
Abrasions	2
Burning	1
Infection	1
Eyes irritated by wetting and soaking solution, alleviated when solutions were switched to Consil	2

the recommended solutions are replaced with others. Photophobia rarely occurs, and spectacle blur is minimal.

RESULTS

Tables 14-1 to 14-3 summarize my findings in fitting 72 patients with the silicone lens.

Initially the supplier had problems of determining the parameters of the lens. Small and thin lenses were usually displaced in the lower fornix. Thin large lenses resulted in variable vision. Finally the thickness was resolved. The lenses are essentially one third thicker than the conventional hard corneal lenses. As to positioning, in most powers the downward displacement of the lens did not appreciably reduce the efficacy of the lens. The problem of the shape of the bevels and edge was finally resolved, but not until a few cases of stippling and corneal abra-

Table 14-2. Reasons lenses discontinued or not delivered

Discomfort	20
Visual acuity	5
Five diopters of astigmatism	1
Stippling	1
Allergy	1
Removal problem	1
Keratoconus	1
Poor centering	2
Abrasion	1
Conjuctival infection	1
Believed hard lenses more comfortable	5

Table 14-3. Length of time wearing lenses

Months	Patients
Less than 1	4
2	3
4	1
7	1
8	4
9	1
10	3
11	2
12	2
13	6
14	2
15	2
18	1
23	1

sions occurred. These cases are included in the results. For a period of time the supplier was slow in executing orders and thus the numbers fitted are small.

An outline of Silcon fitting procedures follows.

SILCON FITTING PROCEDURES

The fitting procedures outlined here follow the experiences with 1,200 clinical patients. In general, fitting and testing procedures are similar to those with hard conventional lenses. These procedures can be modified for individual patients where indicated.

Composition and characteristics of silicone elastomer material

The material from which the lens is fabricated is transparent silicone rubber, more particularly hydrocarbon-substituted polysiloxane rubber. The material has a hardness of 80 to 85 on the Shore A durometer scale and a refraction index of 1.439. The transmission of light is about equal for all colors of the spectrum, measuring 91% when the lens is in the eye. The lenses have some birefringence to the silica filler in the material. The lens takes up less than 0.5% of water by weight, and keeps its softness and flexibility when dry. The amount of water it absorbs is less than what the hard conventional lens absorbs. The material is permeable to oxygen and carbon dioxide, sufficient quantitatively for daily requirements of the cornea.

Selection of patients

Prospective patients for Silcon are representative of the normal contact lens population and should be screened and limited to those with the following:
1. Eyes with corneal astigmatism under 2.00 diopters (except aphakes; see the procedure of correction of corneal astigmatism, p. 135)
2. Eyes and adnexa free of pathology

Good prospective patients for Silcon are also unsuccessful hard lens wearers whose symptoms result from a deprivation of oxygen to the cornea, such as edema, and those unsuccessful because of irritation and discomfort resulting from wearing hard lenses.

Contraindications

The following contraindications are essentially the same for Silcon as for the hard plastic contact lens:
1. Pathological disorders
2. Systemic disorders
3. Poor patient hygiene
4. Poor manual dexterity
5. Environmental conditions
   a. Extremely dusty atmosphere
   b. Noxious chemical vapors, etc.
6. Emotional and/or psychological problems

Patient examination

The physical and optical examination of the patient is performed in the same manner as when fitting a hard lens. Keratometer readings are taken and a manifest refraction test is given. A trial set of Silcon is unnecessary but can be used where preferred. Trial sets are not available at present.

Radius (base curve) of Silcon

The highest percentage of patients have been fitted with a radius parallel to the flatter of the two principal meridians of the cornea—they have been fitted "on K." A few patients have been prescribed radii ranging from 0.1 mm. (0.50 D.) flatter than K to 0.1 mm. steeper than K. Therefore the suggested starting point for radius is parallel to the flatter K.

Base curves can be ordered to a 0.01 mm. to match the K reading. Silcon base curves are not standard or universal curves but are custom made to fit the exact eye curvature.

Size (diameter)

Lens sizes of 10.0 and 10.5 mm. are being fit. The 10.0 mm. size is for small, steep corneas and the 10.5 mm. size is for normal to flat corneas.

In explanation of why these larger sizes are used, there is a relationship of size to thickness, weight, and lag of the lens. To effectively correct corneal astigmatism it has been necessary to make the central area of Silcon thicker. In comparison, a hard lens may have a central thickness of 0.008 inch (0.2 mm.), whereas, Silcon will have a central thickness of 0.012 inch (0.3 mm.). To overcome lag caused by the weight of the lens, which comes from the thickness, a larger overall size is used.

Edges

The edge is 3 to 4 thousandths of an inch thick and well rounded. A thinner edge will fray.

Peripheral curves

Silcon has peripheral curves progressively flatter than the base curve, with flattening from the base curve to the edge of the lens. The junction between the base curve and the peripheral curve is well blended. During clinical tests lenses that had peripheral curves not well blended caused corneal disturbance.

Optics

Optical clarity of the material is excellent and measurement of Silcon lenses on the radiuscope or lensometer is comparable to hard lenses. The index of refraction is 1.44.

Power

The power is determined from the patient's spectacle prescription and base curve relationship to K. An overrefraction is recommended to determine exact power.

Data required for Silcon contact lens prescription

1. *K* Reading—both meridians with axis
2. Spectacle prescription, with vertex distance where needed
3. Horizontal diameter of cornea
4. Any unusual conditions of lids, fissure, pupil, cornea, and so on

Insertion

Use the same technique as with hard lenses.

Removal

Use the same technique as with hard lenses. Do not pinch lens off eye.

Lens positioning

Silcon lenses usually ride low and position inferiorly. Hard minus lenses usually ride high since the minus lens has a "thick" edge, which the upper lid grasps and holds superiorly. With hard lenses the plus lens has a thin edge and has bulk in the center and rides low. The upper lid does not grasp and hold the thin edge of the plus lens but passes over it, striking the central bulk and pushing the plus lens downward. Because all Silcon lenses are thicker in the center, a minus power Silcon would have extra edge thickness; minus lenses are given an outside lenticular edge cut. In effect, minus Silcon lenses are of plus construction, which account for low riding and inferior positioning. To have the low riding lens optically adequate, Silcon has an optical zone size of 9.0 mm.

Motion. The lens should move freely after a blink. The rate of movement is similar to that of hard lens motion.

Optical zones. Optical zones are available in 8.00 mm. or 9.0 mm. However the 9.0 mm. is recommended.

Fluorescein test

Fluorescein patterns may be used to determine lens relationship to the cornea. Silcon fluorescein patterns approximate those of the hard lens. For example, if the lens is tight, a steep fluorescein pattern will be present. Fluorescein will not penetrate or discolor the lens and will wash off as with a hard lens.

Correction of the aphakic eye

The aphake is fit in the same manner as other Silcon patients. Where the astigmatism is less than 2.00 D., "on *K*" fitting is usually satisfactory. Where the astigmatism exceeds 2.00 D., a steeper than *K* radius is indicated, similar to hard lens prescribing in such instances.

Though the high plus lens is necessarily thicker, with the lenticular design the functioning is similar to lower power lenses.

Correction of corneal astigmatism

To effectively correct corneal astigmatism, one must make the central area of Silcon thicker than that of a hard lens with comparable power. Where a hard lens would have a central thickness of 0.008 inch (0.2 mm.) a Silcon lens of the same power would be 0.012 inch (0.3 mm.) central thickness. This added thickness results in a degree of central rigidity of the silicone material, which, when combined with its elastic properties, maintains central sphericity and may correct astigmatism up to 2.00 D.

Patient comfort

The physical feeling of the Silcon lens is very much like the feeling of a well-fitted plastic lens. Even though the lens is soft and flexible, the extra thickness is felt at first by the upper lid. However, adaptation is fast, and usually by the end of the first week full adaptation is achieved. Ordinarily, after a week of wear, lens comfort and feeling should be grade 2 or better according to the following scale:

Grade

0—Unaware that lens is there

1—Aware that lens is there; No foreign body feeling

2—Foreign body feeling but unable to locate its position (as at 9 o'clock)

3—Foreign body feeling and able to locate position; tolerable; no tearing.

4—Foreign body feeling and able to locate position; tearing; not tolerable for long

Patients with comfort of grades 0, 0.5, 1, and 1.5 are the rule rather than the exception.

Adjustments

Silcon lenses cannot be adjusted or altered. A remake should be ordered for any changes.

Patient complaints and symptoms

Patients have gone to sleep forgetting to take the Silcon lenses out. Upon awakening, patients experience none of the usual overwear symptoms of sleeping with a hard lens, that is, injection, photophobia, crusted lid, discomfort, pain, or edema.

Burning and stinging. Burning or stinging or discomfort is not a normal symptom. It is usually caused by contaminated fingers, or objects touching the lens, or by not following the hygienic care instructions. Nicotine, lighter fluid, gasoline, oil, photographic darkroom chemicals, and turpentine are some of the contaminants that have been transferred from the hands onto the lens and then into the eye. Burning, stinging, and irritation result. It is of the utmost importance to maintain a well-functioning lens by keeping the lens clean. If after the hands and lens are washed and stinging and burning persists, return lenses for proper treatment to remove contaminants. If storage solution is not washed off the lens before preparation for insertion, stinging will also occur.

Discomfort. Foreign bodies as towel lint or dust specks will cause discomfort and tearing, and the lens should be removed from the eye, rinsed well in running water (put lens in Porta-Flow case and hold under running faucet), and then wetted with Consil wetting solution and reinserted. Torn or chipped lenses will cause discomfort. Dry spots on a lens are due to improper care and will cause discomfort or fogging of vision. Lens may be contaminated with hand oils, and so on, and proper care with Consil wetting solution as instructed will wet the lens. If dry spots persist, return lens to lab for removal of contaminants.

Photophobia. Complaints of photophobia have been very rare with Silcon. Photophobia with hard lenses is usually a result of eye irritation. Since Silcon is soft, the usual cause of photophobia is not present.

Other symptoms. Symptoms that usually are associated with hard methylmethacrylate lenses, such as overwear syndromes, Sattler's veil, edema, tearing on initial insertion, positioning up of the head and partial closure of the lid, less than all waking-hour wearing time, and persistent foreign body feeling, do not usually occur with Silcon.

Care and handling and preparation of lenses for insertion

Silcon should be handled with more than ordinary care. Silcon can tear, chip, or crack unless precautions are taken. Sharp objects such as fingernails can penetrate the material and cause it to crack. Rough unnecessary handling can cause the edge to chip. When lens is placed in storage case, care should be taken to keep lens out of way of cover when it is snapped shut. Edge chipping would otherwise result. Frequent gross bending of the lens in half upon itself will cause it to crack.

Lenses should be stored in Consil storage solution for silicone lenses. On preparing to insert lenses, one must rinse off the storage solution with tap water, apply Consil wetting solution to the lens, and place the lens on the cornea. Upon removal of lens from the eye, store the lens in Consil storage solution.

WARNING: Contact lens solution containing chlorobutanol will bind to the surface of the lens and become irritating. Solutions on the market that are not compatible with the lens surface for adequate wetting can become a source of eye irritation. Consil solutions are the only solutions that have tested out compatible both for wetting and for irritants. Other solutions have either become sources of irritation, or have affected the wettability of the surface, or both.

Lenses are stored overnight in Consil storage solution in the Porta-Flow lens case.

The Porta-Flow case is a very satisfactory case for Silcon because of easy lens removal, protection of lens from breakage, adequate space to contain a sufficient volume of storage solution for hygiene, and good method of washing lens off with tap water without handling the lens. This case has been tested for leaking from case to lens, with negative results. Instructions for using Consil solutions are available and are furnished to doctors for distribution to patients.

The laboratory will send with each prescription the following care items:
1. Consil storage solution
2. Consil wetting solution
3. Patient guide to Silcon lens care and use of solutions
4. Porta-Flow case

Lenses are available in all radii to 0.01 mm. and in powers from −20.00 through +20.00 D.

Bifocals, torics, tints, or trial sets are not now available.

REFERENCES

1. Hill, R. M.: Effects of a silicone rubber lens on corneal respiration, J. Amer. Optom. Ass. **37:**1119-1121, 1966.
2. Hill, R. M., and Schoessler, J.: Optical membranes of silicon rubber; and their effects on respiration of human corneal epithelium, J. Amer. Optom. Ass. **38:**480-483, 1967.
3. Burns, R. P., Roberts, H., and Rich, L. F.: Effect of silicone contact lenses on corneal epithelial metabolism, Amer. J. Ophthal. **71:**486-489, 1971.

PART IV

Aphakic correction

Chapter 15

Correcting the aphakic patient

Thom J. Zimmerman, M.D., and Antonio R. Gasset, M.D.

The best way to optically correct an aphakic patient is with contact lenses. The contact lens alleviates many of the spectacle-corrected aphake's problems (tunnel vision, ring scotoma, "Jack-in-the-box" phenomena, and magnification). For the binocular aphake, contact lenses are a great boon; for the monocular aphake, a contact lens is a necessity if the patient is to enjoy binocular vision. In fact, in the "bad old days," monocular aphakia was considered "second only to cancer." The monocular aphake wearing a spectacle correction has a 25% magnification, whereas the contact lens decreases this to 7% magnification and the patient usually experiences no difficulty with sensory fusion.[1] Now that we've decided that contact lenses offer the optimal optic benefit to the aphakic patient, which contact lens should be used?

After a contact lens has been decided upon, the problems outlined above are essentially solved and attention can now be focused on two other aphakic maladies: frequent high cylinders and no means of accommodation.

The conventional hard contact lenses very nicely correct the corneal astigmatism by altering the effective corneal surface and rendering it essentially spherical. In regard to astigmatism, the fact has been pointed out that total astigmatism equals the sum of corneal astigmatism plus lenticular astigmatism ($TA = CA + LA$). With the lens gone, total astigmatism is equal to corneal astigmatism and can be read directly from the keratometer. Keeping this fact in mind helps us greatly in correcting our aphakes as we will point out later. Meanwhile let us return to the problem of high cylinders. Although the hard lenses correct the astigmatism, there is still a necessity for reading glasses, and many of our elderly aphakic patients are unable to insert and remove hard lenses. For this and several other reasons, we now prefer to fit aphakic patients with the soft (hydrophilic) contact lenses.

Although the soft contact lens does not alter the corneal astigmatism (and therefore the total astigmatism), we feel that it offers many advantages. The most important perhaps is that soft lenses do not have to be inserted and removed daily. Although it is optimal to remove and clean any contact lens daily, we have many patients who have worn, without difficulty, their soft lenses for months at a time. Special care, however, needs to be taken to assure a "perfect fit" in patients who wear their soft lenses for extended periods. If the patient has nimble-fingered family or friends, they can be taught to remove, clean, and reinsert the soft lenses on a weekly or bimonthly schedule. Otherwise the ophthalmologist can see the patient every month or so, and at that time the lenses can be removed, cleaned, and reinserted. The corneas are carefully checked on these visits also.

Table 15-1. Trial lens selection for hydrophilic lenses (Griffin Naturalens)

Corneal Keratometer Readings	Lens base curve	Lens diameter
40.0-41.5	8.4	14.5
41.5-43.0	8.1	14.0
43.0-44.5	7.8	13.5
44.5-45.0	7.5	13.0

In fitting aphakic patients with soft lenses, we get keratometer readings first, which tells us how much cylinder and where. Retinoscopy is done to estimate the amount of plus needed and then a soft lens is chosen from a trial set. To choose a soft lens from the trial set, three parameters are considered: base curve, diameter and power. By using K readings, one obtains the lens base curve and diameter from the table provided with the soft lens (Table 15-1). For the power, the spherical equivalent is calculated and then a diopter or so is added to the spherical equivalent to compensate for the vertex distance change (vertex distance from phoropter to corneas). Then, for reasons that are not quite clear to us, we have found that we must empirically add 2 more diopters to the above obtained sum to correct the patient to the 20/60–20/30 range with the soft lens alone. In summary, to obtain the power of the soft lens, we add approximately 3 diopters to the spherical equivalent of our phoropter refraction. The selected soft lens is inserted, the fit inspected, and an overrefraction done. If the overrefraction axis does not agree with the previously taken K readings, something is wrong and the fit should be carefully checked.

Here is an example to show that the procedure is not as complicated as it sounds: It is 1:00 on Wednesday afternoon and you are checking over the afternoon's schedule. You have two aphakes to correct, one new patient, and an important tennis match at 5:00 (it's not going to be easy). You start your first aphake:

1. Keratometer readings 43.25/−45.75 cyl. axis 90; so there is a +2.50 cyl. axis 90. [15-love]
2. Retinoscope broken. [15-15]
3. Maybe we can get along without retinoscope. Place the patient behind the phoropter and "crank in" the cylinder and axis (we know that's right from the K reading). Start at +12.00, and without touching the cylinder, subjectively click in different spheres until the best visual acuity is achieved. The patient now reads 20/25 with +11.00 + 2.50 cyl. axis 90. [30-15]
4. Follow calculations to choose a soft lens.
   Get the base curve and diameter from the table and K readings:
   Base curve 7.8
   Diameter 13.5
   Calculate power:
   Spherical equivalent   12.25
                              + 3.00
   Power of soft lens   15.25

So choose a lens:
   Base curve 7.8
   Diameter 13.5
   Power 15.25
Insert lens; inspect for proper fit.
Patient reads 20/40. [40-15]
5. Refract over soft lens (the nurse fixed the retinoscope).
Patient reads 20/20.
Write prescription for glasses. Don't forget add.
Give the patient an appointment of 1 week to check glasses and soft lens
fit. [Game]

With aphakic patients, we have found the use of soft lenses very gratifying.

This study was supported in part by USPHS grants EY-52868 (Gasset) and EY-00446 from the National
Eye Institute.

Chapter 16

Aphakia and Griffin Naturalens:
Case reports

Joseph A. Baldone, M.D.

Most of the aphakic patients in my series (29 eyes) are those who have been considered hard contact lens failures.

A 70-year-old lady had an uncomplicated cataract extraction of the right eye and could not adjust to the presence of a hard contact lens. She could obtain good visual acuity with a soft gel lens but *would not* learn the application and removal procedures. Since this patient resides in the same hotel-apartment building that I do, I could gradually increase her soft lens wearing time to 24 hours per day, and eventually to wearing the lens for at least 2-week periods. After enjoying good vision for several weeks, her motivation increased to the point that she was able to master application and removal.

In the next case, a 72-year-old man developed bullous keratopathy 8 weeks after bilateral cataract surgery. He had edema and large bullae over both corneas and was referred for fitting with bandage lenses. He was fitted with Griffin lenses (8.1 14.0 +13.25 right eye and 8.1 14.0 +16.00 left eye) and obtained immediate comfort. He was able to use soft lenses without the addition of 5% saline solution, and I did not need to replace lenses because of crystal build-up. I am not implying, that, in my series, there is definitely a cause-and-effect relationship between crystal build-up and the use of 5% saline solution, but there is a definite *association*. It is believed that compression alone from the Griffin lens is sufficient in most cases. His visual acuity was adequate, and he wore these lenses continuously for 9 months, at which time the lenses were removed to determine if his bullae would return. Currently, 9 months after discontinuing soft lenses, his corneal epithelium remains completely normal in appearance, and the patient is using spectacle correction.

A 63-year-old bilaterally aphakic engineer complained of a tear deficiency and frequent foreign bodies beneath his hard contact lenses. His K readings were 43.00/43.00 (right eye) and 44.50/43.50 (left eye). Griffin soft lenses, 8.1 14.0 +16.25 = 20/25 (right eye) and 8.1 14.0 +15.25 = 20/20 (left eye), were delivered to the patient. The base curves in this case were flatter than K in the right eye by 1.38 diopters and in the left eye by 1.88. The patient was instructed to use 0.45% saline as needed because of the deficiency of his tear production. After 2 months of daytime wear, the patient's lenses suddenly steepened, requiring −2.25 (right eye) and −1.75 (left eye) to attain visual acuity of 20/25. By applanation tonometry, intraocular tensions, which normally were 12 mm. Hg in both eyes, had elevated to 22 mm. Hg in each eye. We now plan to refit the patient with the base curves of 8.4 or 8.7 mm.

A 46-year-old oil company president came to us with an aphakic left eye and light perception in his right eye from a childhood injury. He had been unable to adjust to hard contact lenses. K readings were 45.00/45.75. Whether a 7.5 or 7.8 mm. lens should have been used was immaterial because on the day of the patient's office visit, the steepest lens in my inventory was an 8.1 mm. lens (3.50 diopters flatter than K). When 8.1 14.0 +12.50 was placed on the eye, the patient had a visual acuity of 20/20. He was elated with the comfort and stability of vision. His intraocular tension was normal and remained so after 3 months of wearing this lens daily.

Another patient, a 58-year-old unilateral aphakic male, was unable to tolerate a hard contact lens. A number of Griffin lenses were tried, but good visual acuity could not be attained with the lens alone, nor with overrefraction. However, when this patient was fitted with a "cushion lens" (soft lens under a hard lens) 8.1 14.0 −0.25 0.37, he had complete comfort. K readings were made over the lens and found to, be 44.50/42.00. A hard contact lens base curve 42.50 +12.00 8.3 mm. was fitted over the soft lens, and a visual acuity of 20/15 obtained. Original K readings on his aphakic eye were 46.00/43.25. This patient has worn the combination of cushion lens and hard contact lens for 5 months, sometimes up to 3 weeks at 24 hours per day, with complete physical and optical comfort. This case definitely proves that the combination of hard and cushion lenses will be of use in some cases.

Another patient recently fitted has a history of traumatic cataract and central retinal damage to his left eye at age 6. Some 30 years later his remaining eye was severely damaged when a soft drink bottle exploded. He sustained corneal and lens damage and subsequently received a combined keratoplasty and cataract extraction. The patient wore a hard contact lens for approximately a year and then developed a retinal detachment. He had retinal detachment surgery and discontinued the hard contact lens. Good visual acuity could not be attained with a Griffin lens alone, but when fitted with a hard contact lens over a cushion lens, he obtained visual acuity of 20/30+ and complete physical comfort.

The Paragon bifocal lens is made to have the reading segment invade well into the pupillary area. This does not interfere with distance vision as happens with the DeCarle bifocal and the Centrad bifocal. Their reading segments are located in the central pupillary area. The segment of the Paragon bifocal covers the lower third of the pupillary area. Based on this principle, attempts are being made to design a hard plastic reading segment to be worn on the distance soft lens. Proper shapes and sizes will have to be determined to provide adequate adhesion and the necessary upward displacement by the lower lid border when the eye is in the downward gaze. That such a portion of a lens will seek good position and can be comfortably worn has been established. Good, immediate near vision is still an unreached goal. This technique may serve some purpose until the problems of bifocal soft lenses are otherwise solved.

A 64-year-old woman (unilateral aphake) was fitted with a Griffin lens 8.1 14.0 +18.00 and attained a visual acuity of 20/20 *and* Jaeger 1 (J1). Good near visual acuity in some of the hyperopic lenses is probably attributable to different powers being present over the different areas of the soft lenses. This is also demonstrated by a +2.00 hyperope who requires a +2.00 add in spectacles, but is able to see 20/20—*and* J1 with an over-plus of only +0.75 diopter sphere in her Griffin lens.

Of the cases of aphakia with normal corneas in my series of 29 eyes, I was able to attain visual acuity of 20/20 in 10 eyes and 20/25 or better in another 10 eyes. Four eyes had a visual acuity of 20/30 or better, 3 eyes had 20/40 or better, 1 eye had 20/50, and 1 eye had 20/100, but, with overfitting of a hard contact lens, the eye was able to obtain a visual acuity of 20/30+.

Chapter 17

Use of hydrophilic contact lenses for correction of aphakia

Jack Hartstein, M.D.

LENS HISTORY, TYPES, AND CHARACTERISTICS

Hydrophilic aphakic contact lenses have many characteristics in common with hydrophilic phakic contact lenses. Therefore, an understanding of the basic materials, problems, and fitting characteristics of hydrophilic contact lenses are discussed first.

Hydrophilic contact lenses have been introduced under various names and some of them are as follows:

1. Gel contact lenses
2. Gel contact flexible lenses
3. Hydrogel contact lenses
4. Hydragel contact lenses
5. Soflenses
6. Gelatin contact lenses

They were first developed by Professor Wichterle from the Institute of Macromolecular Chemistry in Prague, Czechoslovakia. They are made of hydrogel polydiazethylene methacrylate, which is hydrophilic. Of the lens weight, 50% to 60% is water when fully hydrated. It can be compressed and water removed from it in the same manner as one would squeeze moisture from a sponge. The lenses must be kept in an aqueous solution (a solution of 0.5% sodium chloride and 0.5% sodium bicarbonate in distilled water is recommended). When hydrated, the lens can be bent into any form and still return to their original shape. When dry, the lenses become flat and brittle and must be soaked in solution for several hours after they are worn again. These lenses are thicker than standard hard contact lenses. A -10.00-diopter hard lens may be 0.1 mm. thick, whereas a -10.00-diopter soft lens may be 0.3 mm. thick.

Basic problems

In the early days some basic problems were noted and these problems still exist today: (1) Visual acuity is not usually as good as in methylmethacrylate lenses. (2) Eyes with corneal astigmatism of 1.50 to 2.00 diopters cannot be fit with soft lenses since the lenses follow the corneal shape. (3) Fluorescein cannot be used to evaluate the fit since the lens absorbs the stain.

In elaboration on point 2 just mentioned, when a soft lens is placed on the cornea, its curvature is altered by the corneal scleral topography and also by lid pressure. Because of its flexibility, the posterior surface of the lens tends to assume the shape of the underlying anterior surface of the cornea and sclera. This change is transmitted to the anterior surface of the lens, which may be further altered by lid pressure. The transformed anterior surface curvature often has a different central radius and overall shape; that is, a given spherical anterior curve of a given radius may be transformed into an aspherical anterior curve of another radius. The quality of the surface may also be altered; that is, a regular surface may be transformed into an irregular surface.

Hydrophilic potential

The hydrophilic potential of the hydrogel lens can be varied by altering certain steps in the production of the gel material. As a result, the water-holding capabilities may be changed from 5% to more than 90%. The problem has been and still is to determine exactly what the hydrophilic potential of the finished lens should be. Theoretically, the material should have a 75% water-holding capability if our intent is to match the water content of the cornea. This would in theory ensure equilibrium between the lenses and the cornea. In the early days of the gel lens they were made of a water-holding potential of 80%; this, however, proved unsatisfactory. From a practical point of view one cannot work with a plastic mesh of less than 40%, thus allowing only 60% fluid, which is 15% out of balance with the cornea. The fluid potential of 60% was used until about 1965 when it was dropped to about 50% by investigators then working with the lens in the United States. At the present time most manufacturers experimenting with this material have been dropping the water-holding potential steadily to the point where it now falls somewhere between 35% and 50%. There are three reasons why the water holding potential is being reduced:

1. The harder it is, the more resistent it is to damage.
2. As the water content is reduced and the lens becomes flexible, one is able to fit more corneal astigmatism. When the lens was 60% hydrophilic, astigmats above 1.00 diopters could not be fitted. When the water-holding content is reduced to 40%, one is able to fit up to 1.75 diopters with the gel lens.
3. The third reason for reducing the water potential is thickness. As fluid is taken up by the soft lens, it swells and thickens the lens. A thick lens is generally not as comfortable nor as well tolerated as a thin lens.

When the soft lens has a water-holding potential of 80%, its average hydrated thickness will be 0.5 to 0.6 mm. If the potential is dropped to 50% or 60%, the average thickness will be 0.3 to 0.4 mm. less. When water-holding potential is reduced to 35% to 40%, the same power range will have a thickness of 0.2 to 0.3 mm. A thickness of 0.4 to 0.6 mm. cannot be tolerated by the average contact lens patient.

GRIFFIN LENS COMPOSITION AND CHARACTERISTICS

The lenses that I have used in this study have been the Griffin Bionite lenses and the following discussion relates to certain characteristics of a properly fitted Griffin Bionite Lens:

1. It should center on the cornea and follow eye movements with little or no lag even on upward gaze.
2. It need not move when the lid blinks over it.
3. It should glide easily over the eye when it is slightly touched by the finger.

The diameters of the lenses vary from 13 to 16 mm., and in my experience the average diameter that works best is 14.0 mm. I believe that one should try and fit a diameter 2.0 mm. larger than the cornea.

The base curve of the lens varies from 7.5 to 8.7 mm. and is available in 7.5, 7.8, 8.1, 8.4, and 8.7 mm. I have found that the most common base curve for aphakic patients is now 8.1 and 8.4 mm. Originally, as will be pointed out later, I did fit some 7.8 mm. base curves, but here I ran into some problems with tightness.

The base curve should be flatter than the radius of the cornea in the central region, and can vary from 0.3 to 0.7 mm. flatter than the flattest meridian of the corneal curve. The lens thus rests on the eye in two regions, the central corneal region and a circular peripheral region on the sclera. The inside radius vaults the region of the limbus.

LENS WEARING
Blinking

Normal blinking is said to be important in the comfortable wearing of the hard contact lenses. It is also important for the wearing of soft contact lenses, but for other reasons:
1. The pumping action of the lids produces a good tear flow into the lens.
2. It is essential that the front surface as well as the back surface be kept in a hydrated state, which again is accomplished by a good blink rate.

If symptoms of irritation arise, one should consider the following three reasons:
1. Incorrect saline solution
2. A tear or nick in the lens
3. Particles of dust or debris under the lens

Sometimes a patient will appear with injected eyes, experiencing no feeling of the lens and having no subjective complaints. This would probably be associated with sluggish movement and poor vision and would indicate tightness.

Limbal injection

Injection around the limbus is generally considered a universal symptom of tightness and may be accompanied by other tight symptoms such as sluggish movement, irritation, and poor vision.

Scleral indentation

One final observation before considering our cases is that of scleral indentation. One sometimes finds an indentation on the sclera in the form of a ring around the cornea where the edge of the lens has been resting. This may indicate one of two things:
1. The lens is too tight.
2. The patient has an unusually soft sclera.

FITTING APHAKIC PATIENTS (CASE HISTORIES)

In discussing the application of hydrophilic lenses for the correction of aphakia, I have selected certain cases to point out specific observations.

A 56-year-old monocular aphakic had a cataract removed from his right eye on May 11, 1970. On June 3, 1970, he was fitted with a hard lenticular cataract contact lens that had the following dimensions:

Base curve	Front vertex power	Diameter	Optical zone
8.10 mm.	+ 14.00	10.0 mm.	7.6 mm.

Thickness	Secondary curve radius	Color
0.45 mm.	9.10 mm.	Light blue

He could wear the lens well and his vision was excellent, but he had great difficulty handling this lens, that is, inserting and removing it, since he had no one to help him and was frequently out of town. On this basis he was refitted with a Griffin soft contact lens of the following measurements:

Base curve	Diameter	Power
8.1 mm.	14.0 mm.	+ 14.25

Vision achieved with the Griffin lens ranged from 20/40 to 20/30, unimprovable with additional spectacles, but the patient is quite happy.

I emphasized that he should remove his lens each night to clean it and sterilize it, but when he returned several months later, he informed me that since November 1970 he had been wearing the lens 4 to 6 days at a time before removing, recleaning, and reinserting it. He stated that he did this because he was in situations where he did not have the solutions with him when he was out of town and had found that he could tolerate the lens for these periods without any discomfort. In fact he told me that the only reason he removed it once or twice a week was for *my* benefit, not because of any visual or subjective discomfort.

This case demonstrates two things:

1. The hydrophilic lens is more practical for those who are unable to handle the regular hard contact lens even though they can wear either, once they are in the eye.
2. The aphakic eye can apparently accept this lens for a period longer than 24 hours without any apparent pathological damage.

The second case is that of a 52-year-old bilateral aphakic who had surgery on the left eye in 1969 and on the right eye in 1970 and with the following spectacle prescription was corrected to 20/20 in each eye:

O.D. + 12.25 − 1.25 cyl. axis 90 = 20/20
O.S. + 11.50 − 1.25 cyl. axis 135 = 20/20

I elected to fit him directly with soft contact lenses, and Griffin lenses were ordered as follows:

	Base curve	Diameter	Power
O.D.	8.1 mm.	14.0 mm.	+ 11.50
O.S.	8.1 mm.	14.0 mm.	+ 11.75

Upon receiving these lenses, the patient found that he could only wear them for 1 hour before developing severe burning and redness in both eyes.

Examination revealed tight lenses with conjunctival blanching at the edges of the lens.

New lenses were then ordered according to the following dimensions:

	Base curve	Diameter	Power
O.D.	8.4 mm.	13.5 mm.	+13.00 = 20/30
O.S.	8.4 mm.	13.5 mm.	+13.50 = 20/30

The patient found that he could immediately wear these lenses comfortably with no reaction. An overrefraction showed the following:

O.D. Plano −1.00 cyl. axis 90 = 20/20
O.S. +0.75 sphere = 20/25

Glasses were dispensed as executive bifocals with a +2.25 add to be worn with his contact lenses, which he wears comfortably now during his entire waking hours.

This case demonstrates that the soft lenses just as the hard contact lenses can be fitted too tightly and will result in an inability to wear the lenses. This inability should be noticeable within a short period of time.

The third case is that of a 51-year-old monocular aphakic who had cataract surgery performed on his right eye in 1969. He was fitted with a Griffin soft contact lens of the following dimensions:

Base curve	Diameter	Power
8.1 mm.	13.5 mm.	+9.00

An overrefraction showed the following:

+0.50 −1.00 cyl. axis 90 = 20/30

This overrefraction was prescribed as an executive lens with a 2.50 add. He is able to wear the lens comfortably all day without symptoms, but he is not able to achieve 20/20 vision even with the contact lens plus the overrefraction, whereas he can achieve 20/20 vision through glasses. Nevertheless he is happier wearing the contact lens.

The fourth case is that of a 59-year-old monocular aphakic who had cataract surgery performed on his right eye in 1970. His aphakic refraction is as follows:

O.D. +10.00 −1.00 cyl. axis 90 = 20/20

He was fitted with a Griffin Lens according to the following measurements:

Base curve	Diameter	Power
8.1 mm.	14.0 mm.	+11.00 = 20/30

Note that the best vision obtainable with the contact lens alone was 20/30. An overrefraction showed the following:

Plano −1.00 cyl. axis 90 = 20/20

With this overcorrection, he is able to achieve 20/20 vision; note that this is the exact same cylinder and same axis, that he required in his original manifest refraction. He is able to wear this lens confortably all day without symptoms.

The fifth case that I have chosen to illustrate is a 37-year-old monocular aphakic who had a dense cataract removed from her left eye in 1963. A manifest refraction showed the following:

O.S. +13.00 +1.50 cyl. axis 75 = 20/40 to 20/50

(Best obtainable)

Note that the best vision obtainable is in the range of 20/40 to 20/50.

She was fitted with a hard contact lens, and this also resulted in a vision of 20/40 to 20/50 rather than a similar range to spectacles.

She was fitted with a Griffin lens in October 1970 with the following measurements:

Base curve	Diameter	Power
8.1 mm.	14.0 mm.	+14.50 = 20/50 to 20/40

Again, the vision with the soft contact lens is comparable to that in the hard contact lens and also to that with the glasses.

The sixth, and final, case that I have chosen is that of a 22-year-old diabetic female whose best corrected vision was, as follows:

O.D. 15/200

O.S. 20/200

Cataract surgery was performed on the right eye in 1969 by incising the capsule and by repeated aspiration and irrigation.

She was then fitted with the Griffin lens according to the following dimensions:

	Base curve	Diameter	Power
O.D.	7.8 mm.	13.5 mm.	+14.00

She achieves 20/40 vision not improvable with additional spectacles. This vision also is not improved beyond 20/40 by spectacle refraction alone. She is able to wear this lens comfortably all day without symptoms.

In summary, I find that aphakic soft contact lenses offer the following advantages:

1. They can be worn comfortably for extended periods of time.
2. They are actually easier to handle by the patients.
3. Though the vision achieved by the contact lens alone may not in many cases be as good as that vision achieved by hard contact lens alone, the difference can be made up in spectacles to be worn over the contact lenses, and therefore this deficiency proved to be no additional problem.

Although not discussed in this particular presentation, information is being gathered to show that aphakic soft contact lenses will have particular application in aphakic infants as contrasted to our present methods of handling these particular patients.

PART V

Treatment of keratoconus

Chapter 18

Hydrophilic contact lenses
in management of
keratoconus

Antonio R. Gasset, M.D., and Edward L. Shaw, M.D.

Although patients with keratoconus of significant degree generally cannot see well without contact lenses, the fitting of such patients with hard contact lenses has produced serious problems. It is generally impossible to find a contact lens that fits all of the distorted corneal surface. Steep contact lenses seal out tears and oxygen and cause edema, whereas flat lenses, which must be used, rest on the apex of the cone and may not be well tolerated. There is also some evidence that contact lens's rubbing on the apex of the cone may produce scarring more rapidly than might otherwise occur and that some types of scleral lenses may encourage rapid growth of the cone. If soft contact lenses could be used for the optical corrections of patients with keratoconus, the lenses might permit vision and eliminate the need for surgery in a significant portion of patients who cannot tolerate hard contact lenses. In addition, there is the theoretical possibility that a flexible soft lens might produce less scarring than has been attributed to hard contact lenses.

At first, it seemed unlikely that a soft lens, which molds to the cornea, could produce optical correction in these distorted eyes, but clinical experience with this modality has been extremely encouraging. Our experience, described in this report, clearly indicates that patients with keratoconus can be comfortably fitted and optically corrected with soft contact lenses and that, in many of them, surgery caused by intolerance to hard lenses can be avoided. It is not yet clear and will not be clear for many years whether, in fact, such lenses avoid or minimize corneal scarring.

MATERIALS AND METHODS

In this study, only Griffin hydrophilic lenses were used because preliminary experience with some other types of lenses did not produce adequate optical corrections. Griffin lenses are different from other soft lenses,[1-3] and these differences appear extremely important in the optical correction of keratoconus patients.

In these patients keratometer readings were always taken to determine steepness of the cone, astigmatism, and axis, but were not used as a guide to fitting the lenses.

The lens initially selected for fitting was as flat as possible, usually an 8.4 or

8.1 mm. radius base curve. It was inserted and the fit was immediately evaluated. A lens steeper than the eye resulted in an air bubble trapped under the lens, generally near the lens center. A lens flatter than the eye resulted in an edge that lifted away from the eye at its margin, or tended to fold. Since it was easier to tell when a lens was too flat rather than too steep, it was our practice to begin with the flattest lens and then try progressively steeper lenses if necessary. To increase adhesiveness and promote proper centering, lenses with diameters of 14.0, 14.5, and 15.0 mm. were frequently used.

After this rather simple trial lens procedure, keratometer readings were usually done on the surface of the lens. Any astigmatism measured by the keratometer was an indication of residual corneal astigmatism and was corrected with subsequent refraction if necessary.

Refraction over the lens was done by standard techniques, but the spherical errors in these patients were often large, and it was necessary to explore a considerable range to find the right correction.

If a spherical correction provided adequate vision, the proper lens was given, and the fitting was ended. In some patients, especially those who had very high errors, we could obtain adequate vision only with an astigmatic correction in addition to the contact lens. In most cases, the contact lens alone provided adequate distance vision, and the astigmatic correction was used in spectacles as a reading glass. In some patients whose vision could not be corrected by any other way, the astigmatic correction was sufficiently large to warrant their wearing spectacles in addition to the soft contact lenses. As a rule, only half of the measured astigmatism was prescribed in spectacles at the start, but this depended on patient tolerance and the improvement of visual acuity.

RESULTS

Keratoconus patients were selected at random from persons referred to the University of Florida Eye Clinic, and a total of 24 eyes were fitted with Griffin hydrophilic lenses. Seventy percent of these patients had discontinued hard lenses because of discomfort and intolerance, or because the cone appeared too large to adequately fit with a hard lens. In this series 25% of the previous hard lens wearers had developed keratoconus while wearing hard lenses (Fig. 18-1).

Despite the fact that keratometer readings were taken routinely in all follow-up visits, the effect of the soft contact lenses on the prevention of keratoconus cannot be properly ascertained at the present time. In evaluating the follow-up keratometer readings in these patients, we must divide them into two main categories: (1) Patients with keratoconus who wore hard acrylic contact lenses for optical correction up to the time they were refitted with the soft contact lenses make one category. We must emphasize that these patients were hard contact lens failures for one of the following reasons: inability to tolerate these lenses, corneal edema, corneal vascularization, and hard lenses that failed to remain in position. This group represents 70% of the total number of patients fitted with these new soft lenses. (2) The second group represents the remaining 30% of the patients and are composed entirely of patients who never wore hard acrylic contact lenses. To evaluate K readings in the first group would be an error, since it

HYDROPHILIC CONTACT LENSES IN MANAGEMENT OF KERATOCONUS

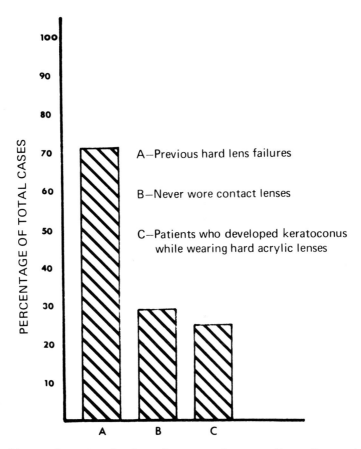

Fig. 18-1. Incidence of previous hard acrylic contact lens use. (From Gasset, A. R., and Kaufman, H. E.: Hydrophilic contact lenses in the management of keratoconus, J. Amer. Optom. Ass. **43**:334-337, 1972.)

is well known that spectacle blur and changing of keratometer readings occur in keratoconus patients as they do in normal patients wearing hard lenses. These changes are unpredictable and most difficult to evaluate. In the second group of patients, those who have never worn hard acrylic contact lenses, we have found little or no change in the keratometer readings. However, in the absence of a control group (patients with keratoconus of the same severity that have never worn any type of lenses and followed for the same length of time), no attempt will be made to claim that soft contact lenses could delay conical progression in patients with keratoconus.

Until recently most practitioners unequivocally accepted views such as those of Mandell,[4] who stated that hard acrylic contact lenses acted as a transparent pressure bandage that is constantly reshaping and inhibiting the progression of the cone. "However in view of our findings that 25% of the previous hard lens wearers had developed keratoconus while wearing hard acrylic contact lenses," and similar findings by Hartstein,[5] I feel that we can now state that (1) corneal

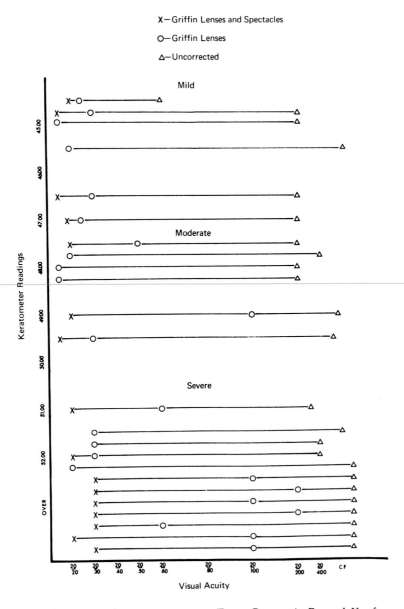

Fig. 18-2. Visual acuity in keratoconus cases. (From Gasset, A. R., and Kaufman, H. E.: Hydrophilic contact lenses in the management of keratoconus, J. Amer. Optom. Ass. **43**:334-337, 1972.)

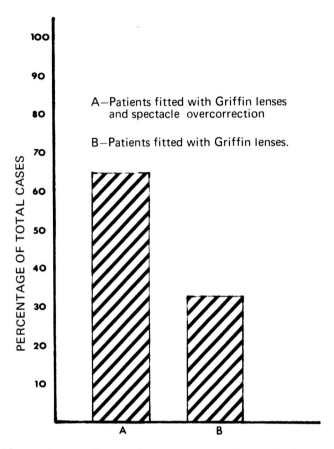

Fig. 18-3. Incidence of required spectacle correction over the Griffin lenses. (From Gasset, A. R., and Kaufman, H. E.: Hydrophilic contact lenses in the management of keratoconus, J. Amer. Optom. Ass. **43:**334-337, 1972.)

contact lenses do not retard cone progression, (2) keratoconus can develop in patients who, prior to wearing hard acrylic contact lenses, showed no signs of this condition. Although at the present time there is no sufficient evidence that keratoconus can be produced by wearing hard acrylic contact lenses, the increasing number of such reports,[6] particularly in patients who have worn hard acrylic contact lenses for a significant length of time, from 5 to 15 years, should not be readily discarded, and further studies must be carried out.

The visual acuity attained in these patients is illustrated in Fig. 18-2. The uncorrected visual acuity was less than 20/200 in all cases. In many patients, usually those with the less steep keratometer readings, lenses alone were sufficient to improve visual acuity to between 20/20 and 20/30. In others, generally those with keratometer readings up to 52 diopters, lenses alone were considered adequate in 50% of the cases, with the remaining 50% needing some spectacle overrefraction for satisfactory reading vision. In a third group of cases, generally those with keratometer readings greater than 52 diopters, 75% required spectacle overcorrec-

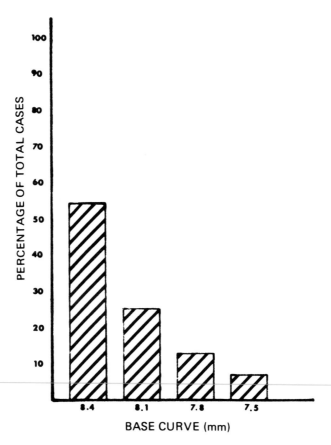

Fig. 18-4. Incidence of base curve used in keratoconus. (From Gasset, A. R., and Kaufman, H. E.: Hydrophilic contact lenses in the management of keratoconus, J. Amer. Optom. Ass. 43:334-337, 1972.)

tion to achieve visual acuities of 20/30 or better, but this group would generally be considered impossible to fit with hard acrylic lenses.[7] In all of these cases spectacle correction over the lenses improved visual acuity to 20/30 or better, and this combination was well tolerated.

In all, two thirds of the cases required spectacle overcorrection to improve visual acuity to acceptable levels (Fig. 18-3). In some cases spectacle corrections as high as −8.75 +7.75 cyl. axis 120 were given and well tolerated by these patients.

The base curves used in obtaining the best optical performance are shown in Fig. 18-4. More than 75% were fitted with very flat lenses (8.4 or 8.1 mm.), and almost 90% of the patients were fitted with lenses 14 mm. or more in diameter (Fig. 18-5). These lenses have now been worn continuously during waking hours from 5 to 24 months (Fig. 18-6).

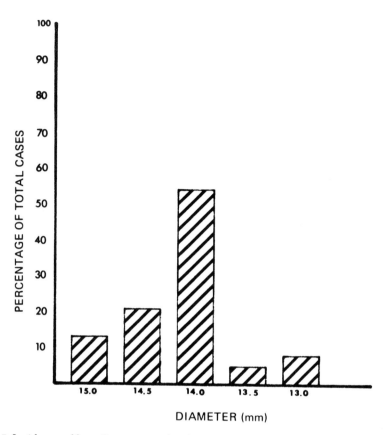

Fig. 18-5. Incidence of lens diameter used in keratoconus. (From Gasset, A. R., and Kaufman, H. E.: Hydrophilic contact lenses in the management of keratoconus, J. Amer. Optom. Ass. **43:**334-337, 1972.)

DISCUSSION

Although soft contact lenses mold to the eye, the fact is clear that Griffin hydrophilic lenses can be used to optically correct patients with keratoconus and are especially valuable in patients who cannot tolerate hard lenses.

At first we were shocked at the thought of giving patients both contact lenses and spectacles, but experience with patients who could not see well without this combination, indicates that both can be extremely well accepted. In addition, any changes in refraction can be handled simply by changing the spectacles. The soft contact lens is used to provide spherical correction, generally for the myopia that is present, and to correct the irregular astigmatism, while the spectacle provides the necessary correction for any residual regular astigmatism.

As a rule, hard contact lenses cannot perfectly fit the configuration of a cone and must be fitted flat to prevent pressing on the peripheral cornea, which seals

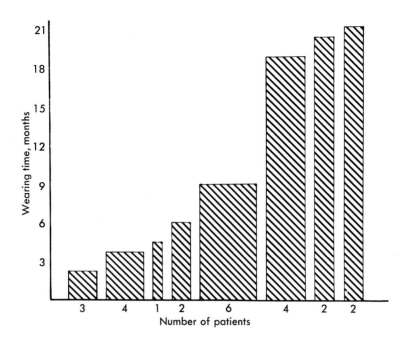

Fig. 18-6. Duration of Griffin lens therapy. (From Gasset, A. R., and Kaufman, H. E.: Hydrophilic contact lenses in the management of keratoconus, J. Amer. Optom. Ass. **43**:334-337, 1972.)

out the tear flow and oxygen from the area of the cone. Some investigators believe that over a period of years hard lens rubbing on the cone may increase scarring and accelerate the need for corneal surgery.[7] Even if this problem with hard lenses is true, we are not certain that soft contact lenses avoid corneal scarring and prevent this problem. There is some theoretical reason to believe that a soft lens would not produce the same kind of corneal scarring that an acrylic hard lens resting on the apex of the cone would cause, but prolonged follow-up over a period of a decade is needed to determine the true effects of soft and hard lenses on apical scarring.

Our experience indicates that soft contact lenses can be extremely valuable in the optical correction of keratoconus patients. It is important to emphasize, however, that the success rate depends largely on the use of the proper lenses, and meticulous attention to detail in fitting these patients.

SUMMARY

Concerned about their difficulties encountered in hard contact lens therapy for keratoconus, 24 keratoconus patients were fitted with soft hydrophilic contact lenses (Griffin). The patients were followed for over 2 years and soft contact lenses appeared especially useful in patients in whom hard lenses could not be tolerated. Large, flat lenses were generally used, and in many cases, spectacles were used in addition to the lenses to correct residual astigmatism.

It is possible that the use of soft contact lenses may avoid some of the corneal scarring attributed to the rubbing of hard contact lenses on the corneal surface, but only prolonged follow-up will establish whether this is significant.

Although skill and patience is required in fitting these patients, this study indicates that patients with keratoconus can be comfortably fitted and optically corrected with soft contact lenses and that in many of them surgery because of intolerance to hard lenses can be avoided. However, it is not yet clear and will not be clear for many years whether, in fact, such lenses avoid or minimize corneal scarring.

This study was supported in part by USPHS grants EY-52868 (Gasset), EY-00446, and EY-00266 from the National Eye Institute and RR-82 from the General Clinical Research Centers Programs of the Division of Research Resources, National Institutes of Health.

REFERENCES

1. Gasset, A. R., and Kaufman, H. E.: Therapeutic uses of hydrophilic contact lenses, Amer. J. Ophthal. **69:**252-259, 1970.
2. Kaufman, H. E., Uotila, M. H., Gasset, A. R., Wood, T. O., and Ellison, E. D.: The medical uses of soft contact lenses, Trans. Amer. Acad. Ophthal. Otolaryng. **45:**361-373, 1971.
3. Morrison, D. R., and Edelhauser, H. F.: Permeability of hydrophilic contact lenses, Invest. Ophthal. (In press.)
4. Mandell, A.: Keratoconus and contact lenses, Contacto **13:**101-104, 1959.
5. Hartstein, J.: Keratoconus that developed in patients wearing contact lenses, Arch. Ophthal. **80:**345-346, 1968.
6. Nauheim, J. S.: Corneal curvature changes simulating keratoconus in patients wearing contact lenses, Contact Lens Med. Bull. **2:**7-12, 1969.
7. Benton, J. W., and Chambers, F. E.: Indications for surgery. In Advances in keratoplasty, Int. Ophthal. Clin. **10**(2):197, 1970.

Chapter 19

Correction of keratoconus with hydrophilic contact lenses

Jack Hartstein, M.D.

Keratoconus is still a much misunderstood condition as far as etiology, progression, and evaluation of the disease is concerned, and I can safely say that there is much conjecture at this point as to just how these cases are helped by fitting them with a hydrophilic lens.

It has been stated that astigmatism greater than 1.50 to 2.00 diopters is a contraindication for the hydrophilic lens and yet these cases of keratoconus with their steep and sometimes indescribable astigmatisms are benefited tremendously, as the following cases will illustrate.

LENS SELECTION

Since keratometer readings in these cases are unreliable and in many cases unobtainable, I have used the following criteria in selecting the initial lens:
1. The cornea should be measured and a lens selected that should be at least 2 mm. larger than the measured horizontal corneal diameter.
2. I would then arbitrarily select a lens with a base curve of 7.5, which is the steepest curve I have available in my trial set, and use that as a starting point. Should this lens appear to be too steep, either because of blanching of the vessels at the edge of the lens or if too large an air bubble encroaches on the pupil, a lens with a base curve of 7.8 mm. would then be selected. Because these lenses are quite large averaging 13.50 to 14.00 mm. in diameter, their steepness-rightness relationship is determined as much by the sclera as by the cornea.
3. The lens is then rinsed in sterile saline and inserted into the eye.
4. A few moments are allowed for the lens to become compatible with the tears of the patient's eye.
5. As soon as the redness has cleared and the patient quits tearing or loses the feeling of the lens in his eye, the fitter then holds the lids wide open and instructs the patient to look straight ahead. He then moves the lens on the cornea with the forefinger so that one portion of the edge of the lens is midway between the apex and the periphery of the cornea.
6. The lens is then released with the lids still kept open, and if properly fitted, the lens should center itself.
7. If it does center, this is a fair indication of a good fit.

CASE HISTORIES

I have selected five patients who illustrate what happens when a soft contact lens is placed on a keratoconic eye.

The first case is that of a 50-year-old female with bilateral advanced keratoconus, with the left cornea worse than the right. Her best corrected vision was 20/200 (right eye) and she could count fingers at 3 feet (left eye). Keratometer readings were unobtainable. She was fitted with the following Griffin soft contact lenses:

	Base curve	Diameter	Power
O.D.	7.8 mm.	14.0 mm.	− 2.50 sphere
O.S.	7.8 mm.	14.0 mm.	− 2.00 sphere

An overrefraction showed the following:
O.D. +2.00 −2.25 cyl. axis 85 = 20/30
O.S. +2.00 −3.50 cyl. axis 50 = 20/100

The patient states that she is now able to see in the distance, something that she has been unable to do for many years.

Note that the vision in the right eye comes up to 20/30 and that the vision in the left eye is 20/100, but they could not be improved beyond that level. I might mention at this point that this patient as well as the others are those who were unable to be fitted with hard contact lenses and it was only on that basis that they were selected to be fitted with the soft contact lenses.

The next patient is a 60-year-old white female with bilateral severe keratoconus. Keratometer readings are unobtainable. Her best corrected vision in the right eye was 20/200 and in the left eye less than 20/400.

She was fitted with the following Griffin lens in her right eye only.

	Base curve	Diameter	Power
O.D.	7.8 mm.	14.0 mm.	− 3.50 = 20/100

You will note that this gave her 20/100 vision, but an overrefraction of plano −3.75 cyl. axis 125 brought this vision down to 20/40 −2. She finds that she can read for the first time in years and loves to see in the distance. She wears this lens without symptoms her entire waking hours.

The third case is that of a 22-year-old law student with bilateral keratoconus. Slit lamp examination revealed the typical signs of keratoconus, including Vogt's stripes. His keratometer readings showed the following:
O.D. 41.75/44.00
O.S. 43.00/49.00

He was then fitted with the Griffin lenses as follows:

	Base curve	Diameter	Power
O.D.	7.5 mm.	13.5 mm.	− 3.00 = 20/30
O.S.	7.5 mm.	13.5 mm.	Plano = 20/40

Note that he obtained 20/30 vision in the right eye and 20/40 vision in the left eye and they were not improved with spectacles. He wears his lenses comfortably his entire waking hours. Note that he shows 2.25 diopters of astigmatism in the right eye and 6.00 diopters of astigmatism in the left eye. With the soft lenses in place his vision improves remarkably, and yet no additional cylinder can be prescribed in spectacles.

The fourth case is that of a 31-year-old priest with bilateral keratoconus who had a transplant performed in his right eye and has subsequently developed a cone in the transplant. The K readings for his right eye show the following:

O.D. 48.00/44.00

The best corrected vision is 20/100 with the following prescription:

O.D. −8.50 −2.50 cyl. axis 150

He was fitted with one Griffin contact lens for the right eye as follows:

	Base curve	Diameter	Power
O.D.	7.5 mm.	13.5 mm.	−10.50 = 20/40

Additional lenses or glasses do not improve this vision. He wears the lens comfortably his entire waking hours. Note that with this lens he is able to obtain 20/40 vision.

The fifth case is that of a 52-year-old white female with severe keratoconus who was presented with the following glass prescription:

O.D. +5.00 cyl. axis 100 = 20/30

O.S. +8.75 −11.00 cyl. axis 100 = 20/100

Her keratometer readings were as follows:

O.D. 46.75/52.00

O.S. Unobtainable

Trial soft contact lenses were inserted as follows:

	Base curve	Diameter	Power
O.D.	7.50 mm.	13.0 mm.	−1.75
O.S.	7.50 mm.	13.0 mm.	−1.75

An overrefraction surprisingly showed the following and resulted in remarkably good vision:

O.D. +1.00 −1.25 cyl. axis 150 = 20/25

O.S. −7.00 −2.00 cyl. axis 15 = 20/40 −3

Note how the soft contact lens reduces the amount of required cylinder by three to four times. In the right eye she went from a −5.00 to a −1.25 diopter cylinder and actually had an improvement in the vision from 20/30 to 20/25. In the left eye she went from a −11.00 cylinder to a −2.00 cylinder and had a remarkable visual improvement. Her acuity improved from 20/100 to 20/40 −3.

COMMENT

As I mentioned earlier there has been much conjecture as to just how the soft contact lens corrected the vision in these grossly astigmatic eyes. One suggested explanation is that the cone is not ordinarily centered over the apex of the cornea but rather is found to be decentered down and in (most often) or up and out and perhaps the patient now peers through a different portion of his cornea. Another explanation might be that the soft lens bridges the cone and to some extent fills in the irregularities in the cornea to provide a new refracting surface. In any case, this question is certainly far from answered but does offer exciting prospects for further investigations.

Chapter 20

Keratoconus and use of Griffin Naturalens

Joseph A. Baldone, M.D.

The Griffin Naturalens can be of great help in some cases of keratoconus. Good visual acuity can be obtained with these alone or combined with a forward spectacle correction. Time may prove, perhaps, that the Griffin lens should be reserved for only those cases that cannot be fitted with rigid lenses.

One patient in this series has had keratoconus for over 24 years. As of this date, she has worn Griffin lenses daily for 2 years. The right lens has never been replaced, an indication of the potential durability of these lenses. There is no objective or subjective evidence that her condition has progressed. She is much more comfortable physically and optically than she was during 4 to 5 years of hard contact lens wear. Another patient is now at 18 months of daily wear without objective or subjective evidence of progression of the keratoconus.

Some cases show a marked reduction of the refractive cylinder, and this reduction may be due to a compensating cylinder created on the anterior lens surface. Whether a particular cornea can be fitted with regard to the amount of cylinder read by the keratometer is determined not by how much *cylinder* is present, but by how much of the corneal surface is involved in the cone. One patient has 13 diopters of cylinder in her refraction and with a hard lens there is 3 diopters of residual cylinder. This is reduced to 0.75 diopter with her Griffin lens. Another patient has 4.00 diopters of cylinder in his refraction and this is reduced to 2.00 diopters of residual cylinder with his Griffin lens and completely corrected by the addition of spectacle correction.

A 26-year-old medical resident had bilateral keratoconus and received corneal transplants in both eyes. The right eye attains a visual acuity of 20/20 −1 with a hard contact lens. The left graft shows neovascularization at each attempt to use a hard contact lens. The vessels shrink when the hard contact lens is discontinued and topical steroid treatment instituted. The left eye K readings are 51.00/49.00. This patient was fitted with a Griffin lens 8.4 14.0 −7.00 and with an overcorrection of −0.25 +1.00 cyl. axis 75. He attained visual acuity of 20/25. It is hoped that he will be able to tolerate this soft lens without further neovascularization of the graft.

An ophthalmology resident who was recently fitted plans, if possible, to become a 24-hour-per-day wearer. He reasons that the restraining effects of the semirigid lens should be ever present over his corneas. Other patients generally are wearers during waking hours only.

Anisometropia was so great in one patient with keratoconus after bilateral corneal transplants that a Griffin lens was used on only one eye and this lens almost perfectly equalized the errors of refraction of both eyes. This patient has been able to return to her duties as a bookkeeper, with a combination of one Griffin lens and a pair of spectacle lenses.

The next case may not be a true keratoconus. She had worn hard contact lenses for 13 years. When she was seen in March 1971, K readings were not possible on the right eye. Left-eye K readings were 52.00/56.00. Both corneas showed markedly irregular anterior and posterior surfaces. Her visual acuity unaided was 20/100 -1 (right eye) and 20/100 (left eye). When fitted with Griffin lenses (O.D. 8.1 14.0 $+2.50$; O.S. 7.8 13.5 $+3.25$), her acuity was 20/80 (right eye) and 20/40 (left eye). The patient is very pleased with this visual acuity, but it cannot be improved with overrefraction or with hard contact lenses fitted over the soft lenses.

A 22-year-old woman was able to attain visual acuity of 20/40 in each eye with hard lenses, but by correcting residual astigmatism of 1.00, it was correctable to 20/25 in each eye. When Griffin Naturalenses were fitted, best visual acuity attainable was 20/30 in each eye with overrefraction. Some patients are not able to attain as good a visual acuity with soft lenses and overrefraction as they can with hard lenses and overrefraction.

A 27-year-old male patient with keratoconus with hard lens wear had a visual acuity of 20/150; with soft lens his visual acuity was limited to 20/70. With the soft lens this could not be improved with overrefraction, but when the curvature of the soft lens was measured and the patient was fitted with a hard contact lens onto the surface of the soft lens, he attained visual acuity of 20/20.

Several different soft lenses (even of the same parameters) should be tried if good visual acuity is not obtained. Different lenses will give widely varying results with overrefraction.

Chapter 21

Fitting flexible contact lenses in keratoconus

Victor Chiquiar Arias, O.D.

During my training in fitting hydrophilic contact lenses (Griffin Naturalens) in March and April 1970, I saw my professor Dr. Antonio Gasset fit several cases of keratoconus with surprisingly good results. The fact that Griffin lenses bend to the shape of the cornea, limiting their effectivity in high astigmatism, would seem to preclude them from use in keratoconus. However, we must keep in mind that:

1. When a flexible contact lens is placed on an astigmatic cornea, they *transmit part* of the astigmatism to its anterior surface; but they also *mask part* of the corneal astigmatism.
2. Keratoconus differs greatly from astigmatism in that in many cases only the ectasia and part of the surrounding cornea have an irregular shape. The rest of the cornea, especially *the periphery is generally more spherical than one would suppose.*

Out of almost 10,000 contact lens patients, we have close to 700 keratoconus cases, and out of these, we have 35 that have frequently ruptured and have epithelial staining and 2 that have slow healing ulcers. We decided to use hydrophilic lenses in the percentage of keratoconus cases (5%) that could not be fitted properly or use safely hard contact lenses.

In the course of our investigation we found that the Griffin lenses could be worn comfortably and safely in several cases of keratoconus with the following conditions:

1. Excessive epithelial fragility (all 35 cases must have this)
2. Persistent staining of the epithelium (all 35 cases must have this)
3. Corneal topography, or lid shape that would not allow stable corneal contact lenses to be fitted (12 cases) (sclerals could have been used).
4. Slow healing ulcerations (2 cases)

The main problems were sterilization, breakage, and vision. We had expected the last problem and utilized two methods previously proposed to improve vision:

1. Prescribing a pair of spectacles (eyeglasses) to be used in conjunction with the soft lens.

2. Fitting a hard contact lens on top of the hydrophilic one (cushion lens).

We found that Dr. Gasset's method of prescribing the full amount of cylinder measurable on the anterior surface of the hydrophilic lens in situ gave good results in terms of vision. However, several patients complained of asthenopia and dizziness while using these full-cylinder-correction spectacles in conjunction with their hydrophilic lenses, especially while walking or driving. In these cases we suggested that they use their hydrophilic lenses alone for activities that did not need critical vision, reserving the additional spectacles only for the cinema, television, and so on. Some cases agreed to this limitation. We experimented with the cushion lens method proposed by Dr. Baldone in several cases, but were unable to have the stable lens hold on top of the hydrophilic lenses in any case. Dr. Baldone has now personally explained his method of fitting the hard overlens and we will reevaluate this method.

The "piggyback" (double cushion lens)

Based on the above observations and noting the problem of fitting a stable contact lens on top of the hydrophilic one, Dr. Daniel Vargas, an associate in my practice, suggested trying the use of *two* hydrophilic lenses (one on top of the other) on each eye. The reasoning was this:

1. If the hydrophilic lens fitted on a patient's cornea with 4 diopters of astigmatism masks approximately 1 to 2 diopters of astigmatism, could not a second hydrophilic lens fit on top of the first one and mask a substantial portion of the transmitted astigmatism?
2. And further, if the first hydrophilic lens, fitted on a conical cornea, will transmit some of the irregularity to its anterior surface but also mask a percentage of it, would not the second hydrophilic lens fitted on top of the first one further mask part of the remaining irregularity?

We decided to try this on several keratoconus patients who were previously fitted with hydrophilic lenses but were unable to obtain good vision. The results of this trial were positive:

1. In several cases the visual acuity (VA) of a keratoconus patient fitted with one pair of hydrophilic lenses was further improved when we fit a second pair of lenses on top of the first.
2. The amount of astigmatism and distortion measured on the anterior surface of the second hydrophilic lens (fitted on top of the first one) was significantly less.
3. The second hydrophilic lens holds well on top of the first one. Generally, the first and second hydrophilic lens are not absolutely concentric. However, this does not seem to be a problem as far as VA or comfort is concerned. Most patients reported that they can wear both lenses, one on top of the other, on the same eye without discomfort, and most are quite satisfied with the VA obtained.

How we fit hydrophilic lenses in keratoconus

Probably as a carry-over or "conditioned reflex" of our years of experience hard (stable) lenses in keratoconus, we initially selected the steepest radius in our inventory of hydrophilic lenses. However, we found that the 7.2 radius was generally too steep (short), and when it was combined with a diameter of 14.0 or even 13.5 mm., a central bubble would form.

In others, even though the 7.5 radius combined with a 14.5 diameter seemed appropriate, patients complained of foggy vision, variable vision, conjunctival injection, blanching of conjunctival vessels, indentation of the conjunctiva where the edge of the lens rests, and stinging or burning sensations. (This last symptom is generally more related to materials used in the various chemical sterilizing methods than to lens fit).

Generally speaking, the second hydrophilic lens (the one that goes on top of the first one) is fitted with a smaller diameter and shorter (steeper) radius than the first hydrophilic lens (the one that rests on the patient's cornea). As in almost everything else regarding flexible lenses, trial and error is the procedure. We look for a combination of diameter and radius that will hold on top of the first lens and the one that will give the least distortion, as measured with the keratometer on the anterior surface of the second lens. This generally gives the best VA.

In most cases, we have obtained the best results by putting most of the negative power on the first lens.

Based on our experience of fitting conventional hard (stable) contact lenses on keratoconus for over 20 years and with flexible contact lenses for nearly 2 years, we conclude the following:

1. In cases of keratoconus, where stable lenses can be used, this is our method of choice because it gives the patient:
   a. The best visual acuity than with any other method.
   b. All-day tolerance in most cases.
   c. Excellent performance, in most situations.
   d. Can be used safely all day, for many years, in the majority of cases.
2. In the cases of keratoconus where stable contact lenses cannot be used because of excessive fragility of the epithelium, recurrent ulceration, and so on, the cases should be handled with hydrophilic contact lenses.
3. Where vision with the hydrophilic lenses on is deficient, three methods should be tried:
   a. Prescribe in spectacles the full-cylinder (or spherocylindrical) correction that gives the best VA possible. These spectacles are to be worn in addition to the hydrophilic lenses to improve vision. They should be worn in every situation where the patient tolerates them.
   b. Try to fit a stable lens on top of the hydrophilic lens, as Dr. Baldone suggests.
   c. An additional pair of hydrophilic contact lenses should be tried on top of the first ones in an effort to improve VA.

By preserving the integrity of the patient's cornea, whichever method gives the best visual results in most circumstances and gives the patient the best, more comfortable vision for all activities, should be the method of choice.

FUTURE RESEARCH

We plan to conduct long-term research with keratoconus patients fitted with hydrophilic lenses to clarify:

1. Preservation of the health of the ocular tissues of the patient
2. Absence of complications

3. Effect of wearing hydrophilic contact lenses in advanced keratoconus, comparing it with:
   a. A group of patients wearing stable lenses
   b. A group of patients with keratoconus not wearing any lenses
   c. Some patients where the hydrophilic lens is used on only one eye and the other eye with no contact lens
   d. Some patients wearing a hydrophilic lens on one eye and a stable lens on the other

We will present a preliminary report as soon as feasible and progress reports periodically. We would like to invite other colleagues, especially those attached to research centers to start similar research programs on keratoconus patients. This way the results we obtain will be confirmed or modified by other reports in an effort to find best overall therapy for keratoconus.

Perhaps this work will help spark the enthusiasm necessary to conduct the greatly needed and long overdue investigations into the etiology of keratoconus and pave the way not only for the curative treatment of the condition, but most important, its preventive treatment. As the benefit and welfare of so many patients afflicted with keratoconus is at stake, we fervently hope that our plea will be answered by a vigorous aggressive research program now!

PART VI
Therapeutic uses

Chapter 22

Medical uses of soft contact lenses

Herbert E. Kaufman, M.D., Maija H. Uotila, R.N., Antonio R. Gasset, M.D., Thomas O. Wood, M.D., and Emily D. Varnell, B.S.

At present, there are a variety of soft contact lenses under investigation. Most of these lenses are different from each other, and it is essential to recognize these individual characteristics. Lenses vary in composition, tolerance, absorption and release of medication, and also differ in the availability of a variety of sizes (radii and circumferences). Although these differences are significant in cosmetic treatment, they are crucial in therapeutic use. Therefore, it is essential to consider each lens type separately. Although we have practical knowledge of other types, this report will consider primarily our experience with the Griffin soft lens.

BANDAGE LENSES

The use of a Griffin lens as a bandage for corneal disease has been described in the literature.[1]

Distinct advantages of the Griffin bandage lenses, in addition to the safety factor, include their use in the treatment of bullous keratopathy, drying syndromes, and corneal ulcers.

Safety factor. As bandages, the most remarkable and significant aspect of these lenses is their safety factor. For example, when placed on corneas with large bullae and edema, the bandage lenses do not break the bullae or cause ulceration. They can be worn on corneas with scars and gross irregularities without causing ulceration and are tolerated so well that many patients wear them 24 hours a day for a period of weeks or months without removal. The Griffin lenses differ from the flush-fitting lenses in that they are well tolerated, relatively easy to fit, and safe. If there is any change in the eye, or if the lens rotates, there is no danger of ulceration, whereas the movement of hard, flush-fitting lenses results in lens pressure on the cornea and possible damage.

Bullous keratopathy. Many investigators have found Griffin lenses valuable in the treatment of bullous keratopathy. By rendering the anterior surface of the cornea optically smooth, they eliminate much of the anterior irregular astigmatism. Unlike the epikeratoprosthesis, they do not provide an impermeable anterior membrane, which can promote stromal swelling as fluid leaks through the endo-

Presented in part at the Seventy-fifth Annual Meeting of the American Academy of Ophthalmology and Otolaryngology, Las Vegas, Nevada, October 5-9, 1970, and published in the March-April, 1971, issue of Transactions of the Academy.

thelium. On the contrary, the lenses enormously augment osmotically active agents, permitting not only the smoothing of the anterior surface but a much greater effect of osmotherapy on dehydration. Thus, visual improvement resulting from osmotherapy plus the use of the Griffin lens can be significant and, as with potentiation of other drugs, is different from that seen with other lenses. In almost all instances, such lenses relieve the pain of bullous keratopathy. The details of management of this problem are discussed elsewhere in the literature.[2]

Drying syndromes. In treating the terrible drying syndromes, exacting care is required.[3] In these patients, chronic blepharitis is the rule and lid hygiene is important. In several patients with dense corneal scarring caused by severe keratitis sicca, the bandage lenses have provided corneal protection after surgical intervention and have permitted us to perform lamellar or penetrating keratoplasties.

Corneal ulcers. Ulcers that will not heal and severe recurrent erosions are serious clinical problems. Much research has been done in the study of the production of collagenase by such chronic ulcers, and there is a possibility that this enzyme is involved in corneal and stromal melting. However, the efficacy of present collagenase inhibitors in man has not been clinically established. It is clear that this enzyme is produced by ulcerated rather than healed epithelium, and an alternate approach to the treatment of such ulcers is an attempt to heal the epithelium. Griffin lenses protect the epithelium from the lids and promote healing by holding it in place. The detailed management of erosions and ulcers will be considered elsewhere, but cycloplegia is of critical importance for comfort.

COMPLICATIONS

Patients with corneal disease clearly are more prone to develop complications. The use of antibiotics (without preservatives) such as chloramphenicol (Chloromycetin) can assist in the control of chronic conjunctivitis or blepharitis, but the importance of lid hygiene, expecially in the severe drying syndromes, cannot be overemphasized. Although a patient with bullous keratopathy and Stevens-Johnson syndrome may wear the lens constantly for weeks or months at a time, it is vital that every patient be taught the techniques of insertion and removal. If conjunctivitis does occur, this lens should be removed (as should any contact lens in the presence of infection) and every patient must know how to remove the lens if the eye becomes red or uncomfortable.

In this series, two patients with severe corneal ulcers developed some vascularization under the lens. Since it was not clear whether the lenses might be contributing to this vascularization, they were removed.

Infection has been a problem in only four patients. Two patients developed chronic bacterial conjunctivitis and despite a purulent discharge continued wearing the lens for a full week. They developed corneal ulcers, which, fortunately, responded to therapy, and there was no significant decrease in visual acuity. One patient had a lens inserted on an open ulcer. A technician had placed the lens in unsterile saline solution and had not cleaned or sterilized it. An infection resulted. Another patient with bullous keratopathy and keratitis sicca had a corneal infiltrate, which was noticed and considered inactive. The lens was inserted, but it was obvious by the next day that this infiltrate was active and *Candida* was isolated from the lesion. Apparently this infection was probably present before the lens was inserted.

Complications from soft lenses have been minimal, and the fact has become apparent that under normal circumstances neither bacteria, fungi, nor viruses penetrate into the Griffin lens, which has an extremely small pore size.

LENS USE WITH SUPPLEMENTARY DRUGS

As mentioned previously, one of the most remarkable properties of soft contact lenses is the ability to take up medication and release it to the eye, thus providing a tremendously potent drug effect over a long period of time. Since the prolonged delivery of relatively high concentrations of a preservative can damage the cornea, lenses should never be soaked in a solution that contains preservative. If eye drops that contain a preservative are used in conjunction with the lens, they will sometimes produce ocular irritation and punctate corneal staining. Although we have not seen any significant corneal damage in patients who have used customary eye drops, the employment of such medication should be avoided. On the other hand, the use of soft lenses as a therapeutic method for drug delivery is an exciting possibility.

The idea of using lenses or pledgets in the eye for the prolonged release of medications is not new. However, previous attempts to insert gelatin and other substances into the cul-de-sac have neither met with general success nor proved clinically useful.

Although Waltman and Kaufman[4] already described the precise effect of hydrophilic contact lenses on the entry of fluorescein into the eye, this substance might be bound by the lens and could behave differently from other drugs. Our present studies were carried out to evaluate the effect of the Griffin hydrophilic contact lens on the action of medication instilled into the eye. Experimental studies were done both in animals and humans.

Antiviral agents. Twenty-five New Zealand white rabbits were infected in both eyes with McKrae herpesvirus, and 3 days later Griffin lenses were placed in one eye of each animal. Both eyes were treated with 0.1% 5-iodo-2-deoxyuridine (IDU) staining with fluorescein; a blind study was conducted when the eyes were examined with the slit-lamp. Corneal ulcers were graded on a basis of 0 to 4, as follows: 0—no ulcer; 1—one fourth of cornea ulcerated; with progression to 4—total corneal involvement. The eyes treated with the lenses plus IDU drops improved significantly faster than those which received IDU drops alone.

Antibiotics. In order to test the effect of lenses on antibiotic therapy utilized in ulcers experimentally induced with *Pseudomonas,* 22 New Zealand white rabbits weighting 2 to 4 kg. were inoculated in both eyes with a 10^9 suspension of *Pseudomonas aeruginosa.* After 36 hours most of the corneas had large ulcers and were randomly divided into three groups. The first group served as controls and received no treatment. The second group received topical polymyxin B, 0.25%, four times a day. The third group was treated with hydrophilic contact lenses (which had been soaked in polymyxin B, 0.25%) and polymyxin B, 0.25% drops, four times a day.

After 17 days, the experimental *Pseudomonas* ulcers were divided into five categories, varying from small, 1 to 2 mm. ulcers (grade 1) to large ulcers that resulted in perforation and endophthalmitis (grade 5). The course of the ulcers was similar in both treated groups, with peak severity of symptoms being reached in the first 2 to 3 days. Vascularization of the corneas began at the end of the first week. Improvement of the ulcers was noted in the second week, and at 2½ weeks resolution of the process was obvious. The untreated control ulcers progressed after stabilization of the treated ulcers had occurred.

The final evaluation was made 1 month after the onset of the infection. The eyes treated with polymyxin B alone had results similar to those treated with polymyxin B and the Griffin contact lens. The lenses did not alter the course of the disease. All of the control eyes developed severe ulcers, resulting in loss of one third of the eyes. Vascularization of the cornea occurred in all three groups and correlated with the severity of the initial ulcer. Although the lenses showed no beneficial effect on the outcome of the infections, they had no deleterious effect on the corneas when kept in place for 2½ weeks during an active infection.

The results of this experiment suggest that in treating bacterial corneal ulcers the usual antibiotic concentration is sufficient, and once effective antibiotic levels are obtained, a higher concentration has no beneficial effect on the infection.

Phenylephrine in human studies. Ten human volunteers were fitted with a Griffin lens in one eye and the size of both pupils were measured, by use of a television monitor in a brightly lighted room. After initial measurements, two drops of 5% phenylephrine in saline solution, without a preservative, were instilled in both eyes. Hourly measurements were carried out for the first 8 hours, with additional measurements at the tenth and twelfth hours. Measurements were stopped in each subject when the pupillary size of both eyes had returned to normal (Fig. 22-1).

For evaluation of the possibility that any lens might have a similar effect, the same ten subjects in the Griffin lens experiment were used to evaluate the effect of phenylephrine in persons wearing a hard contact lens in one eye and a soft contact lens (Bausch & Lomb Soflens) in the other. The Bausch & Lomb lens is thinner, is composed of a different plastic, and has lower water permeability than the Griffin lens. After the initial measurement, two drops of 5% phenylephrine were instilled into both eyes and hourly measurements of pupil size were carried out as in the first phenylephrine experiment.

The results of phenylephrine instilled into the cul-de-sac of volunteers wearing Griffin soft lenses are shown in Fig. 22-1. The effect of phenylephrine is greatly augmented by the presence of the Griffin soft lens, both in terms of extent and duration. A hard methacrylate contact lens had no effect on the action of the phenylephrine, and the presence of another soft lens (Bausch & Lomb Soflens) only slightly augmented the phenylephrine effect, as revealed in Fig. 22-1.

Pilocarpine in human studies. Pilocarpine was tested in human volunteers by first using pupil size and then intraocular pressure as an indicator.

The first experiment was carried out to determine if pilocarpine would affect an eye wearing a lens differently from a control eye where no contact lens was worn. Five volunteers were fitted with Griffin soft lenses in one eye. The lenses were hydrated in a normal manner with saline and exposed to tears. Both pupils

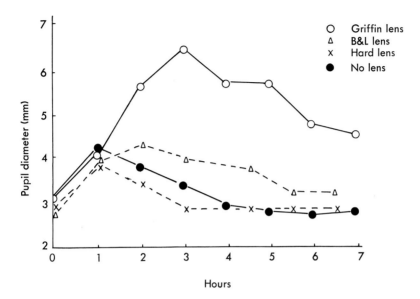

Fig. 22-1. Pupil diameters of volunteers with normal eyes shown after installation of two drops of 5% phenylephrine. (From Kaufman, H. E., Uotila, M. H., Gasset, A. R., Wood, T. O., and Ellison, E. D.: The medical uses of soft contact lenses, Trans. Amer. Acad. Ophthal. Otolaryng. **75:**361-373, 1971.)

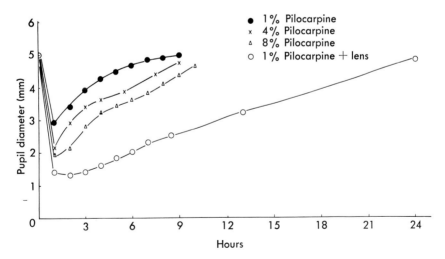

Fig. 22-2. Dose-response curves of pilocarpine in normal eyes as measured by pupil diameter. Addition of 1% pilocarpine to eyes wearing Griffin soft lenses produces miosis greater than that elicited by 8% pilocarpine and lasts approximately 24 hours instead of usual 5 to 6 hours. (From Kaufman, H. E., Uotila, M. H., Gasset, A. R., Wood, T. O., and Ellison, E. D.: The medical uses of soft contact lenses, Trans. Amer. Acad. Ophthal. Otolaryng. **75:**361-373, 1971.)

then were measured by the following method: The subjects were placed in a dark room, a television camera with an infrared light source was focused on the eye, and the size of the pupil was measured directly from a television monitor located in the next room; the unit of measure then was converted into millimeters by appropriate calculations.

After the initial measurement, two drops of 1% pilocarpine hydrochloride without preservative were instilled into both eyes, and the size of both pupils was measured. Subjects were examined to be certain there were no corneal epithelial defects. The dose-response curves of varying concentrations of pilocarpine hydrochloride and the effect of 1% pilocarpine hydrochloride used in conjunction with the lens were all measured on the same subjects, but eyes with the lenses were alternated (Fig. 22-2).

Patients with glaucoma then were studied. After removal of the lenses, intraocular pressures were measured both by Schiøtz and applanation tonometers. In several patients, the pressures were measured at the time of lens removal, and one-half hour, and 1 hour later to be certain that the manipulation of removing the lens did not transiently affect the pressure. No significant changes were seen.

Finally, dose-response measurements of intraocular pressure were made on glaucoma patients with and without soft contact lenses. An examination of dose-response relationships in the same subjects clearly indicates that two drops of 1% pilocarpine in an eye with a lens has a pupillary effect that is significantly greater

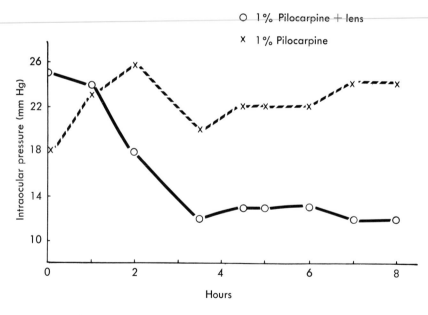

Fig. 22-3. Intraocular pressure measurements in patient with glaucoma. Use of 1% pilocarpine in one eye shows no effect on lowering pressure. In combination with soft lens in other eye, pressure is lowered to 12 mm. Hg. (From Kaufman, H. E., Uotila, M. H., Gasset, A. R., Wood, T. O., and Ellison, E. D.: The medical uses of soft contact lenses, Trans. Amer. Acad. Ophthal. Otolaryng. **75**:361-373, 1971.)

and more prolonged than the pupillary effect of 8% pilocarpine in an eye without a lens (Figs. 22-3 and 22-4).

Preliminary studies performed on patients with glaucoma indicate that the intraocular pressure effect of Griffin lenses on pilocarpine activity is equally great. Fig. 22-5 illustrates a patient with mild glaucoma. The pressure is brought to a lower level with the lens, and pilocarpine effect is detected for 20 hours after a single administration.

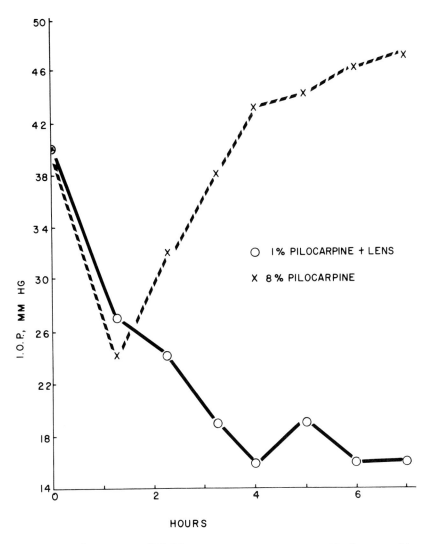

Fig. 22-4. Intraocular pressure **(I.O.P.)** measurements in patient with glaucoma. Use of 8% pilocarpine in eye wearing lens previous day does not lower pressure in same patient shown in Fig. 22-3, whereas 1% pilocarpine plus lens lowered pressure to 15 to 18 mm. Hg. (From Kaufman, H. E., Uotila, M. H., Gasset, A. R., Wood, T. O., and Ellison, E. D.: The medical uses of soft contact lenses, Trans. Amer. Acad. Ophthal. Otolaryng. **75:**361-373, 1971.)

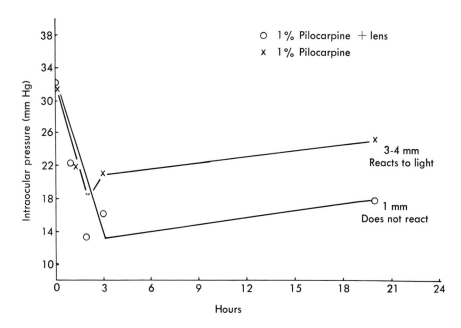

Fig. 22-5. Intraocular pressure brought to a lower level in patient with mild glaucoma with lens plus pilocarpine than the level in treatment with 1% pilocarpine alone. Drug is still effective for 20 hours. (From Kaufman, H. E., Uotila, M. H., Gasset, A. R., Wood, T. O., and Ellison, E. D.: The medical uses of soft contact lenses, Trans. Amer. Acad. Ophthal. Otolaryng. **75:**361-373, 1971.)

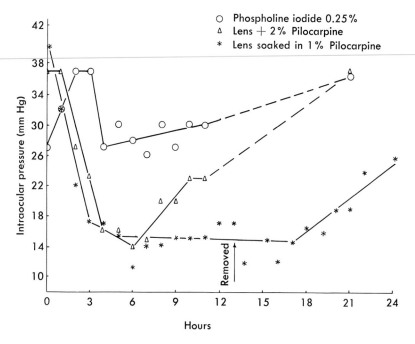

Fig. 22-6. In more severe case of glaucoma, 2% pilocarpine drops used with soft lens is more effective than 0.25% phospholine iodide. Soaking the lens in 1% pilocarpine produces an even greater effect. (From Kaufman, H. E., Uotila, M. H., Gasset, A. R., Wood, T. O., and Ellison, E. D.: The medical uses of soft contact lenses, Trans. Amer. Acad. Ophthal. Otolaryng. **75:**361-373, 1971.)

With more severe glaucoma, administration of 1% pilocarpine alone may have little effect, whereas with the soft contact lenses in place a significant and prolonged lowering of pressure is seen (Fig. 22-6). In this patient, 2% pilocarpine drops used with a lens are clearly more effective than echothiophate iodide (Phospholine Iodide); lenses soaked in pilocarpine are especially effective.

We have had several other patients with uncontrolled pressures (despite echothiophate iodide, pilocarpine, acetazolamide [Diamox], and epinephrine therapy) that were dramatically lowered to normal with use of the lenses. This finding is consistent with the work of Drance and Nash[5] that indicates that higher concentrations of pilocarpine can be more effective in treating glaucoma than those usually employed.

SUMMARY

It would be false to assume that Griffin lenses are a panacea for the treatment of glaucoma and other ocular diseases. Our present data indicate favorable results in erasing astigmatism and in potentiating osmotherapy in bullous keratopathy, the drying syndromes, corneal ulcers, and other corneal conditions requiring protection. However, our studies do not permit us to be certain what proportion of patients (such as patients with glaucoma who are resistant to conventional therapy) will be controlled with the help of these lenses. Nor can we be certain that when a tremendous pilocarpine effect is observed, some toxicity of this generally safe drug is not present. However, the mechanism of action of this drug is quite different from that of echothiophate iodide, and there is a clear possibility that some types of toxicity from the cholinesterase inhibitors could well be avoided by the use of this type of approach.

This study was supported in part by USPHS grants EY-00033, EY-00446, and EY-00007 from the National Eye Institute.

REFERENCES

1. Gasset, A. R.: Epikeratoprosthesis versus the Kaufman bandage lens. In Polack, F. M., editor: Corneal and external eye diseases, Springfield, Ill., 1970, Charles C Thomas, Publisher, pp. 213-225.
2. Gasset, A. R., and Kaufman, H. E.: Bandage lenses in the treatment of bullous keratopathy, Amer. J. Ophthal. **72:**376-380, 1971.
3. Gasset, A. R., and Kaufman, H. E.: Hydrophilic lens therapy of severe keratoconjunctivitis sicca and conjunctival scarring, Amer. J. Ophthal. **71:**1185-1189, 1971.
4. Waltman, S. R., and Kaufman, H. E.: Use of hydrophilic contact lenses to increase ocular penetration of topical drugs, Invest. Ophthal. **9:**250-255, 1970.
5. Drance, S. M., and Nash, P. A.: The dose response of human intraocular pressure to pilocarpine, Canad. J. Ophthal. (In press.)

Chapter 23

Scleral lenses and soft lenses

Keith A. Whitham

In reflecting on my experiences fitting scleral lenses over the last 10 years, there are many contrasts and comparisons to be evaluated. There are 1,980 patients and 2,434 eyes involved. All lenses or shells in this study were made from an impression of the eye. The majority of the cases were done with two doctors, John Espy, of Columbia Presbyterian Hospital, and Herbert Gould,[1-3] of Manhattan Eye, Ear and Throat Hospital.

The first cases were done at Massachusetts Eye and Ear Infirmary under the direction of Dr. William Stone, Jr., using equipment sent from Moorfields Eye Hospital in London; I was trained to make Ridley Lenses. Through the ensuing years, the principles laid down by Frederick Ridley,[4] proved to be valid and were followed closely. A great deal of credit also must go to Charles Trodd of Moorfields, who was the "golden hands" behind Mr. Ridley. When I left Massachusetts and went to New York, I left an excellent laboratory behind. Ingenuity brought about the attache-case flushfitting shell-manufacturing set-up, and at one time I was serving 12 hospitals with a flushfitting shell service.

In 1965 a generous grant sponsored a laboratory at Manhattan Eye, Ear and Throat Hospital. As the years rolled by, a great deal of knowledge was gained into the indications and contraindications in the fitting of scleral lenses.

With the advent of hydrophilic lenses, I embarked on the fascinating new modality. I started as a skeptic in 1966, working with Allan Isen, and soon became one of its most vocal exponents. In this paper I make a comparison between hard acrylic scleral lenses and the use of soft lenses in many of the same types of conditions.

METHODS AND MATERIALS

The eye is desensitized with a topical anesthetic. An impression is taken by using a molding tray, which is a perforated scleral lens with a hollow shaft. The tray is inserted under the lids. An alginate is injected through the shaft and into the space between the eye and tray. The patient is fixated as though looking down the shaft of the tray. A little over a minute is required for the alginate to set. The impression is removed, and a positive model of the eye is made by pouring dental stone into the impression. The stone is allowed to harden. All imperfections are removed from the model and a clear acrylic shell is pressed over the model.

If it is to be a therapeutic flushfitting shell, promptness is imperative. The shell should be inserted within as short a time as possible. As an example, in symblepharon surgery, it is possible to have the shell inserted in the recovery room before the patient is conscious.

The follow-up of a pathological case with a flushfitting shell is relatively simple but sometimes intensive. In many cases, because of the inherent dangers involved, a patient is admitted to the hospital where he can be medicated and observed more efficiently. It is the rule, rather than the exception, that a patient gets worse before getting better. There is a rejective symptom in most cases at first. The ulcer or staining area gets larger at first but after a day or two, it recedes. As the edema subsides, the shell usually loses its integrity. A tight lens can be handled by utilizing fenestrations, but a loose lens must be discarded and a new impression made. In one case, there was so much chemosis I made a total of nine shells before complete resolution.

During treatment of a patient's only eye, when one makes the final shell, the posterior surface can be lightly buffed or polished and a curve lathed and polished on the anterior surface. The patient is then overrefracted. A spectacle prescription can be provided or, if the prescription is spherical, the appropriate curve can be cut on the lens itself. As long as the posterior surface is clear, regardless of aberration, amazing results have been achieved. Dr. Gould and I have achieved these results time and time again. Dr. Whitney Sampson stated, "Therefore, if this interface is grossly irregular as it is in the flushfitting lens, the optical result on the eye is of necessity going to be very poor."[5] I also had the pleasure of working on a patient of Dr. Charles E. Iliff, who had the same phenomena. In this interstitial keratitis case, a lady had been wearing a flushfitting shell with a front curve for 6 years at the occasion of her visit to our office. We could get no reading through this lens on a lensometer, yet she had 20/30 vision. I attempted to get an equal result on her other eye, but because of a central leukoma, it was not achieved.

The pathological flushfitting shell is usually worn 24 hours from the outset. When the epithelial integrity has been established, the patient goes on to a daytime wear only. There are exceptions such as trichiasis and exposure, where there is no alternative.

The optical scleral lens starts out in the same manufacturing process. After the plastic has been pressed over the model, a base curve is fashioned, which should be slightly flatter than the cornea. In grossly irregular corneas, one needs to keep this curve with no more than 0.25 mm. clearance at its deepest point. If this clearance is greater, a persistent bubble will reside there, despite a fenestration. This bubble will usually interfere with the patient's vision, and sometimes a drying of the cornea will occur at this site. In these grossly irregular cases, except for the optical zone, the base curve must be sculped by hand. There is also a method called "foiling," in which an appropriate layering of plastic or lead is laid over the corneal portion of the model prior to pressing the acrylic over it.

Although I have seen many fluid or conventional scleral lenses, I have never fit one. I have, however, adjusted or copied these lenses, and in some cases, converted patients from fluid lenses to fenestrated sclerals or corneal lenses. Usually I would merely polish the fluid lenses and send the patients on their way.

Except in my early years, I fitted fenestrated lenses almost exclusively. It did not make my job easier, but I always wanted a patient to wear lenses all waking hours, without breaks. This was nearly unheard of in fluid or channeled lenses.

Scleral lenses do accomplish many results that cannot be accomplished any other way. I still fit a few, as few as possible. Compared to corneal or soft lenses, there is no way to charge the patient what your time is worth. The labor involved is at least 10 times as much as a corneal or soft lens. If I thought I could get 10 times as much money, I would be glad to go at it full time and so would most other technicians.

Table 23-1. Optical considerations of scleral lenses

Condition	Patients	Lenses
Keratoconus	283	510
After keratoplasty	108	117
Aphakia	40	68
High myopia	21	39
High astigmatism	21	33
Low correction (sport lenses)	16	32
Decentered pupil	11	11
Albinism	8	16
Lid crutch lenses	4	4
High minus telescope	3	3
Painted with clear pupil	21	21
Painted shells to mask disfigurement	262	262
	798	1116

Table 23-2. Therapeutic considerations of flushfitting shells

Condition	Patients	Lenses
Bullous keratopathy	312	328
Surgical splints	208	217
Neuroparalytic keratitis	203	207
Exposure keratitis	175	176
Ulcerations	86	96
Dystrophies	60	62
Trichiasis or lid scarring	37	51
Stevens-Johnson syndrome	27	55
Other sicca conditions	20	40
Pemphigus	16	32
Chemical keratitis	10	17
Herpes	8	8
Radiation keratitis	8	8
Interstitial keratitis	6	10
Mustard gas keratitis	3	6
Acne rosacea keratitis	1	2
Lupus vulgaris	1	2
Leprosy	1	1
	1182	1318

The last category belongs to the cosmetic cover shell. Using a faithful reproduction of the flushfitting shell in white plastic and painting it, gives the most satisfactory result in a disfigured globe or eviscerations. Patients wear them 24 hours a day with no excessive mucus. The motility is outstanding. This is an established efficient use for the flushfitting shell, which, for the near future, will remain the treatment of choice. Tables 23-1 and 23-2 summarize my experience with scleral lenses.

COMPARISON OF GRIFFIN LENSES WITH MOLDED SCLERAL LENSES

Availability. With the approval of the Griffin Naturalens, a great void will be filled. Most of the varied forms of treatment afforded by scleral lenses would then be available in every community.

Ease of fitting. Griffin soft lenses require less skill or time when they are compared to scleral lenses. Certainly, there are many steps to learn in this new mode of therapy, but it is much simpler.

Effectiveness. In bandage lens therapy, it is certainly better, because of the lack of trauma, to use soft lenses. Reports indicate that the cornea starts to heal immediately without the rejective symptoms spoken of earlier.[6,7] In use as an optical lens, the Griffin lens is much easier to fit and has no discomfort from the start.

Table 23-3. Comparison of scleral lens with Griffin lens

Condition	Visual acuity	Comfort	Wearing time	Photophobia	Flare	Mucus	Injection	Infection	Ease of fitting	Availability	Scarring	Healing	Vascularization
Keratoconus	s	G	G	G	G	G	G	G	G	G	G	-	-
Aphakia	X	G	G	G	G	G	G	G	G	G	G	-	-
Hi minus	G	G	G	G	G	G	G	G	G	G	G	-	-
Hi astigmatism	s	G	G	G	G	G	G	G	X	G	G	-	-
After keratoplasty	s	G	G	G	G	G	G	G	G	G	G	-	G
Cosmetic (low prescription)	X	G	G	G	G	G	G	G	G	G	G	-	-
Bullous keratopathy	G	G	G	G	G	G	G	G	G	G	G	G	-
Dystrophies	X	G	G	G	G	G	G	G	G	G	G	G	G
Neuroparalytic keratitis	X	-	G	G	G	G	G	G	G	G	G	G	G
Exposure keratitis	X	G	X	G	G	G	G	G	G	G	-	G	G
Stevens-Johnson syndrome	G	G	X	G	G	G	G	G	G	G	-	G	G
Pemphigus	s	G	X	G	G	G	G	G	G	G	-	G	G
Sicca conditions	s	G	G	G	G	G	G	G	G	G	-	G	G
Trichiasis and lid scarring	X	X	X	G	G	G	G	G	G	G	-	X	-
Indolent ulcers	G	G	G	G	G	G	G	G	G	G	-	G	-
Chemical keratitis	G	G	G	G	G	G	G	G	G	G	G	G	G

s, Scleral lens superior. G, Griffin lens superior. X, No discernible difference. –, Not pertinent.

In higher astigmatism, until toric soft lenses are available, sclerals are superior optically.

Safety. After these years of accepting all the insult that a patient suffers with scleral lenses, I must say, this is the greatest motivating reason to switch to Griffin lenses. Bearing in mind that many of the eyes we managed had no alternative treatment, we went through an impressive list of complications: corneal scarring, severe photophobia, severe edema, abrasions, ulcerations, uveitis, and sometimes conditions that resulted in enucleation. Most of these complications were grudgingly accepted as part of the system. There is one very important complication that was not mentioned. Vascularization, by continuous wear of a flushfitting shell, is almost inevitable. In some conditions it was welcomed as a nutritional aid to a flagging cornea. In most cases, it was viewed with disdain because of the possibility of complicating future keratoplasty. Table 23-3 outlines the differences between the scleral lens and Griffin soft lens.

SUMMARY

Although for the near future there are some indications for acrylic lenses, soft lenses seem to be superior in most categories.

One must remember that soft lenses form a new technology. Despite this newness, they are already superior in many ways. As we gain experience, more uses will be found. Hard acrylic lenses have been in use for over 30 years and have shown a history of constant improvement. We are near or have reached a plateau where improvement of any degree is improbable. Soft lenses do not have this luxury of time. The Griffin Lens is a good lens and it does do the job. There has been a very rapid upgrading of quality over the last 3 to 4 years. It is already in a position to challenge all hard lenses. It is time to recognize that soft lenses, which have been through the discipline required for FDA approval, are safe. They have been scrutinized far more, in every aspect, than hard lenses ever were.

The future is bright for soft lenses. They will bolster the ophthalmic practitioner's ability to treat visual and pathological problems to a degree never before possible.

REFERENCES

1. Gould, H. L.: The therapeutic role of scleral contact lenses. Presented at the Contact Lens Symposium, Ohio State University, September 24-26, 1964.
2. Gould, H. L.: Molded flushfitting acrylic shells in ocular surgery. In Smith, B., and Converse, J. M., editors: Proceedings of the Second International Symposium on Plastic and Reconstructive Surgery of the Eye and Adnexa, St. Louis, 1967, The C. V. Mosby Co., pp. 412-431.
3. Gould, H. L.: Corneal and scleral contact lenses. In Girard, L., editor: Proceedings of the International Congress, St. Louis, 1967, The C. V. Mosby Co.
4. Ridley, F.: Scleral contact lenses, Arch. Ophthal. **70:**740-745, 1963.
5. Sampson, W. G.: Role of scleral lenses in ocular therapy, current status and new developments. In Smith, B., and Converse, J. M., editors: Proceedings of the Second International Symposium on Plastic and Reconstructive Surgery of the Eye and Adnexa, St. Louis, 1967, The C. V. Mosby Co.

6. Gasset, A. R., and Kaufman, H. E.: Bandage lenses in the treatment of bullous keratopathy, Amer. J. Ophthal. **72:**376-380, 1971.

7. Kaufman, H. E., Uotila, M. H., Gasset, A. R., Wood, T. O., and Ellison, E. D.: The medical uses of soft contact lenses, Trans. Amer. Acad. Ophthal. Otolaryng. **75:**361-373, 1971.

8. Waltman, S. R., and Kaufman, H. E.: Use of hydrophilic contact lenses to increase ocular penetration of topical drugs, Amer. J. Ophthal. **9:**250-255, 1970.

Chapter 24

Bionite hydrophilic bandage lenses in treatment of corneal disease

James V. Aquavella, M.D.

The use of a Griffin Bionite lens as a bandage in cases of corneal disease has been described by Kaufman and others[1] and Gasset.[2] Additionally Leibowitz[3] and Buxton[4] have related their experience in the use of another hydrophilic material (Bausch & Lomb Soflens) in the treatment of certain corneal conditions. Aquavella, Jackson, and Guy[5] have attempted to elucidate some of the factors involved in bandage lens therapy. The detailed management of corneal disease with the Griffin Bionite hydrophilic bandage lens is presented here.

MATERIALS AND METHODS

All lenses employed in this series were composed of the Bionite hydrophilic polymer and supplied by Griffin Laboratories (Buffalo, New York). Before insertion, each lens was sterilized with hydrogen peroxide, neutralized with sodium bicarbonate, and flushed in normal saline solution.[1] Lenses were inserted directly over the underlying corneal ulceration (Fig. 24-1). All patients in the series wore the lenses on a 24-hour-a-day schedule, and the lenses were not removed until the termination of therapy unless refitting was indicated.

CASE SELECTION

Table 24-1 illustrates the wide variety of disease entities represented in this series of 205 eyes. Basic refractive problems such as keratoconus, aphakia, leukoma, and healed corneal grafts have been excluded.

The mechanical category includes erosions secondary to lid surgery, lid pathology, and those cases directly resulting from trauma such as lacerations with or without loss of substance. Recurrent erosions have also been placed in this group, since the original insult was usually traumatic.

Alkaline burns of the cornea are included with other cases of chemical injury. The great majority of viral disease was recurrent herpes simplex keratitis.

PRINCIPLES OF LENS SELECTION

Bionite bandage lenses are available in a wide variety of diameters ranging from 12.0 to 15.5 mm., in increments of 0.5 mm. The lenses may also be ordered

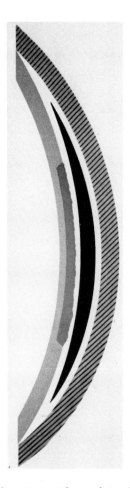

Fig. 24-1. Diagram of corneal ulceration with overlying bandage lens in place. Note relatively large interface area.

in differing curvatures, ranging from 7.5 through 8.7 mm. in increments of 0.3 mm. The general range of thicknesses found in these bandage lenses varies from 0.20 to 0.75 mm., and of course a wide variety of refractive power is obtainable.

In the selection of a specific lens one of the important factors to consider is the stability of the lens on the cornea. A lens that exhibits excessive motility may irritate the underlying corneal lesion, appear "loose," and will not tend to afford a significant degree of pain relief. The criteria for a flat fit are as follows:

1. No central air bubble
2. Stable light reflex
3. Stable acuity with blinking
4. Lens lag with blink and ocular rotation
5. Generally inadequate pain relief
6. Overrefraction consistent with the patient's spectacle manifest refraction

Table 24-1. Etiology of the disease processes treated with the Bionite bandage lens

Disease entity	Number of cases
Viral	32
Postoperative keratoplasty	26
Mechanical	20
Fuch's dystrophy	18
Bullous keratopathy	17
Dry eye syndromes	15
Glaucoma	15
Degenerative	11
Exposure	11
Filamentary keratitis	11
Dystrophies	7
Bacterial	5
Chemical	5
Trophic	4
Epikeratoprosthesis failures	3
Nutritional	3
Fungal	2
Total	205

7. Relatively narrow lens

8. Relatively greater radius of curvature

In general, lenses of wider diameters and steeper curvatures tend to demonstrate a high degree of stability. To properly access this factor, one should allow the lens to "settle" for periods of several minutes. In patients with significant amounts of lacrimation even a wide and steep lens will seem to have excessive motion initially. Often after a delay of 15 or 20 minutes, reexamination reveals that the lens has indeed stabilized and appears "tight." There is very little motion with blinking or ocular rotation.

A second important consideration in lens selection is curvature. Although the cosmetic lenses are usually flat (Aquavella, Jackson, and Guy[6]) in dealing with corneal ulcerations, it is preferable to select lenses of a steeper configuration to obtain a rather large interface area (Fig. 24-1). With the expanded interface area, there is less chance of traumatizing the underlying corneal ulceration with movements of the upper lid. Additionally, a steep curvature is also a factor in achieving lens stability.

In Fuchs' dystrophy and bullous keratopathy it is usually advisable to select a flat lens. In theory the reduced interface will assist in corneal deturgescence.

In general, it is preferable to employ a rather thin lens (0.20 to 0.33 mm.). Although the Bionite polymer has a high degree of fluid and gas permeability, these thinner lenses will demonstrate increased permeability characteristics.

Some routinely employed lens parameters are listed in Table 24-2.

The average bandage lens employed has a plano power, although certain

Table 24-2. Recommended average bandage lenses

	Radius of curvature	Diameter
Flat	8.4	14.0
	8.4	14.5
	8.1	14.0
Steep	7.8	14.5
	7.8	15.0
	7.5	14.0

cases may require a high degree of plus or minus power depending on the refractive status of the eye.

PRINCIPLES OF THERAPEUTIC EFFICACY

The following are main factors involved in therapeutic efficacy:

Protection	Fluid and gas permeability
Splinting	Delivery of medication
Pain relief	Vision

The protection afforded by these lenses is certainly a very important factor. In cases of extensive or deep ulceration a splinting effect is achieved that prevents the wrinkling of the lesion by the upper lid.

Pain relief has been mentioned by various authors and is indeed another significant factor associated with the mode of therapy. The Bionite polymer has been shown to possess a high degree of fluid permeability evidenced by the fact that in its fully hydrated state almost 60% of the lens weight is represented by water. Recent studies at the University of Florida have confirmed a significant amount of oxygen permeability.[7]

Another basic characteristic of this therapeutic modality is the ability of the lens to assist in the delivery of medication to the underlying diseased cornea.[1] The delivery of medication may be further enhanced by the lens pump situation created by the steepness of fit. Thus, the pressure of the upper lid tends to collapse the interface area with the expulsion of tearfilm and medication into the conjunctival fornix (Fig. 24-2). The release of the upper lid results in an active reformation (Fig. 24-3) of the interface. Clinical experience suggests a transfer of medication from the lens surface to the fluid interface and then to the corneal epithelium.

A final consideration should not be overlooked, and that is the ability of this therapeutic system to enable the patient to see while the bandage is in place. This is, of course, more important in monocular cases or even in aphakic cases. A bandage lens may be selected with specific power conforming to refractive status.

TECHNIQUE

In considering the specific technique of initiating this mode of therapy, several steps may be mentioned. It is important to realize that a great number of patients with corneal ulcerations have a significant degree of ciliary spasm, which should be relieved by the administration of a cycloplegic drug. I prefer to instill cyclo-

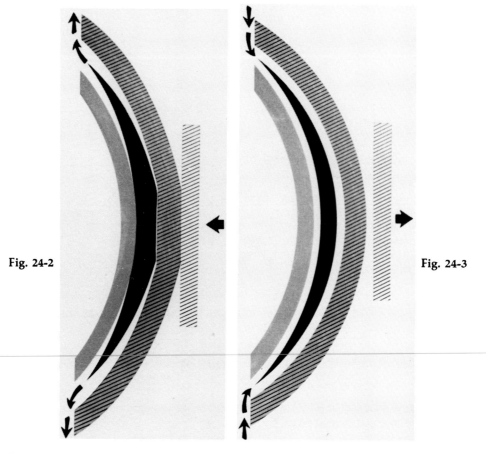

Fig. 24-2. Diagram showing pressure of upper lid being transmitted to bandage lens with collapse of interface area.

Fig. 24-3. Diagram showing reformation of interface area after removal of upper lid pressure.

pentolate hydrochloride (Cyclogyl) prior to insertion of the lens and then to reinforce the cycloplegia with instillation of Cyclogyl twice daily. Because of the generally prolonged action of medications in the presence of a bandage lens, we have preferred not to use atropine or homatropine to routinely initiate or maintain cycloplegia.

There are several methods of actually inserting the lens between the lids. Proficiency is readily developed although one occasionally has to resort to the use of a speculum. Significantly we prefer not to instill a drop of topical anesthetic prior to lens insertion. One can better access the degree of pain relief in the absence of a topical anesthetic. On the other hand, in dealing with infants and very young children, instilling one drop of proparacaine prior to lens insertion may be expedient.

In determining the proper fit, we usually advise employing a lens of relatively wide diameter and relatively steep curvature. When such a lens is inserted, an air bubble will be visible in the lens-cornea interface area and will tend to persist for a period of several minutes. In addition, by 15 or 20 minutes after insertion the lens demonstrating a proper fit should have stabilized.

If a flat fit is desired, there should be no air bubble after insertion and a fair amount of motion with blink and rotation even after a period of several minutes.

The criteria for the determination of a flat fit are summarized on p. 191. Such criteria for a steep fit are as follows:

1. Persistence of a central air bubble
2. Distortion of the light reflex with blinking
3. Variable acuity with blinking
4. Relatively little motion with the blink or ocular rotation
5. Good pain relief
6. Additional minus correction required on overrefraction
7. Wide diameter lens
8. Relatively small radius of curvature

The next consideration concerns the use of topical medication to be instilled over the lens. In cases where the bandage lens has been inserted primarily to perform a protective function, it has been found useful to instill one-half normal saline drops 3 or 4 times daily. This is particularly important over the first 48 to 72 hours of bandage lens therapy. When the underlying pathology is that of a basically dry eye, the same regimen has proved of value. The rationale for the use of one-half normal saline solution is related to the relationship of the concentration of the saline solution to maintaining the proper parameters of the Bionite hydrophilic bandage lens. Although these lenses are stored in an isotonic environment, instillation of normal saline drops over the lens surface may result in producing a relatively hypertonic environment with evaporation of a certain portion of the fluid content.

The use of other specific medications depends on the basic etiology of the underlying disease. Thus the cases of herpes simplex were treated with combinations of IDU and steroids, whereas bacterial infections were treated with the specific antibiotic of choice.

PATIENT FOLLOW-UP

The first 48 hours of bandage lens therapy are extremely important in determining if a proper lens has been utilized and if, in fact, the therapy is proceeding satisfactorily. Therefore, I recommend that the patient be checked at the end of 24 hours and again at the end of 48 hours. Some mild discomfort can be tolerated during these first 2 days, but in general the patient should be comfortable. Other factors to be ascertained at these early follow-up visits are the continuing degree of cycloplegia, the appearance of the lens as far as fit relationships are concerned and the dosage of medications. Here we refer to the fact that topical medications instilled over a bandage lens will often have a greater and more prolonged effect. When dealing with a grossly debilitated and diseased cornea, it is extremely important to recall the necessity for instillation of a prophylactic antibiotic. A

Table 24-3. Effectiveness of bandage lens therapy

Patients	Number	Percentage
Total	205	100
Could not tolerate therapy	5	2.5
Tolerated therapy but demonstrated no improvement	10	5
Did not return for follow-up and developed infection	1	0.5
Improved with bandage lens therapy	189	92

related factor is to avoid the unnecessary removal of the lens by either patient or physician to reduce the possibility of contamination.

RESULTS

Out of a total of 205 cases there were only five complete failures (patients who could not be made comfortable with bandage lens therapy). In 10 other cases, the patients were comfortable, but there was no discernible improvement in the condition of the underlying cornea. Several of them, however, did have better acuity with the lens in place than could be obtained by spectacle correction. One patient with absolute glaucoma demonstrated a reduction in pressure by using pilocarpine over the lens and then did not return for follow-up for several months. During the absence she had lived alone, although totally blind, and had instilled neither pilocarpine nor prophylactic antibiotic. She developed an inflammation that had bothered her for several weeks. When she reappeared for examination, a deep bacterial ulceration (Staphylococcus), which threatened perforation, was present in the central cornea. The ulceration cleared with appropriate antibiotic therapy.

These results are summarized in Table 24-3.

DISCUSSION

In analyzing the results of this series we must recall that the bandage lens constituted only a portion of the total therapeutic regimen and that the majority of patients received concomitant therapy in the form of topical instillation of various medications.

In the glaucoma cases, all 15 patients obtained a greater reduction in intraocular pressure with bandage lens plus topical medication than with the same topical regimen alone.

In 18 cases of Fuchs' dystrophy one patient could not tolerate the bandage lens and five others demonstrated no improvement in visual acuity. The degree of visual improvement in the remaining cases ranged from dramatic to slight. Almost all of these cases received instillations of hypertonic saline solution over the Bionite bandage lens. A few of the cases were able to decrease the frequency of instillation, and two were able to eliminate the drops altogether.

All the cases of bullous keratopathy demonstrated relief of pain with the bandage lens therapy. Occasionally, one of the bullae would rupture under the lens and cause a recurrence of discomfort. In almost all cases vision improved.

Many of these patients were refitted several times with increasingly flat lenses in an attempt to improve visual acuity. A lens that is too flat can cause the rupture of epithelial bullae so that this process must be accomplished slowly and carefully.

There were two failures in 11 cases of filamentary keratitis. Both of them occurred during the early phase of the investigation and were accompanied by excess rather than decreased tear formation. The lenses were never able to stabilize and the patient could not tolerate the therapy.

Many of the degenerative corneal ulcerations seemed to respond nicely to the bandage lens alone, with an occasional drop of prophylactic antibiotic being the only ancillary medication.

In postoperative keratoplasty edema of the graft was controlled by instillation of topical steroids and hypertonic saline over the bandage lens. Several patients without edema but with moderate discomfort from the sutures, responded rapidly to the insertion of a bandage lens.

The exposure cases were among the most difficult to treat, since a very wide and steep lens is required with frequent instillations of one-half normal saline to maintain the hydration of the lens as well as the underlying cornea. Once proper fitting was accomplished, an equilibrium seemed to become established whereby the instillations of fluid could be reduced after the first few weeks. This phenemona was evident in the dry eye syndromes as well. Many of these eyes required surgical lysis of symblepharon prior to lens insertion. In some cases superficial keratectomy followed by lens therapy resulted in greatly increased acuity.

In dealing with alkaline burns it is recommended that the bandage lenses be replaced every 24 hours for the first few days to guard against the possibility of incorporation of alkali in the lens. All of these cases were treated with antibiotics and anticollagenase drugs were administered frequently.

Some of the most dramatic results were obtained in recurrent herpes simplex keratitis. The patients were maintained on bandage lens therapy with instillation of IDU and topical steroids. Progress of the lesion could be easily followed and the drops regulated according to the healing.

SUMMARY

The introduction of Bionite bandage lens therapy in the treatment of corneal disease has been a very significant addition to the therapeutic armamentarium of the ophthalmologist.

The details of this type of therapy are presented, as well as the results of 205 cases representing a wide variety of disease entities. In the final analysis the success or failure of this type of therapy will depend on application of the knowledge of the mechanics involved.

REFERENCES

1. Kaufman, H. E., Uotila, M. H., Gasset, A. R., Wood, T. O., and Ellison, E. D.: The medical uses of soft contact lenses, Trans. Amer. Acad. Ophthal. Otolaryng. 75:361-373, 1971.
2. Gasset, A. R., and Kaufman, H. E.: Therapeutic uses of hydrophilic contact lenses, Amer. J. Ophthal. 69:252-259, 1970.

3. Leibowitz, H. M., and Rosenthal, P.: Hydrophilic contact lenses in corneal disease, Arch. Ophthal. **85**:283, 1971.

4. Buxton, J. N., and Locke, C. R.: A therapeutic evaluation of hydrophilic contact lenses, Amer. J. Ophthal. **72**:532-535, 1971.

5. Aquavella, J. V., Jackson, G. K., and Guy, L. F.: Therapeutic effects of Bionite lenses: mechanism of action, Ann. Ophthal. **3**:1341-1350, 1971.

6. Aquavella, J. V., Jackson, G. K., and Guy, L. F.: Bionite hydrophilic contact lenses used as cosmetic devices, Amer. J. Ophthal. **72**:527-531, 1971.

7. Morrison, D. R., and Edelhauser, H. F.: Permeability of hydrophilic contact lenses, Invest. Ophthal. **11**(1):58-63, 1972.

Chapter 25

Therapeutic uses of hydrophilic contact lenses

Howard M. Leibowitz, M.D.

The hydrophilic or soft contact lens was primarily developed as an optical device for the correction of refractive errors. However, soft contact lenses are not limited to this role. Of equal importance and perhaps even more gratifying to the ophthalmologist is their usefulness as an adjunct in the therapy of various corneal disorders. The observation that soft contact lenses are extremely well tolerated over prolonged periods by many patients with a diseased cornea was of great significance and led to the investigation of their therapeutic potential.

My own experience is limited entirely to the Bausch & Lomb Soflens. In all of the studies that I discuss here the lens was fitted without keratometry and without particular regard to corneal curvature; the soft pliable hydrophilic material molded satisfactorily to the cornea being treated. All lenses were sterilized prior to fitting by boiling in isotonic saline for 15 minutes.

SUPERFICIAL, STERILE, INDOLENT ULCERS

A group of patients having superficial noninfected indolent corneal ulcers that failed to respond to conventional therapeutic modalities were fitted with a hydrophilic contact lens. In most instances, the ulcer was superficial, involving the epithelium, Bowman's membrane, and the anterior stromal lamellae. If, at the time a patient was referred to us, a diagnosis had not been established, then every attempt was made to do so with the aid of smears, scrapings, cultures, and so on. If active infection was suspected, specific therapy was instituted after bacterial and viral cultures were taken. After a course of chemotherapy, attempts were made to promote reepithelialization of the ulcer by the use of a pressure dressing. Because of the uncertainty of the conventional pressure dressing, which uses tape alone, the patch was affixed with tape in the usual manner and then reinforced with a gauze head roll bandage. The pressure dressing was used for a minimum of 72 hours. The eye was examined, and the pressure dressing was replaced every 24 to 48 hours. Only if we were unsuccessful in promoting healing of the ulcer by this approach, was the soft contact lens used. Then, under topical administration of proparacaine hydrochloride anesthesia, the epithelium of the involved eye was removed, generally in toto, by use of a no. 15 scalpel blade. The corneal surface was copiously irrigated with sterile isotonic saline and the hydrophilic contact lens was put in place. A wire speculum facilitated the maneuvers. Ocular pain after epithelial debridement was variable, but usually it was limited to the first 24 hours and was satisfactorily controlled with orally administered codeine.

The soft contact lens was left in place for approximately 1 week. The patient was followed frequently during that week, and with the aid of the slit lamp bio-microscope, the progress of epithelial regeneration often could be seen beneath the contact lens. The epithelium grew in centrally from the limbal area, and re-generation was usually complete within 5 days. Topical chloramphenicol and, where indicated, atropine drops were used. In our initial studies, both of these preparations were compounded without preservatives. We have published the results of our first 18 cases. In this initial group, herpes simplex keratitis was by far the leading cause of the ulcers. These were all chronic cases with stromal involvement and scarring in which the overlying epithelium refused to heal. All of these cases had had previous prolonged courses of IDU. All had negative virus cultures at the time the lens was inserted. Several were unsuccessfully treated with EDTA drops prior to contact lens trial. Additional etiologies encountered in our initial 18 cases included two cases of peripheral keratitis associated with severe reheumatoid arthritis, two cases of peripheral corneal degeneration (Ter-rien's or furrow dystrophy), one case of neuroparalytic keratitis after neurosurgical removal of an acoustic neuroma, two cases after scleral buckling surgery with re-moval of the epithelium at the time of surgery, and three cases of superficial ulcers in which all diagnostic test results were normal and a definitive diagnosis could not be established. Many of these cases were unsuccessfully treated with EDTA drops and subconjunctival heparin injections prior to the use of the hydrophilic contact lens.

Our therapeutic regimen was successful in all 18 cases. By successful, we mean that the superficial ulcer was completely healed, epithelial regeneration was com-plete, and comfort was restored. In a few cases, vision was improved, but this was a result of the restoration of a smooth, continuous epithelial surface and a decrease in density of some of the underlying stromal changes; thus the improvement in vision was only indirectly attributable to the soft contact lens. We have continued to fit the hydrophilic contact lens for the indications described and by the regimen outlined, and our present experience exceeds 75 cases. In our hands, the hydro-philic contact lens has continued to be an extremely useful adjunct in promoting the healing of indolent corneal ulcers. Our success rate in such cases has been more than 90%. The result is usually quite dramatic and the rate of recurrence quite low. The lens is amazingly well tolerated, despite the presence of corneal disease, and no significant complications have been encountered thus far in our patients. Only a short course of wearing the lens is generally necessary to obtain the desired therapeutic effect, although in a small percentage of cases the lens must be worn for a longer period of time.

With regard to the etiological factors most commonly identified in cases of indolent corneal ulcers treated by us, one group of cases has to be separated from the others in terms of response to treatment by the soft contact lens. The one exception is the group of superficial corneal ulcers, or chronic epithelial defects if you will, that follow scleral buckling surgery for retinal detachment. Subsequent experience with this group of patients has led us to conclude that the soft contact lens does not appear to hasten epithelial regeneration in the majority of such cases. The failure to heal is related to ischemia of the peripheral cornea caused by the surgical trauma itself and may represent a *forme fruste* of anterior segment necrosis. The soft contact lens, nonetheless, has proved to be extremely helpful in these cases by protecting the ulcerated cornea from the repeated trauma of blinking lids and other noxious environmental stimuli. All of these cases ultimately underwent reepithelialization, which generally is accompanied by neovascularization of the peripheral cornea. In the interim, a soft contact lens prevents serious involvement of the corneal stroma by inflammatory processes and subsequent permanent scarring.

The mechanism by which the soft contact lens produces its therapeutic effect in superficial corneal ulcers is not definitely known. Apparently, the lens acts as a very efficient protective bandage, shielding the ulcer from the repetitive irritating influences of the eyelids during blinking and from other noxious environmental stimuli. In addition, it is our feeling that the hydrophilic contact lens provides a structural framework under which the regenerating epithelium may grow.

A word of clarification, or perhaps caution, is in order at this point. In regard to the Bausch & Lomb Soflens, this product has been developed primarily as an optical device for the correction of refractive errors and has led to a series of changes in the course of development that has resulted in a smaller and thinner lens. These changes have indeed improved the optical characteristics of the lens and have resulted in a lens that moves about somewhat easier and is less likely to produce corneal edema with prolonged wear. These are desirable properties when the lens is used for correction of refractive errors, but has decreased the effectiveness of the lens in promoting the healing of indolent corneal ulcers. The results reported here were all obtained with older models of the Bausch & Lomb Soflens, which were thicker, larger, and more immobile. We have found the newer product though optically much more satisfactory, less effective in the treatment of indolent corneal ulcers. This point is emphasized to avoid misunderstanding should one attempt to treat indolent ulcers with the new lenses now being released by Bausch & Lomb and find the results somewhat less satisfactory. One can indeed obtain a good degree of success with the commercially available Bausch & Lomb minus lenses, but I doubt that the results reported here can be completely duplicated. It is hoped that, at a later date, a second product, perhaps less desirable from an optical standpoint, but more effective in the treatment of corneal ulcers, will be approved for release by the Food and Drug Administration, specifically for the treatment of indolent corneal ulcers.

This probably would also be a good time to discuss the use of drugs with the hydrophilic contact lenses. Most publications on the subject of soft contact lenses, including my own, state that standard collyria should not be used with the hydrophilic contact lenses. Evidence has been presented that these drugs are concentrated in the lens and that preservatives used in most commercially available collyria may be concentrated along with the drugs. When concentrated, these preservatives are toxic to and may damage the corneal epithelium, thus producing an effect directly opposite to that sought. I think it is safe to say that this concept remains true in theory. Many preservatives used in the preparation of commercial ophthalmic collyria, when concentrated, are epithelial poisons and could injure the corneal epithelium. In fact, however, this is an area about which we know very little and, to date, probably have less clinical experience. Because of the nature of the corneal diseases we have been treating, we needed to make use of standard collyria concomitantly with the hydrophilic contact lens in a large number of cases. The medications that we have been using include antibiotics, mydriatics, potent corticosteroids, and even IDU. We have used these medications in a large number of cases two or three times daily without ill effect. It is our clinical judgment that the instillation of these standard collyria only two or three times daily allows sufficient time between instillations for tears to dilute the medication and produce washout of the medication from the lens. We doubt that any significant concentration of the medication or its preservative in the lens occurs with a 2-or-3-times daily regimen of administration. We have used standard collyria at more frequent intervals, but I think, at this time, our experience has not been sufficient to make a recommendation regarding their more frequent use while a soft contact lens is in place.

BULLOUS KERATOPATHY

Hydrophilic contact lenses have been found to be extremely useful in the therapy of bullous keratopathy. As you know, this disorder may produce severe pain accompanied by lacrimation, photophobia, and conjunctival injection. These symptoms are generally attributed to rupture of the bullae resulting in exposure of the endings of the corneal nerves, or to acute swelling of the epithelium causing stretching of these nerve endings. A series of patients, suffering from chronic advanced bullous keratopathy causing severe discomfort and ocular inflammation, were fitted with a hydrophilic contact lens. In our first series of patients with this disorder, the prime goal of therapy was alleviation of the patient's pain. All of these patients had previously been treated with topical applications of hypertonic agents, and in all instances, medications had been unsuccessful in alleviating pain. As in the therapy of corneal ulcers, the soft contact lens was fitted without keratometry and without particular regard to corneal curvature. The soft pliable material molded satisfactorily to the cornea being treated. The lens was seated directly upon the corneal epithelium, regardless of the severity or appearance of the pathological condition; no attempt was made to alter or to remove the epithelium. Sterilization of the lens was accomplished prior to fitting by boiling the lens in isotonic saline for 15 minutes. Subsequent to fitting, the hydrophilic contact lens was left in place 24 hours a day; in no instance was it removed by the patient. Initially, half of our patients were treated prophylactically with chloramphenicol drops, 0.5%, administered twice daily; the remaining half received no prophylactic antibiotic therapy. No difference was noted between the two groups. Our current regimen calls for the administration of chloramphenicol drops for 1 week and then discontinuation of the medication.

The lens was well tolerated by patients in this group and continuous wear for long periods resulted in no adverse effects. Neovascularization of the peripheral cornea was seen in several of these patients, but either the ocular or the general medical situation was such that this was not a significant problem. When control was necessary, the peripheral neovascularization could generally be controlled by the topical administration of corticosteroids. To date, we have treated approximately 50 patients with bullous keratopathy. Many of these patients have had the lens in place continuously for well over a year, and our longest-termed patient has just passed the 2-year mark. In no instance is the lens being removed by the patient. On occasion, the lens is removed for cleaning, replacement, examination of the cornea, or measurement of the intraocular pressure by the examining ophthalmologist during the course of a follow-up visit. The lens is then replaced before the patient leaves the office. Otherwise, the lens remains in place at all times. In some instances, particularly in patients with oily skin, proteinaceous, meibomian secretions collect on and become an integral part of the lens itself. These deposits cannot be cleaned from the lens but, in most instances, produce no difficulty. On rare occasion, the deposits result in a roughening of the anterior lens surface and become somewhat irritating to the patient. In such instances, we have merely replaced the lens with a new one.

This mode of therapy has produced a rapid dramatic relief of pain and the accompanying symptoms of bullous keratopathy. The lens is extremely well tolerated, and in most patients the relief of pain is almost immediate. The rate of success is well over 90%, and these patients represent one of the happiest and most appreciative groups of patients that I have ever encountered. Their pain, tearing, photophobia, and blepharospasm all cease very rapidly, and they are able to function normally once again. At times, if significant inflammation persists or the inflammation is unusually severe, topically administered potent corticosteroid solutions can be used twice daily for short periods of time with great success. I must emphasize that the lens itself produces no significant improvement of the clinical appearance of the corneal disease. Symptomatic relief is directly dependant on the lens remaining in place on the diseased cornea. Removal of the lens, in our experience, has generally resulted in a rapid recurrence of the symptoms. To date, we have had no significant complications in this group of patients from continuous, prolonged wearing of the soft contact lens.

Prior to contact lens fitting, all cases in our series had diffuse epithelial edema with multiple large bullae or vesicles and areas of epithelial abrasion where bullae had ruptured. This picture changes slightly when the lens has been in place for a time. There are usually fewer vesicles, and one generally sees a picture of diffuse epithelial edema after the lens has been worn for some time. However, the soft contact lens certainly does not prevent the formation or the rupture of bullae. Some of our patients continue to report a transient intermittent very mild recurrence of symptoms. This is often described simply as an awareness that the lens is in place. The sensation clears spontaneously within 24 to 48 hours and generally does not cause the patient sufficient discomfort to warrant his seeking medical attention. On the few occasions we were fortunate enough to examine the patient under these circumstances; the findings led us to conclude that the symptoms were probably attributable to bullae that had ruptured beneath the lens. Seemingly, rupture of bullae with exposure of the corneal nerve endings to drying and other noxious environmental stimuli produce the severe discomfort associated with bullous keratopathy. We may reasonably assume that the Bausch & Lomb Soflens achieves the therapeutic affect we have noted by preventing such exposure.

Emphasis has been placed upon the fact that symptomatic relief in bullous keratopathy is dependent on the lens remaining in place on the diseased cornea and that no significant improvement in the degree of corneal pathology is produced by the lens itself. Consequently, very little improvement in visual acuity ensues as a result of therapy with the use of a hydrophilic contact lens alone. However, if patients with bullous keratopathy are carefully selected, then in some instances, corneal edema will be decreased and visual acuity improved by the instillation of hypertonic saline drops while the soft contact lens is in place. Patients for whom vision can be successfully improved by this therapeutic regimen must have an absence or paucity of stromal scarring; the great majority of these patients represent early cases of Fuchs' dystrophy. We have found it necessary to instill 5% sodium chloride drops into the affected eye every 2 hours while the patient is awake. The contact lens is worn continuously without removal except for periodic cleaning. In this instance, we packaged sterile 5% sodium chloride solution containing no preservative in bottles each containing approximately 2 ml. of solution. The patient is instructed to instill the drops every 2 hours from 8 A.M. to 10 P.M. A fresh bottle of hypertonic saline drops is used every day. When the soft contact lens is worn continuously, 24 hours a day, and 5% sodium chloride drops are administered topically every 2 hours during the day, approximately 50% of the patients selected for this treatment experience a satisfactory response to therapy manifested by decreased epithelial and stromal edema and improvement in visual acuity. Approximately 3 weeks of therapy are required before a clinical improvement can be documented in the successful cases.

The mechanism by which this effect is produced is not clear, but there is ample evidence in the literature indicating that corneal epithelium and endothelium are both semipermeable membranes. The capacity of the epithelium to act as an osmotic membrane is of significance in this situation. Under the experimental conditions, the osmolarity of the corneal stroma is approximately 300 milliosmoles, or equal to that of normal saline. Thus 5% saline is equivalent to 1,500 milliosmoles of osmotic pressure. Applied to the corneal epithelial surface, hypertonic saline results in the establishment of an extreme osmotic pressure gradient. If the patient's epithelium is indeed acting as an osmotic membrane, the possibility exists that this osmotic pressure gradient will be sufficient to draw enough water from the cornea to offset the pathological effects of the malfunctioning endothelial pump. To achieve an optimal clinical result, apparently the hypertonic medium must continuously bathe the epithelial surface, a feat that heretofore could not be attained by any practical means. The advent of the hydrophilic contact lens provided us with a new means of achieving this goal. The Bausch & Lomb Soflens is approximately 40% water. Repeated and prolonged administration of 5% saline to an eye wearing the lens assures that the water content of the lens will approach an ion concentration equivalent to that of the hypertonic saline. This provides a hypertonic reservoir for equilibration with the very thin tear film between the lens and the epithelial surface. Since the lens does not adhere to the cornea but moves on blinking, the topically applied hypertonic saline also bathes the corneal epithelium directly. The ability of the lens to be worn around the clock for prolonged periods enables us to maintain conveniently the hyperosmotic medium upon the corneal surface. The osmotic gradient established by our therapeutic regimen may be sufficient to compensate largely for the effective physiological dehydrating mechanisms of the endothelium and a satisfactory clinical result is at times obtained.

DRY EYES

When there is a deficiency of lacrimal secretions—the well-known "dry eyes," a hydrophilic contact lens can be quite useful. Keratoconjunctivitis sicca patients can be symptomatically improved with a soft lens, and in the more severe cases, normal saline drops may be used concomitantly with the lens. We have not been quite as enthusiastic about this approach as others because, although the patients are symptomatically relieved, we have encountered a good deal of difficulty with mucous and oily deposits collecting on or smearing the surface of the lens and interfering significantly with vision. Moreover, our approach of keeping the lens in place 24 hours a day causes these deposits to become an integral part of the lens after a time and they cannot be cleaned. This is a particularly vexing problem in dry eye patients whose lacrimal secretions may be thick and tenacious. We prefer to tackle the dry eye problem medically with a combination of mucolytic and wetting agents and only when we are unsuccessful in this purely medical approach do we tend to resort to a soft contact lens in the treatment of dry eyes. We have just begun to gain experience with a combined therapeutic regimen consisting of a hydrophilic contact lens and topical instillation of a mucolytic agent with the lens in place. This combined approach has some intriguing possibilities of success, but for the moment it remains quite experimental and our experience with this regimen has not been great enough for me to comment further about it.

KERATOCONUS

As we all know, the decreased vision in keratoconus is caused by irregular astigmatism from a conical distortion of the cornea. Because of the irregular nature of the astigmatism, the disease often progresses to the point where one is unable to correct the astigmatism with spectacles and one must then turn to contact lenses. The rationale for the use of contact lenses involves a therapeutic attempt to provide a new, smooth, regular, spherical anterior refracting surface for the conical cornea. The problems encountered in fitting the hard lens, essentially a spherical hard lens, over a conical cornea are well known and do not warrant discussion here. But sooner or later, as the disease progresses, one runs into significant problems and often cannot fit a hard lens successfully in advanced keratoconus.

With the advent of the soft contact lenses, the possibility appeared, particularly after our initial experiences with other types of pathological conditions, that the soft lens might be the answer. My own particular experience with the Bausch & Lomb Soflens, unfortunately, has been somewhat disappointing in this regard. As you know, the Bausch & Lomb Soflens is quite pliable. It is also quite thin; the current lenses are often less than 0.2 mm. in thickness. Although one can often get what appears to be quite a good fit, the lens itself molds extremely well to the conical shape of the cornea. And so it too becomes conical and does not provide, in our experience, the hoped-for refractive correction.

We tried overrefracting these patients, and in a fair number got some improvement in visual acuity. The improvement was not very dramatic, perhaps a line or two, occasionally a little bit more. But again we were somewhat disappointed because most of these patients ultimately gave up wearing the lens, since they felt that the degree of improvement in visual acuity was not sufficient to warrant putting up with the other problems they were encountering. All in all, our experience with the Bausch & Lomb Soflens in the treatment of keratoconus, at least as the lens is now produced and is presently available to us, has been somewhat disappointing, and we have lost much of our enthusiasm for this device as a therapeutic approach to keratoconus.

CONTINUOUS WEAR OF HYDROPHILIC CONTACT LENSES

My own experience with the fitting of hydrophilic contact lenses for the correction of refractive errors is somewhat limited and is in general agreement with the experience of many other practitioners. There is, however, one additional area that merits serious discussion and that is the possibility that hydrophilic contact lenses fitted for cosmetic purposes might be worn continuously.

My own experience has been limited solely to the Bausch & Lomb Soflens, which, to date, is the only type of hydrophilic contact lens that has been approved by the Food and Drug Administration for use by the practitioner for correction of refractive errors. Instructions accompanying this lens recommend an initial graduated wearing schedule. The instruction manual warns that there is a tendency to overwear the lenses since they feel comfortable from the start and admonishes the practitioner to stress to the patient the importance of strictly following the recommended wearing schedule.

The instructions and recommendations for the Bausch & Lomb Soflens are strangely similar to the standard wearing instructions for the conventional hard methylmethacrylate contact lenses. Presumably, these warnings have been issued in anticipation that the soft lens would produce the same problems encountered when the conventional lenses are worn continuously for too long a period of time. However, there appears to be no well-known documented evidence indicating that this is the case in most instances. In fact, our own experience with the identical Bausch & Lomb Soflens supports just the opposite conclusion. We have found that this device is extremely well tolerated by the cornea, even in the presence of severe corneal disease, and may be worn continuously, around the clock, for prolonged periods without ill effect. We therefore initiated a study to determine the effect of continuous wear of a hydrophilic contact lens on the normal human cornea.

Ten informed volunteers, all associated in some capacity with the Department of Ophthalmology at the Boston University School of Medicine, comprised the subjects for this study. All of the subjects underwent a complete baseline ophthalmological examination prior to contact lens fitting. In addition, corneal thickness measurements were performed on each subject for 3 days prior to contact lens fitting. The right eye of each subject was fitted with this device without keratometry and without any particular regard to corneal curvature. An identical plano lens was simply placed on the right cornea of each subject, and those subjects with significant refractive errors continued to wear their own spectacles over the contact lens. The lens was worn 24 hours a day for the duration of the experimental observation period, which was arbitrarily limited to 10 days. The lenses were not removed during the duration of the study.

Each patient was examined with the slit lamp biomicroscope and his visual acuity was recorded twice daily—in the morning prior to 9:00 and in the afternoon between 5:00 and 5:30. Corneal thickness was measured within 30 minutes of the contact lens fitting and, thereafter, five times daily at 9:00 A.M., 10:30 A.M., 12:00 noon, 3:00 P.M., and 5:00 P.M. The clinical examinations and recording of visual acuity were performed independently of the corneal thickness measurements by two examiners in two geographically separate facilities. Neither examiner was aware of the other's findings during the course of this study.

Continuous wear of the Bausch & Lomb Soflens for a 10-day period was successfully accomplished by eight of the 10 subjects studied. In two subjects, the lens became dislodged and was lost prior to the termination of the experimental observation period. This occurred on the fourth and sixth day after fitting, respectively. Both subjects had been wearing the lens without difficulty prior to its loss and neither was aware that the lens was no longer in place at the time it was discovered by the examiner.

No evidence of serious corneal abnormality was observed. Transient corneal edema was noted, however, in three subjects. In the first, slight edema of the central corneal epithelium was present on the second day when the initial examination was performed at 8:10 A.M. It had not been noted previously. The eye was asymptomatic at the time and the visual acuity was 20/20 +4. The contact lens was left in place and the epithelial edema cleared within 2 hours. In a second subject, slight deep stromal edema with definite folds in Descemet's membrane was noted on the third and fourth days during the initial morning examination. Again, the eye was asymptomatic at the time; visual acuity was 20/30. The lens was left in place and the edema was noted to clear progressively beneath the lens. On both days, it was no longer present at 5:00 P.M. and did not reappear on the fifth day or thereafter. A third subject presented with deep stromal edema and folds in Descemet's membrane on the third, fourth, and fifth days. The degree of severity and daily course of the edema was identical to the above case. On each day, the edema cleared by 5:00 P.M. Edema of the corneal stroma was not noted on the sixth day and the patient thereafter lost his contact lens.

In addition, two subjects were noted to have several fine, gray lines at the level of Descemet's membrane. They differed in appearance from true striae, were not accompanied by clinically detectable edema, and did not produce any visual deficit. In the first subject, they appeared on the second day, were noted during the early morning examination, and were no longer present at 5:00 P.M. that day. They failed to reappear thereafter. In the second subject, these lines were observed on the fourth and fifth days; they persisted throughout the entire fourth day, did not increase in severity overnight, and cleared by 5:00 P.M. of the fifth day. In both cases, the lines took several directions but were largely horizontal and diagonal in direction. They were not reflections of the lashes as has been suggested by other workers.

Most of the subjects noted that under the conditions of continuous wear, visual acuity tended to be somewhat variable. In general, they reported intermittent episodes of slight blurring of vision, lasting several minutes to an hour or two, which then cleared spontaneously. In no instance was the blurred vision marked in degree. Visual acuity of each subject at 9:00 A.M. and 5:00 P.M. documented that at these times, at least, the variability in visual acuity ranged from 20/15 to 20/40+.

The variability in visual acuity could not be correlated with corneal edema, either as noted with the biomicroscope or as measured with the pachometer. It appeared to be attributable to two factors: (1) The first was the tendency of oily, proteinaceous meibomian secretions to deposit on the anterior surface of the contact lens, either in the form of a thin, transparent film, which seemed to have little effect on vision, or in the form of gray translucent or opaque deposits, which measurably decreased the vision and caused the subject to report a blurred image even when he was capable of distinguishing a given line on the Snellen chart. There was an increased tendency to form these latter deposits on the anterior lens surface by those subjects who had a history of and difficulty with oily skin. Within the present limited study period, these deposits tended to be removed within several hours to 1 to 2 days presumably by the combination of tears with the abrasive action of blinking lids. (2) The second factor producing variability in vision of up to two to three lines on the Snellen chart, occurred in the absence of any deposits on the contact lens. Improvement in the visual acuity could be achieved either by overrefraction or by the use of a pinhole disc. This change in refraction was presumably attributable to an alteration in the degree of hydration of the lens and tended to correct itself spontaneously in, at most, several hours.

An increase in the thickness of the corneal stroma, as measured with the pachometer, was noted from the first day of contact wear. The increase in stromal thickness varied slightly from day to day but tended to stabilize within narrow limits and did not progressively increase during the experimental observation period. The maximum degree of edema measured produced an increase of 30% in overall corneal thickness. Generally, the increase in corneal thickness was less, and in most instances it neither could be appreciated on biomicroscopic examination nor did it result in a visual deficit. During each day, all subjects exhibited a regular variation in corneal thickness. The majority of measurements documented that the cornea was thickest in the morning and, with the hydrophilic contact lens in place, steadily decreased in thickness during the day.

Seven of the 10 subjects reported a burning or foreign body sensation limited to the eye with the contact lens. In each instance, this occurred immediately after the patient opened his eyes upon awakening. In all but one instance the symptoms were minor and cleared spontaneously within 15 to 20 minutes. In one instance actual pain that persisted for 2 to 3 hours before it cleared spontaneously was reported. These symptoms were not accompanied by blurred vision, halos, or photophobia. Except in the one severe case, overt epiphora was not present.

In an attempt to determine the cause of this symptom, several patients had a pressure patch applied to their right eye while the soft contact lens was in place. They were examined at 8:00 A.M. the following morning and so, in effect, they had not opened that eye during that day. The symptoms were reproduced in two patients and were described as a burning sensation. No evidence of an epithelial defect or other corneal abnormality was observed. Positive findings were limited to a slight injection of the palpebral conjunctiva. The symptoms cleared within 15 minutes and the conjunctival injection disappeared within an hour or two.

I must emphasize that this symptom was limited to the first 3 days of wearing. In no instance, including the one subject in whom the symptoms had been rather severe, did these symptoms occur after the first 3 wearing days.

Examination of the cornea upon removal of the hydrophilic contact lens at the end of the 10-day wearing period revealed only that the epithelial surface was slightly roughened. Application of fluorescein resulted in some pooling of the stain on the corneal surface. No defects in the corneal epithelium were observed and there was no true staining with fluorescein. The epithelial surface was normal in all cases 24 hours after removal, and corneal thickness returned to baseline levels within the same period. In Chapter 3 Morrison and Edelhauser present their data on the oxygen permeability characteristics of several types of hydrophilic contact lenses and show that the oxygen diffusion rates are many times greater than the estimated corneal consumption, even for the least permeable lens studied. They conclude that the in vitro oxygen diffusion characteristics of the three hydrophilic lenses studied, including the Bausch & Lomb Soflens, indicated that corneal oxygen deprivation should not occur as a result of prolonged wearing and that the "overwearing syndrome" observed with methylmethacrylate lenses should not result with the use of hydrophilic lenses. Our present study supports this conclusion. Each of the subjects studied was able to comfortably wear a hydrophilic contact lens continuously from the outset; no special graduated "breaking in" wearing schedule was required for adaptation. Overwearing abrasions of the epithelium were conspicuously absent. Clinically detectable edema was only noted in three subjects and, in each instance, it was transient and cleared without therapeutic intervention while the lens remained in place.

Problematic areas were encountered but, in general, they were minor. They include the deposition of oily proteinaceous meibomian secretions on the anterior lens surface, variable vision seemingly attributable to a temporary change in the degree of hydration of the hydrogel material, and symptoms on awakening generally limited to a very mild foreign body sensation that cleared spontaneously within 15 to 20 minutes of onset. The latter symptoms were attributed to the decrease in tear production occurring during sleep and adherence of the dried palpebral conjunctiva to the anterior lens surface. On opening of the lids, presumably some of the conjunctival epithelium adheres to the lens surface, producing a symptomatic "conjunctival abrasion." Interestingly, this adherence appeared to be self-limited and did not occur beyond the third wearing day.

This data should not be interpreted as representing our support or endorsement of this continuous wear of the presently available soft hydrophilic contact lenses when they are used solely for the correction of a refractive error. The advantages of this mode of wear are obvious. The results of this study are certainly encouraging and, we think, demonstrate that continuous wear is certainly possible. Problems, for the most part minor, have been encountered, as we have indicated, and remain to be solved or circumvented before continuous wear of cosmetic hydrophilic contact lenses can be routinely recommended. Continuous wear does, however, represent a major potential advance in contact lens technology and should be a primary goal in the future development of these devices.

Chapter 26

Griffin Naturalens (bandage lens) in treatment of bullous keratopathy, dry eyes, and corneal ulcers

Antonio R. Gasset, M.D.

BULLOUS KERATOPATHY

Soft hydrophilic contact lenses provide a simple and often useful method in the treatment of bullous keratopathy. They have improved vision and relieved pain, when they are used as an optical bandage over diseased cornea where other sight-preserving techniques have failed or were not possible. However, it has become evident that the details of proper fitting and management of the patient are necessary to obtain best results.

Physiology

Bullous keratopathy is the most severe form of corneal edema. It always involves all three layers of the cornea and results from diseased corneal endothelium, caused by one or more of the following factors:

1. Fuchs endothelial dystrophy
2. Aphakic bullous keratopathy caused by trauma during surgery, vitreous touch, and so forth
3. Postkeratoplasty bullous keratopathy caused by iris adhesion, retrocorneal membrane, and separation of Descemet's membrane
4. Long-standing uveitis
5. Glaucoma

The natural course of the disease can be divided into the following stages:

Degeneration of the corneal endothelium. The corneal endothelium progressively degenerates until it is not able to carry out its function as a mechanical barrier and pump. The endothelium decompensates and aqueous humor leaks into the corneal stroma.

Stroma edema. The stromal edema usually mirrors the endothelial disease. In some cases it is a small well-localized area and in other cases it involves a diffuse area from limbus to limbus. In some cases stromal edema is present for months or even years without scarring or epithelial edema.

Epithelial edema. The edema begins in the basal cell layers spreading through the epithelium and occasionally forming subepithelial bullae. Often before epithelial bullae are noted, a fibrous overgrowth begins between Bowman's membrane and the epithelium. As first this may be visible as irregular moon-shaped reflections seen by specular reflection. Later this subepithelial overgrowth may be quite hazy and grayish, and occasionally it makes a significant contribution to the reduction of vision. Later epithelial bullae and the irregular astigmatism caused by the bullae appear. Irregular astigmatism is often the major cause of vision loss in bullous keratopathy.

Stromal scarring. Scarring results only after long-standing epithelial edema. Corneal scarring usually begins anterior to Descemet's membrane as a slightly yellowish density or as grayish strands forming a hazy star-shaped area.

Folds in Descemet's membrane. Folds in Descemet's membrane are due to swelling and hydration of the corneal stroma. The stroma as it swells cannot proceed anteriorly and is thrown into folds. When these folds are present for a long time, they scar and become fixed folds in Descemet's membrane. These folds also seem clinically important in reducing vision.

Visual acuity and bullous keratopathy

The fact is generally accepted that epithelial edema and irregular astigmatism are the main causes of a decrease in visual acuity in cases of bullous keratopathy.

Zucker and others[1] have shown that in enucleated eyes a 70% increase in stromal thickness reduces obtainable visual acuity in only 25% of the eyes. Moreover, if the edematous epithelium is removed in enucleated cow eyes, the visual acuity can improve up to 40%.

We have shown[2] that epithelial edema in the absence of folds in Descemet's membrane or stromal scarring are responsible for all or almost all the decrease in visual acuity. However, on the basis of our previous experiments with epikeratoprosthesis and bullous keratopathy and our present experience with the Griffin Naturalenses, patients with folds in Descemet's membrane fail to significantly improve in vision unless the folds in Descemet's membrane were reduced.

Treatment of bullous keratopathy

Bullous keratopathy may be treated by the following techniques:
1. Pressure bandage
2. Osmotherapy
3. Conjunctival flaps
4. Chemotherapy
5. Cauterization
6. Epikeratoprosthesis
7. Corneal implants
8. Keratoplasty
9. Bandage lenses

It is not the purpose of this paper to discuss each of the techniques that have been used in the past for the treatment of corneal edema. However, we should mention that since the introduction of the bandage lenses for the treatment of bullous keratopathy, only such lenses and penetrating keratoplasty are being used by us for the treatment of bullous keratopathy if simple osmotherapy fails.

The beneficial effect of the bandage lens stems from the following facts:

1. Acts as a pressure bandage reducing the epithelial edema. As a matter of fact, it is the most comfortable pressure bandage that can be worn constantly.
2. Replaces the irregular astigmatism with smooth optically perfect surface.
3. Acts systemically with osmotherapy. Hypertonic saline used in conjunction with the lenses is absorbed and released over a long period of time, therefore increasing the effectiveness of this form of therapy.
4. Protects bullae from the lids, preventing rupture.

Materials and methods

Although studies were done with other lenses, it was found that for good results lenses with variable curvature and diameter were necessary.

The lens. Only Griffin Naturalenses were used in this study. A detailed description of these lenses has been presented by Chapters 9, 11, and 12.

Fitting procedure. Fitting patients with bullous keratopathy is significantly more difficult than fitting patients for refractive errors especially if good visual results are required. However, experience in fitting patients for refractive errors is a significant asset in the fitting of pathological corneas. It usually simplifies the fitting procedure and improves the therapeutic results in this type of patient.

Trial lens fitting is the easiest and often the only method by which these lenses can be fitted in patients with pathological corneas. Trial lens testing is done to find the proper dimension, curve, and diameter that will give the best and most stable performance.

The first question that must be answered is how to select a lens of the proper curve and diameter for a given patient that will provide sufficient adherence to prevent movement without inducing too much apical clearance and consequent variable vision. Keratometer readings are generally not available.

The selection of any lens can result in only three possibilities:

1. The lens is too steep.
2. The lens is too flat.
3. The lens is of the proper curve and diameter.

Therefore, if one selects any lens from a trial lens set or an inventory and places it in the eye, one of the conditions should result.

If the lens is too flat (or too small), it will move up and down with each blink or will be displaced laterally on sideward gaze.

If the lens is too steep there is alternate blurring and clearing of vision with each blink. This may be somewhat difficult to evaluate initially in a patient with bullous keratopathy. However, if there is any doubt that the lens might be steep, one should proceed for the next flatter lens (or the next smaller diameter lens). Should the lens be too flat it will move excessively. If the lens moves too much, one can be assured that the proper lens is steeper. If the lens seems to center properly in the eye, one can try for a flatter lens to be certain it is not too steep.

If the proper lens dimensions cannot be determined at first, we have found that a lens of 8.1 mm. base curve, 14 mm. diameter, and 0.35 mm. central thickness lens gives the most satisfactory results.

The constant wearing of these lenses results in dehydration of the cornea and a significant change in corneal shape. The lens that was previous properly fitted no longer is satisfactory. This change usually results in a reduction in visual acuity. It is not unusual to find a patient who was initially fitted with these lenses with an improvement in vision from 20/200 to 20/40 in whom, after a few days, visual acuity decreases to 20/100 or 20/200. Biomicroscopy of the eye usually reveals a significant change in the cornea with disappearance of the big bullae and with diffuse epithelial edema. If in these cases the lens is changed to a properly fitted lens, visual acuity usually improves again to 20/40 after hypertonic saline. In some cases several changes in the lenses are required.

Once satisfied that the proper curve and diameter have been determined, the proper refractive power of the lens should be determined. For the beginner plano lenses will simplify the procedure. The proper power can be prescribed by one of the following two techniques:

1. The power that is prescribed can be determined by using the spectacle refraction and vertex distance and refining the refraction through a trial lens procedure.
2. Plano lenses and refracting over may be used.

Use of medications. The following major steps may be taken to reduce pathological conditions:

1. Lid hygiene, as lid scrubs for 5 minutes daily or twice a day, have decreased the incidence of minor infections to an insignificant level.
2. Pupil dilators can be used in cases of chronic bullous keratopathy, especially with epithelial defects because of the concomitant iritis present in almost every case.
3. Antibiotics are used if secondary infections or chronic blepharitis is present at the time of the fitting.
4. Five percent hypertonic saline without preservative is the most important single medication used in combination with the lenses in cases of bullous keratopathy. Its use produces a significant improvement in vision. It is used in most cases as frequently as needed (p.r.n.). However, it should be avoided in the beginning if patients have significant amount of discomfort.

In these cases application of the lenses and pupillary dilation should result in significant relief of pain within a few days. At that time the patient should be refitted and hypertonic saline used for improvement of visual acuity.

Visual acuity

Visual acuity is often improved after the insertion of the Griffin Naturalens and the application of hypertonic solution. However, in many cases several weeks or even months are necessary before the best visual acuity can be obtained and several refittings may be necessary for optimal acuity.

Visual acuity improves after the application of 5% hypertonic saline without preservative. An effective schedule for the application of hypertonic saline seems to be one or two drops every 2 hours (4.2 hours). Hypertonic saline is most needed during the morning hours. In the afternoon visual acuity clears somewhat even without the application of hypertonic saline.

An unexplained decrease in visual acuity is always a reason for overrefraction or refitting of the lens. In several cases refraction and corneal curvature have changed after wearing the bandage lens for several days or weeks. In all cases refitting of the proper dimension and power of the lens have resulted in improvement of the visual acuity.

Relief of pain

In almost every case total comfort is obtained within 1 week. In the few cases where pain was not relieved by the application of the bandage lenses one or several of the following conditions were determined:
1. Improper fitting of the lens
2. Failure to dilate the pupil
3. Conjunctivitis or blepharitis
4. Elevations in intraocular pressure

Case reports

As one can see from these cases, there were several months and refittings of the Griffin Naturalenses, and the application of hypertonic was necessary before the best visual acuity could be obtained.

The first case is that of a 27-year-old male with monocular bullous keratopathy. Visual acuity with 20/20 in the right eye and he could count fingers with the left eye. The patient had been crippled with ocular pain for several months. The classical method of therapy had failed to relieve the pain or improve visual acuity.

He was first seen in our eye clinic on April 21, 1970, at which time a plano lens of the proper base curve and diameter was inserted, with almost instant relief of pain. He was seen on May 11, 1970, at which time he was free of ocular discomfort. At this time he was refitted with Griffin Naturalenses with improvement in vision to 20/30. Visual acuity was later improved to 20/20 with the use of hypertonic saline and the lens. The patient has been asymptomatic with stable visual acuity since that time. He has been able to return to work and carry out normal activities with visual acuity fluctuating from 20/30 to 20/20.

Again, this case shows the necessity of several fittings as well as the intelligent application of hypertonic saline.

The second case is that of a 48-year-old man who had bilateral bullous keratopathy from Fuchs' endothelial dystrophy. Visual acuity in the right eye was 20/60 and in the left eye 20/80. Although this patient was incapacitated by pain and decreased vision, penetrating keratoplasty seemed undesirable because of his relatively good, if decreased, vision. Other medical treatments, such as hypertonic solutions and the use of a hair dryer, had proved unsatisfactory. In March, 1969, the patient was first fitted with Griffin Naturalenses with an almost instant relief of pain. However, his visual acuity improved only to 20/40 in both eyes. After several refittings and the proper use of hypertonic saline the visual acuity improved more than 20/20 in both eyes. For over 1 year this patient enjoyed a 20/20 visual acuity and complete comfort. For 6 months he was wearing the lenses 24 hours a day for 1 month at a time uneventfully with extreme comfort and excellent vision. However, on April 11, 1970, the patient noticed redness, swelling, and mucous purulent discharge in the left eye. Patient was being treated elsewhere and returned to our eye clinic on April 17, 1970, and the diagnosis of *Pseudomonas* ulcer was made. After the proper diagnosis was made, the ulcer was debrided, the lenses were inserted, and the patient was treated with the lens in place with the proper medication. This resulted in healing of the cornea in 10 days. Patient has returned to full-time wearing of the lens, which he has been wearing now for over 2 years with total comfort and 20/20 visual acuity in both eyes.

The third case is that of a 44-year-old man with congenital glaucoma. The left eye had been enucleated. Visual acuity in the right eye progressively decreased to counting fingers at 2 feet. At this time a Griffin Naturalens was inserted with an instant improvement of vision to 20/40. After the proper base curve and diameter was obtained, the visual acuity improved to 20/20. In this particular case an unusually large and flat lens was required because of the megalocornea. The difference between a properly fitted lens and an improperly fitted lens was between 20/40 and 20/20 visual acuity. Even more, with the properly fitted lens the visual acuity was quite stable, and with the improper lens he suffered from quite variable visual acuity. Since the patient was first fitted, visual acuity has remained at the 20/20 level after the insertion of the lens and the proper application of hypertonic saline solution.

DRY EYES

A rational approach for the treatment of dry eyes should be based on the stage or form of the disease. Obviously the mildest form of dry eyes characterized by the low degree of conjunctivitis should not be treated the same as the most extreme form as present in ocular pemphigus. For practical purposes we divided these conditions into the following three groups.

Keratoconjunctivitis sicca. Keratoconjunctivitis sicca appears characteristically in people over the age of 50. Females are more frequently affected than are males. Patients usually complain of constant itching and burning. Slit lamp examination will reveal rose bengal staining, particularly in the lower half of the cornea and

Table 26-1. Findings in cases of Sjögren's syndrome

Source	Number of cases	Sex		Patients with salivary gland enlargement	Patients with dryness of the mouth	Patients with arthritis
		♂	♀			
Sjögren	19	6	13	2	9	13
Beetham	9	0	9	3	7	3
Bruce	14	2	12	6	9	6
Coverdale	5	1	4	3	5	2
Gifford et al.	33	5	28	2	15	11
McLean	3	0	3	2	3	2
Lutman & Favata	2	0	2	2	2	0
Morgan	5	0	5	3	5	4
Total	90	14	76	23	55	41

conjunctiva with little or no staining with fluorescein. Evaluation of every patient includes Schirmer's test; a positive test is considered less than 5 mm. wetting of the paper in 5 minutes in at least one determination.

Keratoconjunctivitis sicca associated with systemic disease. The findings in cases of keratoconjunctivitis sicca or Sjögren's syndrome are outlined in Table 26-1. The following treatments have been advocated: artificial tears, puncture cautery, moist chambers, mucous liquefiers, and flush-fitting lenses.

Essential shrinkage of the conjunctiva. This group represents the most severe form of the drying conditions. The search for a mode of therapy that will be effective against this condition has been long and frustrating.

Physiology

The fact is generally accepted that different rates of secretion are obtained with different stimuli; therefore it seems reasonable to propose a classification based on the different stimuli:

1. *Essential tear flow.* Essential tear flow is the amount of tear fluid continuously secreted mainly by the accessory and secondary glands under "physiological" conditions.
2. *Reflex tear flow.* Reflex tear flow is the amount of tear fluid secreted mainly by the lacrimal gland in response to cornea-conjunctiva sensory stimulation.
3. *Psychogenic tear flow.* Psychogenic tear flow is the amount of tear fluid secreted mainly by the lacrimal gland in response to changes in the psychological environments.

A single mechanism cannot explain the change in flow under different stimuli; instead different mechanisms for each stimuli should be proposed. An extensive study on the neuroanatomy of the lacrimal apparatus would be of little help in the understanding of such a mechanism and thus is not included here.

Evaporation of tears from the exposed area of the eye might play an essential role in the secretion of tears; this implies the presence of some kind of receptor on the conjunctiva of the cornea; however, such receptors have not been shown. More investigation in this area is necessary before a mechanism or mechanisms can be proposed.

Tear flow determination: its technique and interpretation. Schirmer in 1903 determined the rate of "essential tear-fluid flow" in five subjects who had undergone extirpation of the lacrimal sac and all stimuli producing lacrimation were eliminated. He measured the time needed to form the first drop and its weight, adding to it the amount lost by evaporation from the exposed surface of the eyeball, which he previously calculated. From these data he concluded that the flow was 0.5 to 0.75 gm. of tears in 16 hours, which is the same as 0.5 to 0.8 μl./min.

Schirmer also determined the rate of flow produced in response to different stimuli. He described several methods: The first method consists of the introduction of a filter paper in the conjunctival sac and measuring the wetting of the filter paper in 5 minutes. Therefore the reflex tear flow produced by the corneal-conjunctival stimuli is determined. He reported that on the average in normal cases 30 mm. of the paper strip is moistened in 5 minutes. Schirmer's second test consists of the irritation of the nasal mucosa with a hair brush after the eye was anesthetized. A third method is similar to the second, but instead he had the patient look at the sun.

Recently, with a more sophisticated technique, the total volume of tears present in the eye under physiological conditions was measured. The total tear volume was found to be between 10 to 14 ml., and the essential tear flow was about 10% of the total amount of tears present in the eye.

Because of its simplicity Schirmer's first test has become universally accepted. This test can be performed by any technician and does not require the application of topical anesthetics. As mentioned before, this test is a measurement of the reflex tear flow; in other words, it measures the capacity of the main lacrimal gland to secrete tears in response to a corneal-conjunctival sensory stimulation. Application of topical anesthetics is impractical for the determination of tear flow. Essential tear flow is about 1.4 ml./min. Therefore, the essential tear flow measurement in 5 minutes will be 7 ml., which could hardly be measured with standard techniques for the Schirmer test.

Some confusion has been created in the past regarding average tear flow for normal patients. It is much simpler to think in terms of the minimum low value for tear flow. In our experience a value less than 5 mm. wetting of the paper means dry eyes.

Vital staining. Fluorescein stains epithelial defects yellowish green. It is important to realize that fluorescein does not stain epithelial cells, instead fluorescein will diffuse into the corneal stroma if the epithelium is absent, staining denuded areas of the cornea.

Rose bengal stains degenerated epithelial cells in a typical red color. Also mucus will stain with rose bengal.

Keratoconjunctivitis sicca gives a pronounced staining of the cornea and the free area of the bulbar conjunctiva by rose bengal, whereas it practically never stains with fluorescein. In essential shrinkage of the conjunctiva, mucus threads are absent in the inferior fornix.

In cases of disruption of the precorneal tear film attributable to exogenous trauma, equal amounts of staining with fluorescein and rose bengal will be topically present.

Treatment of dry eyes

There is no other ocular condition in which the results are most satisfactory than in cases of essential shrinkage of the conjunctiva. Previous experience in the management of these patients and a complete and full understanding of the natural history of these conditions is necessary. A complete ocular examination, especially the eyelids, conjunctivae, and corneas must be performed on each patient, as follows:

1. *Eyelids.* Trichiasis and blepharitis are often found in cases of essential shrinkage of the conjunctiva. In such cases hexachlorophene (pHisoHex) scrubs should be instituted before the application of the lens. This routine is repeated daily twice a day until the blepharitis is under control. Trichiasis should be treated accordingly. Removal of the eyelashes is usually unsatisfactory. Electrolysis is often sufficient.

2. *The conjunctivae.* Complete evaluation of the conjunctivae to determine the presence and amount of symblepharon, the condition of the cul-de-sac, and so on.

Symblepharon almost always requires surgical correction. Some cases are simple and just require cutting the symblepharon with scissors. In other cases where there is significant amount of symblepharon with no cul-de-sac, a more complicated surgical procedure is required. In advanced cases we have found the following technique the simplest and most effective: After ocular akinesia is obtained and topical anesthetic applied, exposure of the eyeball is obtained by the application of any lid retractor if possible. In some cases because of the massive scarring and symblepharon, exposure of the eyeball has to be obtained manually. After selecting the best place, one introduces the blades of a small hemostat under the symblepharon and closes the hemostat. The hemostat is then removed and the symblepharon cut with scissors. The procedure is then repeated 360° around the limbus following only one plane. Once all the symblepharon has been cut as mentioned above, a 360° conjunctiva-like tissue should be seen around the limbus. It is important to realize that symblepharon should not be sectioned if forceps or hemostat cannot be easily introduced underneath. At this time a reversed peritomy should be performed. With pick-up forceps, the conjunctiva-like tissue is raised and a reversed peritomy carried out to the center of the cornea. Any instrument such as Castroviejo scissors, paufique knife or any other suitable instrument can be used. This is essentially done as any lamella keratoplasty. At the end of the procedure one finds almost a clear cornea with a few deep blood vessels.

At this point the Griffin Naturalens should be placed over the cornea, Neosporin ophthalmic solution and atropine applied to the eye, and subconjunctival methylprednisolone acetate (Depo-Medrol) injection given.

3. *Postoperative course.* Proper management of the patient during the postoperative course is of the utmost importance. Immediately after surgery the patient should have frequent applications of normal saline, Neosporin ophthalmic solution, and Chloromycetin four times a day, and 1% atropine twice a day. Lenses have to be changed quite frequently because of bloodstain, considerable dehydration, and other factors.

4. *Fitting procedure.* The fitting procedure is done by a trial lens testing. However, as one can expect, it is difficult to predict the proper dimensions. Therefore, the initial lens is selected from a plano lens inventory almost at random. The lenses are subsequently changed until the best visual acuity is obtained. At this time the proper base curve has been determined. Usually there are several changes necessary until the proper lens dimensions are determined.

5. *Wearing time.* In all these cases wearing time should be 24 hours a day, at least. Two sets of lenses are given to the patient and lenses are removed according to the patient's skills and needs.

6. *Use of medications*

SALINE SOLUTION. Saline solution should be applied to the eye quite frequently. Initially, installation of saline is necessary as frequently as every 5 to 10 minutes. Because of these frequent applications, slight chemical dermatitis and maceration of the skin of the eyelids occurred in some patients. Topical application of corticosteroid ointments over the skin of the eyelids was sufficient in these cases. The need for saline diminishes as the time goes on. And eventually the patient selects the schedule that best fits his own requirements.

ANTIBIOTICS. Antibiotics should not be used routinely. However, prevention of secondary infection lies in the proper use of antibiotics.

CORTICOSTEROIDS. Corticosteroids are used during the first postoperative week. Thereafter, we seldom have needed to use any significant amount of corticosteroids. In a few cases diluted dexamethasone (Decadron) 1:20 dilution has been used for a few weeks.

ATROPINE. Dilating drops are necessary only during the postoperative course.

Discussion

The use of the Griffin Naturalenses in the treatment of severe drying conditions is most promising. This lens not only provides protection but also supplies badly needed moisture to the cornea.

In patients with severe dry syndromes, meticulous care of the eye is required. It is necessary to employ moisturizing solution to the lens such as isotonic or hypotonic saline. Evaporation from the lens was reduced by using artificial tears. In severe cases the lens tended to stick to the cornea; therefore, to facilitate removal, both the eye and the lens were well hydrated with a generous application of normal saline prior to removal of the lens.

Patients with mild sicca syndrome are relatively easy to treat and therapeutic benefits are obtained almost immediately. Severe drying conditions require more meticulous care, and therapeutic benefits such as improvement in vision and cornea tearing continued for a period of several months. In this group of patients one can easily understand how the lenses dry out and develop "exposure lentitis." Eventually, patients learn how to manage the drying of the lens with moisturizing solutions and wetting agents.

Not all patients can be helped just with the use of the lenses. In few cases with severe stromal scarring lamellar keratoplasty were performed. Immediately at the end of surgery, even when interrupted sutures were used, the lens was used over the graft to protect the graft. This combined therapy has significantly increased the overall success rate of lamellar keratoplasty in severe drying conditions.

The success of the new mode of therapy in the treatment of severe drying conditions is most important, since former treatment of these conditions has been notoriously difficult. However, the use of these lenses in such conditions is not a panacea.

CORNEAL ULCERS

Ulcers that will not heal and severe recurrent erosions are serious clinical problems. If the cornea is protected adequately, the ulcer will heal with minimal—no stromal—scarring. However, if the condition is allowed to progress, secondary infection and destruction of the corneal stroma will eventually take place. Conventional treatments sometimes fail to produce epithelial repair and the final result may be one of leukoma, deep vascularization, perforation, hypopyon, and loss of the eye.

Traditional methods of therapy such as pressure patching may result in healing when the corneal changes are minimal; tarsorrhaphy and conjunctival flaps, although effective in some cases, offer severe limitations in regard to cosmosis and visual acuity.

Protection of the cornea with hard scleral contact lenses was first proposed by Klein in 1943 for cases of severe neuroparalytic keratitis. Relative success in selected cases have been reported by seven investigators.[1-3]

Fitting techniques

Experience has shown that the most important factor in the treatment of this condition is the careful selection of the proper lens, skill in the insertion and removal of the lens, and most important the intelligent application of medication in conjunction with the lenses.

Keratometer readings are unobtainable in patients with recurrent erosion. Therefore, we are left with the trial lens procedure as the only fitting technique in these cases.

1. Keratometer readings are obtained if possible in the nonaffected eye.
2. The keratometer reading of the normal eye provided the starting point for the trial testing. However, in cases of epithelial erosion we preferred to select a steeper lens by one step.
3. Insertion of the lens was usually conducted without local anesthetic. However, in difficult cases with severe pain from the corneal disease, application of one or two drops of local anesthetic was used to permit the patient to open the eye adequately for fitting.
4. After the lens is inserted, it should not be removed unless it has been grossly misfitted. Manipulation such as insertion and removal in a painful inflamed eye was limited as much as possible.
5. Asepsis was preserved throughout this procedure.

Medications

Iritis was present in most cases. Therefore pupils must be dilated before the lenses are inserted. Atropine 1% was used twice a day until the inflammation decreased. In severe cases there was sometimes a considerable amount of lid swelling and dermatitis. In these cases we have used corticosteroid ointment applied to the skin. In a few cases where there had been significant amount of stromal edema, diluted commercial dexamethasone (0.005%) (Decadron 0.1%, diluted 20 times with normal saline) was used in combination with the lens. Antibiotics without preservative have also been used with the lens.

Clinical follow-up

Although no major complication has been encountered with the use of the lenses in the treatment of this condition, patients were examined daily for any sign of infection.

Since the lens takes up fluorescein, the use of fluorescein was avoided until complete reepithelialization had occurred, and the lenses were not needed. Evaluation of the degree of reepithelialization was possible in most cases, with the lens in place without the application of fluorescein. Should fluorescein be used, the lens must be removed prior to the application of fluorescein. We prefer to wait for the reinsertion of the lens rather than trying to irrigate fluorescein from the cul-de-sac. The latter usually results in significant amount of irritation and trauma to the corneal epithelium.

Removal of the lenses in the early stage of reepithelialization may also produce trauma to the healing epithelium. Should this be necessary, care was taken not to traumatize the healing epithelium.

In some cases a slight amount of epithelial edema could be seen with the slit lamp. This was due to the fact that steep lenses, which do not move, are used for the protection of the ingrowing epithelium whereas a flat lens moves over the cornea and disturbs the corneal epithelium, which at this time is poorly attached to Bowman's membrane. When it occurs, this slight amount of epithelial edema is not an indication for removal of the lens and disappears upon removal of the lens. It can also be prevented by fitting an extremely thin lens.

Comfort after the application of the lenses generally was seen in about 1 hour and there was almost total relief of pain in almost all cases within the next 24 to 48 hours.

Clinical results

Table 26-2 summarizes the results of the effect of Griffin lenses in the treatment of 34 patients with ulcers that failed to heal with other modes of treatment.

Of the 34 patients, all but two reepithelialized completely under the contact lens. In this study the ulcer is considered healed or reepithelialized when all grossly visible stain has disappeared. One of the two patients who failed to reepithelialize under the lenses was a case of lye burn that was treated elsewhere for approximately 2 weeks with the conventional treatment and failed to reepithelialize. The patient received this type of contact lens and reepithelialization took place under the lens. However, melting of the corneal stroma was seen and the patient was treated with a conjunctival flap. Another patient has neurotropic keratitis with involvement of fifth and seventh cranial nerves and developed a superimposed bacterial infection. The infection was treated without any permanent damage to the cornea, but the lens was discontinued. From the time the lens is first inserted the patient starts experiencing a significant relief of pain. As a rule, within 12 to 24 hours after beginning of therapy, appreciable subjective relief of pain was experienced by the patient. Within 24 to 72 hours, almost total relief of pain was obtained.

Healing varied according to the cause. After removal of the epikeratoprosthesis, application of the bandage lens resulted in healing in an average of 3 days. After herpes zoster or metaherpetic erosions, healing usually took place in about a week to 10 days. Cases of neuroparalytic keratitis and ocular pemphigus in some cases took over 2 weeks to completely reepithelialize. Most of the other conditions reepithelialized entirely within 4 to 7 days.

Complications during this study were limited to superimposed bacterial infec-

Table 26-2. Epithelial erosion syndrome

Cause	Total number of patients	Results		Lenses		Recurrences (after lenses were discontinued)	Complications
		Healed	Not healed	On	Off		
After removal of epikeratoprosthesis	6	6	0	5	1	None	Stromal infiltrates
After use of graft	2	2	0	1	1	None	None
After herpes zoster	1	1	0	0	1	None	None
After herpes simplex (metaherpetic)	3	3	0	0	3	None	None
Neuroparalytic keratitis (fifth and seventh cranial nerves)	3	2	1	2	1	None	Bacterial corneal ulcer
Corneal insensitivity (fifth cranial nerve)	2	2	0	2	0	—	Bacterial corneal ulcer
Bullous keratopathy	3	3	0	3	0	—	None
Chemical	3	2	1	2	1	None	None
Keratitis sicca	3	3	0	2	1	One	Marginal ulcers
Stevens-Johnson syndrome							
Keratinization	2	2	0	2	0	—	None
Scarring and trichiasis	2	2	0	2	0	—	None
Ocular pemphigus	4	4	0	4	0	—	None
Heat	1	1	0	0	1	None	None

tions, which occurred before we realized the importance of good lid hygiene for the prevention of infection, particularly in cases of neuroparalytic keratitis, keratitis sicca, and essential shrinkage of the conjunctiva. Staphylococcal blepharitis was extremely common in our patients and its management was essential to good results. Small aseptic stromal infiltrates were frequently seen under the glued-on lenses. In one case of bullous keratopathy, after the removal of the epikeratoprosthesis and the application of the bandage lenses a similar infiltrate was seen. This patient was treated with antibiotics. Mild epithelial edema was seen during this study in a few patients. However, they usually disappeared spontaneously.

The mechanism for the failure of a corneal ulcer to reepithelialize seems to be a deficiency in the adhesion of the corneal epithelium to its base because of the damage to the base and stromal edema. Normally, the epithelium is attached to Bowman's membrane with submicroscopic cellular bridges (desmosomes), visible in the electromicroscope.

The therapeutic effect of the Griffin bandage lenses in the treatment of this condition is unique. First, it not only protects the healing epithelium from the mechanical trauma of the of the upper lids, but also has a tendency to maintain the ingrowing epithelium in contact with the underlying tissue. Second, it results in almost immediate relief of pain, eliminating the harmful effects of lacrimation and rubbing. Finally, it seems to prevent or decrease recurrence of this condition.

It is very important to realize that marked iritis usually accompanies cases of recurrent erosion syndrome. Therefore, ciliary spasm should be treated with dilating drops. Atropine 1% twice a day has been used in our patients. Swelling of the eyelids and dermatitis from epiphora is a frequent finding in these patients. Corticosteroid ointments have been used on the skin of the eyelids in these conditions. Cases with a significant amount of stromal edema have been treated with diluted dexamethasone (Decadron) 0.005% over the lenses and antibiotics have also been used in cases with possible infection.

Summary

A simple but effective technique for the treatment of ulcers that do not heal is presented. The Griffin soft plastic contact lens have been used as a corneal bandage in 34 patients with this condition, resulting in relief of pain in all cases and reepithelialization in 32 cases.

This study was supported in part by USPHS grants EY-52868 (Gasset), EY-00446, and EY-00266 from the National Eye Institute and RR-82 from the General Clinical Research Centers Programs of the Division of Research Resources, National Institutes of Health.

REFERENCES

1. Zucker, B. B.: Hydration and transparency of corneal stroma, Arch. Ophthal. 75:228, 1966.
2. Kaufman, E. K., and Gasset, A. R.: Clinical experience with the epikeratoprosthesis, Amer. J. Ophthal. 67(1): 38-45, Jan. 1969.
3. Waltman, S. R., and Kaufman, H. E.: Use of hydrophilic contact lenses to increase ocular penetration of topical drugs, Invest. Ophthal. 9:250-255, 1970.

Chapter 27

Treatment of the alkali-burned cornea with soft contact lenses

Stuart I. Brown, M.D., Michael P. Tragakis, M.D., and David B. Pearce, M.D.

Recent studies have proved that ulcers and perforations of the alkali-burned rabbit cornea are the result of a collagenolytic enzyme produced by the cornea. Part of the proof that these perforations were caused by collagenase was that known in vitro collagenase inhibitors prevented the usually inevitable development of perforations in the totally burned cornea. Apparently when the cornea is exposed to alkali, all the cells of the cornea, as well as the majority of its ground substance, are immediately destroyed. After 7 to 10 days, regrowing epithelium and invading stromal inflammatory cells produce collagenase. This is the danger period when collagenase inhibitors must be initiated to prevent corneal ulcers. It is necessary to continue the use of the inhibitors until the epithelium has completely covered the alkali-burned cornea. At that time significant collagenase production by the epithelium stops and it is unlikely that these burns will ulcerate.

During the past 3 years we have treated several cases of alkali-burned corneas (65 eyes). From these only severely totally burned eyes were chosen to receive collagenase-inhibitor therapy. In all of these cases (33 eyes) the cornea and surrounding sclera were burned, and the corneas were opaque and completely denuded of epithelium. Therapy consisted of three drops of the collagenase inhibitor (cysteine 0.25 M.) applied topically six times a day. Of 33 total burns treated, 30 healed without ulcers, two developed shallow ulcers that later reepithelialized, and one became perforated during a break in the regimen when cysteine was unobtainable. There was a small control series when five of eight total burned corneas not treated with cysteine became perforated.

In 15 of these 33 total burns, soft lenses (Griffin bandage lens) was used in addition to cysteine. These eyes healed an average of 4½ months after the alkaliburn. Eyes treated with cysteine but without the lenses healed an average of 5½ months after the burns. This difference in the healing rate may not be significant, since in six of the 15 eyes the lenses had to be removed because progressing symblepharon or progressing conjunctival overgrowth did not permit proper approximation of the lenses to the eye. This indicated that the soft lenses do not prevent progressing symblepharon or progressing conjunctival overgrowth of the cornea.

The lenses, however, were shown to be of unquestionable value in promoting corneal epithelialization when it was slowed by either trichiasis, incomplete lid

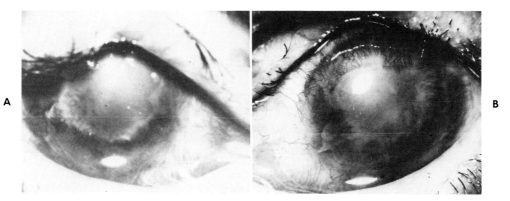

Fig. 27-1. A, Severely burned eye before bandage lens therapy; **B,** After bandage lens therapy.

closure, or reduced tears (Fig. 27-1). It also proved valuable in improving vision just enough to allow these patients to move around their wards unaided. Finally, the treatment of the totally burned cornea with the soft lens relieves the need for constant patching until the eyes are completely healed, which may take up to 14 or 15 months. Presently, we fit soft lenses to every totally alkali-burned eye when the reduction of chemosis permits the contact lens to fit properly.

Seven alkali-burned eyes were treated after they developed ulcers. The progress of the ulceration stopped immediately after treatment with cysteine and all eventually healed. Five of these latter corneas had only partial burns.

Partial burns, if treated with topical antibiotics and patching until the epithelium heals will rarely ulcerate. However, ulcers can occur if these eyes are not carefully patched and are most likely to occur if the partial burn is also associated with the burn of the adjacent limbus and sclera, with total necrosis of the overlying conjunctiva. In addition, ulcerations in partially burned corneas frequently occur after the cornea has healed. Repeated epithelial erosions are common in these eyes and, if not treated immediately, go on to form stromal ulcers. We have found that the soft contact lens quickly heals this type of ulcer and keeps them free of recurrent erosions. The lens must be worn for a minimum of 6 weeks after healing of the epithelium to prevent further episodes of epithelial erosions.

Soft lenses were also used to treat other types of ulcers caused by other types of burns of the eye, such as mustard-gas and tear-gas burns. Such ulcers have healed rapidly and have been maintained free of further episodes of epithelial erosions or ulcers.

CORNEAL TRANSPLANTATION IN THE ALKALI-BURNED CORNEA

As previously mentioned, over 95% of the total burned eyes treated with cysteine will heal. However, these eyes are essentially blind because of dense corneal opacifications. Attempts at visual rehabilitation of the alkali-burned eyes by corneal transplantation has generally failed because the grafts heal poorly and almost invariably become opaque. Recently, we have performed corneal transplants in

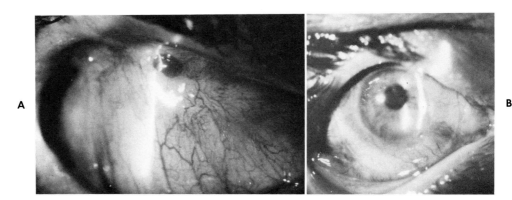

Fig. 27-2. A, Severe alkali-burned eye before keratoplasty; **B,** Corneal graft epithelium is protected by a bandage lens.

13 severely alkali-burned eyes. Twelve had total conjunctival overgrowth and one had a corneal perforation. Six of the 13 eyes had symblepharon of one or both lids to the cornea. Eight of the 13 grafts have remained clear some 12 to 36 months postoperatively. The surgical technique utilized was rather extensive, involving resection of the conjunctival overgrowth, excision of all subconjunctival connective tissue, recession of the conjunctiva, repair of the symblepharon by flaps of the host conjunctiva and corneal transplantation. In six of the eyes cataract extraction was also performed. This was accomplished in one operative procedure.

In the first eight eyes, the donor epithelium was removed from the donor corneas. In four of these eyes, the host epithelium quickly grew over the donor graft, which healed and remained transparent. However, in the remaining four eyes, despite treatment with cysteine and the soft lens, the host epithelium never completely covered the wounds, which did not heal, and the corneas became opaque. These results indicated that an intact eipthelium was essential for the grafts to remain transparent. Consequently, the donor epithelium was left on the grafts in the last five eyes. The donor epithelium not only remained on the grafts but bridged the wound to meet the host epithelium progressing from the recessed conjunctiva. These corneal grafts healed and remained transparent. The authors found that in order for the epithelium to remain on all the grafts they had to be protected with the soft contact lens (Fig. 27-2). Without these lenses, there were repeated epithelial erosions followed by superficial vascularization and eventual opacification. With the soft contact lens, the epithelial erosions were prevented (lenses had to be changed frequently within the first 4 months after the surgery to maintain the necessary proximity to the cornea).

In summary, the collagenase-inhibitor cysteine with bandage lens therapy seems to offer an improved treatment for severely alkali-burned eyes.

This study was supported in part by USPHS grant EY-00502 from the National Eye Institute.

Chapter 28

Pilocarpine delivery with soft contact lenses

Steven M. Podos, M.D., Bernard Becker, M.D., and Jack Hartstein, M.D.

The ability of soft contact lenses to imbibe great quantities of fluid has led to therapeutic implications regarding concomitant topical drug use. Topical preparations utilized with soft contact lenses must be sterile solutions free of potentially toxic preservatives. The Griffin Bionite lens, presoaked in fluorescein, has been found to produce greater ocular penetration of fluorescein than the administration of drops.[1] Drops of 1% pilocarpine instilled in human eyes wearing a Bionite lens provoked greater miosis than did 8% pilocarpine drops alone.[2] An enhanced effect of pilocarpine on intraocular pressure was noted in a few patients when utilized with soft contact lenses.

In vitro pilocarpine uptake by soft contact lenses was five times greater for Bionite than for Soflens (Bausch & Lomb) lenses of average size (Table 28-1). Although the Soflens is a smaller lens, a significant difference in uptake existed per milligram of lens substance, and these two polymers of 2-hydroxyethylmethacrylate have been shown to be structurally dissimilar.

In a prior report pilocarpine therapy with the Bionite lens was studied.[3] The amount of pilocarpine uptake varied with the concentration of soaking solution and duration of immersion. Efflux of pilocarpine from the soft lens was rapid in vitro and in vivo, approximating a half-life of 30 minutes. Essentially all pilocarpine had left presoaked lenses after 4 hours of either elution into water or eye wear. In 10 ocular hypertensive patients, mean intraocular pressure was significantly diminished during the 23 hours that pilocarpine-presoaked lenses (0.5% pilocarpine for 2 minutes) were worn. Pilocarpine 0.5% drops given three times a day alone or over a soft lens in these same eyes had little effect on intraocular pressure. After it was demonstrated that pilocarpine left the lens during the first few hours of wear, shorter wearing times were employed. Diurnal reduction of intraocular pressure was produced by wearing a Bionite lens for at least 30 minutes that had been previously soaked for 2 minutes in 1% pilocarpine.

To date, pilocarpine delivery by means of soft contact lenses has been attempted clinically in 16 patients with open-angle glaucoma. Many of the patients in this series had primary open-angle glaucoma that was not controlled satisfactorily despite treatment with strong and weak miotics, epinephrine, and carbonic

Supported by USPHS Grants EY00004 and EY00336 from the National Eye Institute.

THERAPEUTIC USES

anhydrase inhibitors. Others had intolerable side effects attributable to one or more of the drugs. All of these patients were hospitalized for diurnal measurements of intraocular pressure while the most efficacious therapeutic regimen was sought. Special sterile solutions without preservatives were used. Baseline values were obtained. Bionite lenses were presoaked in lower concentrations of pilocar-

Table 28-1. In vitro pilocarpine uptake*

Pilocarpine concentration (%)	Soak time* (min.)	Mean pilocarpine (5 lenses)	
		Soflens (mg.)	Bionite (mg.)
0.5	2	0.07	0.40
0.5	10	0.15	0.94
1	2	0.20	1.07
1	10	0.26	1.51

*Soaked in 12 drops of pilocarpine by immersing lens in designated percent solution for listed soak times.

Table 28-2. Treatment of open-angle glaucoma with Bionite soft contact lenses presoaked for 2 minutes in 1% pilocarpine

Patient	Regimen	Diurnal intraocular pressure (mm. Hg)
1	Pilocarpine 4%, epinephrine 2%, dichlorphenamide (Daranide)	20-30
	Lens soaked q.24h. and worn 30 minutes	20-42
2	Pilocarpine 4%, epinephrine 2%, acetazolamide (Diamox)	15-32
	Lens soaked q.24h. and worn 30 minutes	16-36
	Lens soaked q.12h. and worn 1 hour	16-23
3	None	24-38
	Pilocarpine 4%, epinephrine 2%	14-32
	Lens soaked q.24h. and worn 30 minutes	19-26
	Lens soaked q.12h. and worn 1 hour	16-22

Table 28-3. Therapy of bullous keratopathy and secondary glaucoma with Bionite lens presoaked for 2 minutes in 1% pilocarpine

Regimen	Intraocular pressure (mm. Hg)	Condition
Pilocarpine or echothiophate, epinephrine, methazolamide, and prednisolone 1% t.i.d.	22-48	20/70 to 20/400 Uncomfortable
Lens soaked b.i.d. and worn while awake; prednisolone 1% at bedtime	20-22	20/50 to 20/60 Comfortable

pine for 2 minutes and inserted once a day for 30 minutes to 1 hour. If this treatment failed, higher percentage solutions and longer or more frequent insertions were attempted.

The soft contact lens mode of therapy has been found to be helpful in approximately half of these patients. However, others could not manipulate the lens without tearing it, a few complained of pilocarpine side effects, and in six satisfactory intraocular pressure control could not be attained.

It became obvious early that this new technique was no panacea; it could not effectively replace maximal medical therapy (Table 28-2). For example, one patient had higher diurnal intraocular pressures while using a 1% pilocarpine–soaked soft lens once a day than while on multiple medications. A second patient had an eye with severe field loss and uncontrolled pressure on pilocarpine, epinephrine, and acetazolamide, too. However, a soft contact lens presoaked for 2 minutes in 1% pilocarpine twice a day and inserted for 1 hour each time, in addition to the acetazolamide given orally, produced good diurnal intraocular pressure control. The utilization of soft lens therapy obviated the need for filtering surgery. A third illustrative case demonstrated that a twice-a-day presoaked lens regimen could promote intraocular pressure control not obtained by weak miotics and epinephrine. Thus a patient who previously had developed toxic manifestations secondary to acetazolamide could be controlled without using a carbonic anhydrase inhibitor.

Finally, the case described in Table 28-3 demonstrated how a soft contact lens can provide dual therapeutic success. Bullous keratopathy and labile glaucoma had resulted in field loss, poor vision, and 2 years of discomfort despite sundry medications. A Bionite lens soaked for 2 minutes in 1% pilocarpine twice a day and worn during waking hours led to remarkable improvement of all parameters.

Drug effects of greater magnitude and duration may be achieved by using a soft contact lens reservoir. There is evidence that the Bionite material binds pilocarpine. Yet, large doses of pilocarpine are being pulsed into the eye in a relatively short time period. The potential toxic effect of such administration is unknown. Alterations of the polymer, enabling slower release, would seem desirable in order to deliver drugs evenly over longer time periods. Moreover, ocular inserts of other sizes or shapes may be more efficient or better tolerated. The present experimental nature of glaucoma drug delivery by soft contact lenses is to be emphasized.

This study was supported in part by USPHS grants EY-00004 and EY-00336 from the National Eye Institute.

REFERENCES

1. Waltman, S. R., and Kaufman, H. E.: Use of hydrophilic contact lenses to increase ocular penetration of topical drugs, Invest. Ophthal. 9:250-255, 1970.
2. Kaufman, H. E., Uotila, M. H., Gasset, A. R., Wood, T. O., and Ellison, E. D.: The medical uses of soft contact lenses, Trans. Amer. Acad. Ophthal. Otolaryng. 75:361-373, 1971.
3. Podos, S. M., Becker, B., Asseff, C., and Hartstein, J.: Pilocarpine therapy with soft contact lenses, Amer. J. Ophthal. 73:336-341, 1972.

PART VII

Cleaning and storage

Chapter 29

A new hygienic regimen for gel lenses

Russell E. Phares, Jr., Ph.D.

FACTORS FOR CARE AND EVALUATION

Many papers have appeared in the literature over the last few years dealing with the therapeutic and cosmetic uses of gel lenses.[1-5] Most of these papers describe procedures of hygenically caring for the lenses and often point out that there are shortcomings in the patient-care procedures. The statement has frequently been made that one of the biggest disadvantages of hydrophilic lenses is the lack of a reliable, convenient, and practical method of lens care. This study was undertaken to determine what is needed for proper lens care and to critically evaluate a new hygienic regimen.

The following major factors must be considered:
Dimensional stability of lenses
Absorptive properties of lenses
Prolongation of drug contact by lenses
Lens porosity
Dilution of system by water absorbed in lenses
Physiological compatibility of the care system
Safety of the care system

Dimensional stability of lenses

To date, all common hydrophilic lenses are principally composed of 2-hydroxyethylmethacrylate (HEMA), which has been cross-linked to varying degrees. Some of the lenses contain other additives in small quantities such as polyvinylpyrrolidone (PVP). Depending on the amount of cross-linking and the amount and type of additives, the dimensions of a hydrophilic lens can be influenced by such factors as pH, tonicity, and molecular or ionic species. The actual percentage change in dimension of the lens depends on the original size and shape of the lens. One way of comparing the effect of various solutions independent of the original dimensions of the lens is to look at the percent hydration of the lens. Table 29-1 shows the effect of several media on the percent hydration of some experimental lenses.

Adsorptive properties of lenses

The ability of hydrophilic lenses to adsorb or concentrate chemicals has been discussed several times in the literature.[6,7] This phenomenon plays a significant role in determining the choice of chemicals that can be used in lens care. Ger-

Table 29-1. Media effect on gel lens hydration

Media	Percentage of hydration
Isotonic saline (25° C.)	38.6
Isotonic saline (50° C.)	40.8
Distilled water	41.7
pH 8.0	42.9
pH 7.4	42.9
pH 6.5	37.5
Isotonic glycerin	40.4

Table 29-2. Binding to hydrophilic lenses*

Chemical	Maximum amount bound per lens (mg.)	Concentration of solution to cause 50% of maximum binding (mg./ml.)
Benzalkonium chloride		
Lens A	4.1	0.405
Lens B	3.8	0.79
Chlorobutanol	1.8	2.48
Phenylethyl alcohol	0.3-0.4	2
Benzyl alcohol	0.3-0.4	2
Methyl paraben	0.67	0.2
Propyl paraben	0.27	0.008
Phenylmercuric acetate	0.25	0.76

*From Phares, R. E., Jr.: Pharmaceutical aspects of soft contact lenses. Presented at the Eleventh Annual Instructional Course in Contact Lens Fitting by the Ophthalmologist, New Orleans, Louisiana, The Rudolph Ellender Medical Foundation, Inc., New Orleans, Louisiana.

micidal agents are chemicals that are toxic to bacterial cells but can normally be used at concentrations low enough to be nontoxic to the eye. If significant amounts of germicide is adsorbed at the microbiologically effective concentration, its use with gel lenses might result in toxic amounts of the chemical being transferred to the eye from the lens. Examples of adsorption of chemical preservatives by gel lenses are presented in Table 29-2.[6] The problem can be minimized by selecting, if possible, preservatives that are not adsorbed or by selecting compounds that are effective against bacteria at very low concentrations and yet remain harmless to the eye even if they are greatly concentrated. Compounds of the latter type might be harmless to the eye, even if some degree of adsorption occurs. A third approach would be to potentiate very low concentrations of preservative with a nontoxic ingredient. This approach might permit low enough concentrations of preservative to be used so that the amount of adsorption would either be negligible or at least safe.

Prolongation of drug contact

Another interesting property of gel lenses is their ability to prolong the contact time between drugs and the cornea. There have been at least two examples of this reported in the literature.[8] From a therapeutic point of view, this could be desirable, but when designing sterilizing solutions for the hydrophilic lens, it can be a source of trouble. Some antibacterial agents such as thimerosal are very slow in action and must be in contact with cells for a long time to be toxic. This slowness can be an advantage since the compound would normally only be in contact with ocular tissues for a short time and therefore have little chance to cause damage. Of course, this slowness in action means that a long time is needed to achieve resterilization of the lens. Such antibacterial agents, which under normal conditions of usage might be considered harmless to the eye, could be potentially damaging or irritating if gel lenses prolonged their contact time with the cornea. Attempts have been made to minimize the irritation caused from increased contact by reducing the concentration of preservatives, for example, from 0.004% to 0.001%. This can help minimize irritation, but it also reduces the antibacterial effectiveness of the system. The problem of prolonged contact can be even more serious in the case of sensitizing compounds such as hexachlorophene and thimerosal.

Lens porosity

There have been numerous articles in the lay press suggesting that bacteria can penetrate the pores of hydrophilic lenses. It is true that gel lenses are porous as is evidenced by the fact that gases and solutions can diffuse through them. One must, however, keep in mind the tremendous difference between the size of molecules such as oxygen, water, and common salts and the size of bacteria. The smallest bacteria are approximately 700 times bigger in diameter than an oxygen molecule. It is generally accepted that bacteria cannot get through pores or holes smaller than 0.22 microns in diameter. Spencer and others[9] examined gel lenses by using a scanning electron microscope at magnifications of 15,000 and 36,000 and could not see any pores. Although the hazard of bacteria invading the pores of lenses might be overemphasized, the porosity of lenses can indirectly increase the chances of microbiological problems. Various components of the tears can be absorbed into the lens through the pores and then serve as a reservoir of nutrient materials, which can be utilized by surface bacteria.

Dilution of system

On the average, hydrophilic lenses contain about 50% water. During wearing, the water is replaced with tears and the various components dissolved in the tears. For optimum comfort, cleanliness, visual acuity, and lens life, these materials should be removed from the lens periodically. This material enters the lens through a slow process of diffusion and must leave the lens by the same mechanism. The speed of the diffusion processes depends on the concentration gradient between the components absorbed in the lens and the solution the lens is soaking in. For material to diffuse out of the lens at a rapid rate, a large concentration gradient should be maintained. This is best accomplished by placing the lens in a volume of soaking solution that is large compared to the volume of water absorbed within the lens. If the bathing solution contains a germicidal agent, this material will diffuse into the lens during soaking. By the use of an adequate volume of soaking solution, the amount of germicide lost by diffusion into the lens is negligible. Diffusion processes take place slowly in viscous liquids, therefore water-thin solutions are preferable for soaking lenses.

Physiological compatibility of the care system

The interrelationship between the hygenic care system and the eye has already been briefly touched upon. Although the physical properties of the lens are important in designing a solution for hydrophilic lenses, the well-being of the eye must be the ultimate consideration. A great deal of care must be given to making the system as physiologically compatible as possible, such factors as tonicity, pH, purity of ingredients, and sensitizing potential of the ingredients must be considered.

Safety of the system

There are several safety factors to be considered in developing a hydrophilic lens care regimen. One of the most obvious and most important facts is the safety of the solutions in the eye. The factors that can modify and affect the safety of the solutions have already been discussed. Another very important aspect of the safety of the solution relates to its ability to perform effectively. The real test of how safe and effective a solution is only comes when the system has been challenged by pathogenic organisms. As long as no problems arise, any solution or lens care program can appear to be safe. A third and most subtle consideration of safety is the ease or simplicity of caring for the lens. Some procedures are safe and effective when followed correctly but become unsafe because of their complexity. The more complicated a procedure, the greater the chances of making errors and therefore the more unsafe the procedure. The ideal lens care system would employ only one solution that would be changed daily.

PROCEDURE

A new lens care regimen that involves a single solution was evaluated. The solution, an investigational drug known as Hexaphen,* contained 0.005% chlorhexidine in a vehicle specially designed to prevent dimensional changes in hydrophilic lenses and to offer maximum patient comfort. The regimen is as follows: After successfully wearing the lens all day, one removes it in the prescribed manner and cleans as directed, using the new solution. A convenient method of cleaning is to place the lens in the palm of the hand, cover it with solution, and then rub it briskly with the finger of the other hand. After cleaning, the excess solution is shaken off and the lens is placed in a suitable storage container, which is then filled with a minimum of 5 ml. of the new solution per lens. Ideally, the lens should float freely in the container so that the solution can have free access to all surfaces of the lens. After overnight storage, the lenses are removed, cleaned once again in the palm of the hand, and then placed directly onto the eye without rinsing.

---

*Barnes-Hind Pharmaceuticals, Inc., Sunnyvale, Calif.

Table 29-3. Corneal effect from lenses soaked in special solution

Percent concentration of chlorhexidine	Soaking time (hours)	Number of eyes	Results	
			Soflens	Bionite
0.004	1	4	−	−
0.004	3	4	−	−
0.004	24	14	−	−
0.005	3	4	−	−
0.005	24	8	−	−
0.01	1	4	−	−
0.01	3	4	−	+
0.01	24	10	−	+

The sign "−" means no corneal staining; "+" means very slight corneal staining.

PHARMACOLOGY

All pharmacological studies for evaluating lens-solution compatibility were conducted on healthy albino rabbits weighing 2.5 to 3 kg. Only animals without eye defects as determined from a thorough eye examination, fluorescein staining, and slit lamp observations were used. Bausch & Lomb's Soflens and Griffin's Naturalens were used in these experiments. Each lens was cleaned and treated according to the manufacturers' recommendations prior to use. In the first series of experiments, the lenses were soaked for 1, 3, and 24 hours in the new formulation containing 0.004%, 0.005%, or 0.01% chlorhexidine. Each lens was soaked in 10 ml. of the approximate test solution. After the prescribed soaking time, the lenses were removed from the solutions and placed directly on rabbits' eyes for a period of 3 to 5 hours. After the wearing period, the lenses were removed and the eyes were examined grossly and with sodium fluorescein and ultraviolet illumination for signs of corneal staining. Table 29-3 shows the results of these studies.

The next study involved a simulated long-term wearing study on rabbits. Animals were selected as for the previous experiment and wore lenses from 7 to 7½ hours a day for 21 days. During this time the same regimen of lens care was followed as previously described for humans. Both Bausch & Lomb and Griffin lenses were involved in this study and both lenses and eyes were examined frequently for any unusual signs. At no time either during or after the experiment was there any difference between the control eyes and those eyes wearing lenses. There were no apparent changes in the physical or chemical nature of the lenses. Their power and dimensions remained constant.

MICROBIOLOGY

One of the biggest challenges in developing a solution for the hygenic care of soft lenses is formulating a product that can be microbiologically effective and yet be well tolerated in the eye. The next series of experiments were conducted to determine if the new physiologically acceptable solution that was developed could in fact effectively kill pathogenic organisms. Only the formulation containing

Table 29-4. Kill rate of the special solution with 0.005% chlorhexidine

Time	Plate counts			
	I	II	III	IV
zero	10	4000	TNTC*	3880
5 min.	0	20	510	—
10 min.	0	5	10	—
15 min.	0	0	—	—
30 min.	0	0	0	—
1 hr.	0	0	0	190
2 hr.	0	0	0	15
4 hr.	—	0	0	0
6 hr.	—	0	0	0
7 hr.	—	—	—	0
24 hr.	—	0	0	0

I, *Pseudomonas aeruginosa* #9027, 6.3 × 10^5/ml.
II, *Pseudomonas aeruginosa* #661322, 1.2 × 10^6 ml.
III, *Escherichia coli* #4352, 3.2 × 10^4 ml.
IV, *Staphylococcus aureus* #6538, 4.8 × 10^3 ml.
*Too numerous to count.

0.005% chlorhexidine was evaluated in these experiments. Table 29-4 shows the kill rate when the solution was contaminated with one of the following organisms: *Pseudomonas aeruginosa* (two types), *Escherichia coli,* and *Staphylococcus aureus.* Notice that in no case was more than 3 hours required to achieve resterilization and that, in most cases, about 15 minutes was adequate. In another experiment simulating overnight storage of solutions contaminated with *Pseudomonas multivorans, Klebsiella* species, or *Proteus mirabilis,* each organism was successfully killed and the solutions were sterile.

CLINICAL STUDIES

Based upon the favorable laboratory studies previously described, clinical studies were initiated throughout the United States. About 15 investigators have clinically followed 400 patients for as much as 5 months. Visual acuity tests as well as biomicroscopy examinations were performed at regular intervals on all patients. A limited number of patients were selected for microbiological testing. All tested solutions were found to be sterile throughout the study.

Slit lamp examinations were done at regular intervals throughout the study and all findings were considered normal for contact lens wearers. There was no evidence of any corneal damage or involvement. It was noticed in a few patients who had been on the new regimen for several months that a slight ocular irritation developed. This problem was found to be caused by an accumulation of mucus and other proteinaceous components of the tears that accumulated in the lens after prolonged periods of wearing. It became apparent that a deep form of cleaning is necessary to remove materials that are absorbed into the matrix of the lens. The use of a specially formulated cleaning preparation seems to alleviate and prevent this problem. Patients found the new hygienic regimen to be convenient and comfortable as long as they kept their lenses clean.

CONCLUSIONS

According to laboratory and clinical studies, it appears as if the daily hygienic care of hydrophilic lenses can be successfully handled by a specially formulated solution containing 0.005% chlorhexidine. The prescribed regimen offers the ultimate in simplicity while minimizing chances for patient error. Patient comfort is achieved without the potential fear of bacterial contamination. Clinical studies show that a periodic cleaning procedure to remove absorbed materials from within the lens might be necessary. This unique cleaning problem is a result of the spongelike nature of the lens and cannot be handled by the surface cleaning, which is carried out in the palm of the hand. Safe and effective deep cleaning methods are currently being evaluated.

REFERENCES

1. Gasset, A. R., and Kaufman, H. E.: Therapeutic uses of hydrophilic contact lenses, Amer. J. Ophthal. 69:252-259, 1970.
2. Watts, G. K.: Hydrophilic contact lenses—a review, The Optician, pp. 10-13, April 23, 1971.
3. Fisher, E.: Hydrophilic contact lenses, Canad. J. Optom. 29:139-144, 1968.
4. Kaufman, H. E., Uotila, M. H., Gasset, A. R., Wood, T. O., and Ellison, E. D.: The medical uses of soft contact lenses, Trans. Amer. Acad. Ophthal. Otolaryng. 75:361-373, 1971.
5. Alexander-Katz, W.: The importance of blinking during the fitting of soft corneal contact lenses, The Contact Lens 2(8):4-5, July 1970.
6. Phares, R. E., Jr.: Pharmaceutical aspects of soft contact lenses. Presented at the Eleventh Annual Instructional Course in Contact Lens Fitting by the Ophthalmologist, New Orleans, Louisiana. Sponsored by The Rudolph Ellender Medical Foundation, Inc., New Orleans, La.
7. Lerman, S., and Sapp, G.: The hydrophilic (Hydron) corneoscleral lens in the treatment of bullous keratopathy, Ann. Ophthal. 2:142-144, 1970.
8. Waltman, S. R., and Kaufman, H. E.: Use of hydrophilic contact lenses to increase ocular penetration of topical drugs, Invest. Ophthal. 9:250-255, 1970.
9. Spencer, W. H. Matas, B. R., and Hayes, T. L.: Scanning electron microscopy of hydrophilic contact lenses. Presented at the Association for Research in Vision and Ophthalmology meeting, University of California, San Francisco, California, August 1971.

Chapter 30

Sterilization of soft contact lenses

Stuart I. Brown, M.D., and Michael P. Tragakis, M.D.

With the recent emergence of soft contact lenses for both cosmetic and therapeutic use, there has been concern as to whether the wearing of the soft lens is
safe from a bacteriological standpoint. The present studies were designed to determine the efficacy of lens cleaning techniques presently available for removal of
microorganisms and to determine if the wearing of the lenses had any adverse
effect on the bacterial flora of the conjunctiva.

MATERIAL AND METHODS

Bacteriological studies. The soft lenses used in this portion of the study were
produced by the Griffin Laboratory and are essentially 2-hydroxyethylmethacrylate
(HEMA) and polyvinylpyrrolidone (PVP).

Lenses were incubated in a nutrient meat infusion broth containing the following organisms isolated from human infections: *Proteus vulgaris, Pseudomonas aeruginosa,
Staphylococcus aureus*, beta-hemolytic *Streptococcus* group A, and *Escherichia coli*. In
addition, other lenses were incubated for 7 days in sterile distilled water with
either *Candida albicans*, two species of *Fusarium, Penicillium, Aspergillus fumigatus*, or
A. niger. All media had colony counts from 10^5 to 10^7 per millimeter of nutrient
media. The soft lenses were then treated with three different cleaning techniques.
The first was soaking in either thimerosal 0.001%, chlorhexidine 0.005%, or a
combination of thimerosal 0.001% and chlorhexidine 0.005%. The second technique
consisted of soaking in 3% peroxide for 5 minutes, followed by a 1-minute exposure
to sodium bicarbonate in 0.9% sodium chloride, and then immersing in 0.9% sodium
chloride for 15 minutes. The third technique was boiling the lens for 15 minutes.
With the first technique, cultures were taken of the lenses and cleaning solutions
at 15 minutes, and 1, 2, 8, and 24 hours after exposure to the cleaning solutions.
Cultures of the lenses were taken immediately after the hydrogen peroxide and
the boiling techniques. After the cleaning procedures, all the lenses that had been
infected with bacteria were reincubated in nutrient broth for 14 days and cultured.

After the cleaning procedures, the lenses previously infected with fungi were
reincubated in distilled water and both the lenses and the water were cultured at
weekly intervals over a period of 1 month. The authors considered that microorganisms were killed when there was no regrowth after reincubation for 2 weeks
or more.

Clinical studies. The conjunctivae of 51 eyes that were wearing soft contact
lenses for either therapeutic or cosmetic purposes were cultured at various times

Table 30-1. Inhibition of bacterial growth by thimerosal and chlorhexidine

Bacterial species	Bacteria per milliliter	Thimerosal (0.001%)					Chlorhexidine (0.005%)					Chlorhexidine (0.005%) and thimerosal (0.001%)				
		15 min.	1 hr.	2 hr.	8 hr.	24 hr.	15 min.	1 hr.	2 hr.	8 hr.	24 hr.	15 min.	1 hr.	2 hr.	8 hr.	24 hr.
Staphylococcus	10^5	++++	++++	++	+	+	++	+	—	—	—	+	—	—	—	—
Streptococcus	10^6	++++	++++	++	++	—	++	+++	+++	+	—	++	+	—	—	—
Pseudomonas	10^6	+++	+++	++	—	—	+	—	—	—	—	+	+	—	—	—
Proteus	10^7	++	++	+++	+	—	++	++	+	—	—	++	—	+	—	—
Escherichia	10^5	+++	—	—	—	—	—	—	—	—	—	—	—	—	—	—

   —   No growth
   +   1 to 10 colonies
  ++   11 to 20 colonies
 +++   21 to 30 colonies
++++ 31 or more colonies

before and after wearing soft contact lenses. Forty-five of the eyes were wearing the Griffin lenses and six eyes wore lenses made by Bausch & Lomb. All lenses were cleaned at least once each week with either the peroxide technique, boiling, or overnight soaking in chlorhexidine. Thirty of the 51 eyes were cultured two or more times at intervals varying from 2 weeks to 3 months. Nineteen of the 51 eyes with soft lenses were being treated with topical corticosteriods or topical antibiotics or both for various types of corneal diseases. All medications were discontinued the evening before the cultures were taken.

For a control group, the conjunctivae of 50 apparently normal eyes were cultured in a similar manner. Twenty-three of the 50 eyes were cultured two or more times at intervals varying from 2 weeks to 3 months.

RESULTS

Bacteriological studies. There was no growth of any of the microorganisms tested after exposure of the contact lens to hydrogen peroxide. Cultures taken after boiling showed no growth of any microorganism except for *Aspergillus fumigatus.*

There was no growth of any of the microorganisms 8 hours after exposure to the chlorhexidine and thimerosal combination (Table 30-1). There was no growth of any microorganisms from the lenses after 24 hours exposure to chlorhexidine. However, *Proteus vulgaris* was cultured from the latter lenses after reincubation in nutrient broth for 48 hours. Chlorhexidine completely inhibited this reemergence of *Proteus vulgaris* when its concentration was reduced to 10.[5]

Exposure of the lenses to thimerosal for 24 hours completely inhibited growth of all microorganisms except *Staphylococcus.*

There was no growth of any of the fungus strains immediately after 2 hours of exposure to either thimerosal, chlorhexidine, or the combination.

With the exception of the reemergence of *Proteus vulgaris* after 24 hours in chlorhexidine, there was no reemergence of any of the bacteria or fungi in lenses that were reincubated for up to 1 month after exposure to the cleaning solutions.

Clinical studies. *Staphylococcus aureus* was the only pathogenic organism in both series. It was found in three of 80 cultures of the 50 eyes in the control series and two of the 103 cultures in 51 eyes wearing the soft lenses.

COMMENTS

The results of the first part of this study show that peroxide or a combination of thimerosal and chlorhexidine killed all the organisms tested. Chlorhexidine appeared to have killed all the organisms except *Proteus vulgaris,* which was only suppressed since it reemerged after reincubation of the lenses. When the rather high concentration of *P. vulgaris* was reduced from 10^7 to 10^5, the organism was killed. Boiling killed all of the microorganisms except for *Aspergillus fumigatus.* Thimerosal was found to be ineffective as a cleaning agent.

From a practical standpoint, the peroxide and boiling techniques are the most valuable. Their effect is immediate. This is obviously important when the lenses are dropped and need to be quickly replaced and when immediate cleaning is necessary during the fitting of more than one patient with the same lens.

In the second part of the study, pathological organisms were cultured from the conjunctivae of 4% of the control eyes. This finding is comparable to most studies of the bacterial flora of normal eyes. The presence of pathogenic organisms in 2% of the eyes wearing soft contact lenses clearly demonstrates that wearing the lenses does not introduce any pathogenic bacteria into the eye nor does it change the environment allowing the emergence of such organisms.

These studies indicate that wearing properly cleaned soft contact lenses should not promote infections of the eye. Nevertheless, infections must be expected when the lenses are used to treat diseased eyes. This is especially true with dry eyes where the lenses have had their most dramatic therapeutic effects. The dry eye has no protective mechanism; that is, the epithelial barrier is either desiccated or eroded and the cornea cannot be cleaned because of insufficient tears or inefficient blinking. In the past these severely dry eyes would loose their vision because of conjunctival overgrowth, symblepharon, corneal opacities, or corneal ulcers. Presently, with the advent of the soft lenses, vision frequently can be retained, but unless the epithelium heals and remains healed, there is a definite risk of infection.

Chapter 31

Microbiology of cleaning and storage solutions for use with Griffin lenses

Emily D. Varnell, B.S., and Herbert E. Kaufman, M.D.

Because commercially available cleaning solutions for hard lenses are not recommended for use with the soft lenses, various solutions were tested for use in cleaning and storing these lenses. Since Bausch & Lomb supplies a boiling unit for cleaning their Soflens, this report deals only with the cleaning of the Griffin soft contact lens.

Although studies in our laboratory and two others have shown that boiling the lenses in sealed glass vials killed all the organisms tested in 15 minutes and produced no apparent degradation of the lens, this procedure has not been recommended for general patient use.

We have tested three other procedures currently in use by patients. They are the use of hydrogen peroxide and two other solutions (Flexsol by Burton-Parsons and Hexaphen by Barnes-Hinds) specially formulated for use with the soft lenses.

Let us first consider the peroxide treatment. Although some question has been raised about the stability and efficacy of commercially available 3% hydrogen peroxide, all of our studies were done using Parke-Davis 3% peroxide, which the company reports has a shelf life of 5 years. Lenses were soaked in a broth culture of actively growing microorganisms containing more than 10^8 organisms per milliliter and incubated for several hours. The organisms, isolated from ocular infections in our eye clinic, included *Pseudomonas, Staphylococcus, Proteus, Candida, Aspergillus,* and *Fusarium.* Lenses were removed from the organisms, placed in 3% peroxide for varying lengths of time, and then placed in fresh broth and reincubated.

When the procedure was carried out with the old white and blue plastic case supplied by Griffin Laboratories for patient use, approximately half of the cultures remained positive even when the lenses were left in peroxide for as long as 2 hours. These cases, however, did not seal tightly and leaked, and organisms possibly entered the case from the uncleaned portions of the case after the peroxide treatment. We have repeated these tests using the new glass vials presently being supplied with the lenses and found that it is possible within 5 minutes to completely sterilize the lenses in peroxide.

Since we believed that no treatment would be able to overcome a really massive inoculum and that we should be testing a system more approximately like the patient encounters in daily use, Flexsol and Hexaphen were tested in a slightly different manner. Organisms were grown in broth cultures for 24 hours. Small amounts of microorganisms were added to the Flexsol, Hexaphen, and saline (control) solution in amounts that would approximate the contamination introduced by lenses during use. At various time intervals aliquots of the solutions were removed, mixed with thioglycollate broth to inactivate any residual thimerosal carried over from the preservative, and then were placed out on agar to enable us to count actual colonies of bacteria present.

Early studies utilizing Flexsol containing only 1:100,000 thimerosal showed that organisms could not be recovered after 2 to 10 hours in contact with the Flexsol. If, however, the solutions were allowed to remain at room temperature for 1 week, organisms could again be cultured, indicating that the preparation was bacterio-

Table 31-1. Colony counts of bacteria after incubation with solutions for use with Griffin soft contact lenses

Incubation time (hours)	Saline		Flexsol IV		Hexaphen	
	No lens	Lens	No lens	Lens	No lens	Lens
Staphylococcus aureus (7.0×10^4/0.1 ml. of original inoculum)						
1	7.0×10^2	2.7×10^3	100	40	0	0
4	4.0×10^4	5.3×10^5	0	0	0	0
6	9.1×10^5	1.9×10^6	0	0	0	0
24	2.5×10^8	1.1×10^7	0	0	0	0
Pseudomonas (3.7×10^7/0.1 ml. of original inoculum)						
1	5.8×10^2	1.3×10^3	10	0	0	0
4	7.1×10^3	4.7×10^5	0	0	0	0
6	8.1×10^3	9.5×10^6	0	0	0	0
24	2.8×10^5	1.2×10^8	0	0	0	0

Table 31-2. Growth of fungi after incubation with solutions for use with Griffin soft contact lenses

Incubation time (hours)	Saline	Flexsol IV	Hexaphen
Aspergillus niger (1.2×10^5/0.1 ml. of original)			
1	+	−	+
4	+	−	+
24	+	−	+
A. fumigatus (3.2×10^3/0.1 ml. of original)			
1	+	−	+
4	+	−	+
24	+	−	+
Fusarium (7.1×10^4/0.1 ml. of original)			
1	+	−	+
4	+	−	+
24	+	−	+

"+" means growth; "−" means no growth.

static and not bactericidal. The newer formulation designated Flexsol IV, which contains chlorhexidine gluconate and EDTA in addition to the thimerosal, does not show this reimmergence of organisms.

The following is a summary of many trials using Flexsol IV and Hexaphen (Tables 31-1 and 31-2).

Studies were done in some cases with lenses in the solution and others with no lenses present to be certain that none of the lens material inactivated the preservatives, and they revealed that the lenses had no effect.

Flexsol IV killed the organisms tested in less than 4 hours, Hexaphen killed all except the *Aspergillus niger* in less than 1 hour (it had no noticeable effect on the *Aspergillus niger*).

These studies have shown that it is possible to make the Griffin soft contact lens aseptic by either of the three methods tested. The final selection of method or combination of methods used by the patient will probably be made by a comparison of the superior cleaning of the lens with the peroxide versus the simplicity of using a single solution.

This study was supported in part by USPHS grant EY-00446 from the National Eye Institute.

SUMMARY AND DISCUSSION OF PART VII

Dr. Isen: I have personally worked on the development of hydrophilic contact lenses for about 10 years and have been boiling lenses since 1963. We have tested every available solution procedure that has come along and have tried to cooperate very closely with the various solution manufacturers. However, I am a little disturbed at the subtle way in which the competitive spirit arises at these meetings. As various companies try to "shoot each other down," a great deal of misinformation is disseminated.

Although it has been reported that the Griffin lens cannot be boiled, our studies have shown that the problems came from the containers and not the lenses themselves. We have boiled large numbers of lenses continuously for 1,000 hours with no adverse effects or changes. This was done in Type I glass containers with silicone rubber stoppers.

My data relate only to the Griffin lens. First, let me point out that the subject is complex. We are dealing not only with the properties of the lens and solutions, but also with the interaction of how their particular solution behaved with the Griffin lens. Now we have completely changed our procedure and do all of our own studies. We have studied every type of solution carefully, and I would like to share our results with you.

To begin with, let me explain the peroxide procedure. Peroxide has a reputation for being unstable. Parke-Davis hydrogen peroxide—3% is very stable (this is not true of all brands of peroxide). Parke-Davis degradation studies show that the cap can be taken off a bottle of peroxide and kept at a temperature of 117° F. for 14 days without any change in activity or strength. Parke-Davis also has data that indicate 5 years of shelf-life stability. In fact, they have data on 9 and 10 years. On the other hand, if one goes into a drugstore, buys a variety of different brands, takes them to the lab, and tests them, some of them are nothing but pure water.

Peroxide has some remarkable properties to offer the Griffin lens. First, it penetrates every aspect of the lens in 30 seconds. If a lens is set up as a filter barrier between distilled water and peroxide, peroxide can be measured on the water side in 30 seconds. It kills microorganisms very fast and we know that there is no toxicity caused by peroxide.

When the lens is placed in peroxide, it swells rapidly, expanding from 14.0 to 17.0 mm. In addition, the peroxide oxidizes any mucoprotein that exists on the surface of the lens. Simultaneously, it kills all bacteria, fungi, and viruses that may be present on the lens surface. The expansion of the lens and the later contraction has the effect of exercising the permeability.

After the peroxide is spilled out, the lens container is filled with a bicarbonate solution. This shrinks the lens rapidly, squeezing the peroxide out of the lens and into the solution where it is more easily neutralized. This bicarbonate solution is replaced with normal saline (lightly preserved) for overnight soaking, and by morning all of the peroxide is eliminated. Occasionally, an additional rinse is required in the morning to complete the cycle. The peroxide remaining in the lens can also be neutralized by using normal saline without the bicarbonate step. Additional changes in solution are required.

There are important advantages to peroxide. First, the lens surface is always clean and surface debris does not accumulate or remain adhered to the lens surface. Microorganisms are killed rapidly. The long-time effects of daily peroxide use do not harm or degrade the lens. There may be a gradual increase in lens strength and perhaps some increase in permeability. This subject needs more study.

The saline solution used is preserved with a low concentration of thimerosal to make the solution bacteriostatic. Higher concentrations used with the lens will cause ocular irritations. There is no binding of thimerosal in the lens. After a lens is soaked for quite a while in preserved saline, it accumulates 2.3 parts per million of thimerosal inside the lens and no more. If this lens is then placed on an eye, there is no thimerosal left in the lens after 2 hours.

Currently, we are studying the in-and-out movement of many of the various preservatives that are used for different medications, and the flow of the medications themselves. I wish we had enough data to present at this meeting, but we are still in the middle of these studies.

Chlorhexidine gluconate has other kinds of problems. We have some evidence to indicate that some chlorhexidine may slowly bind inside Griffin lenses and, for that matter, any hydrophilic lenses. We are not sure what the significance of such binding may be, but it certainly requires a great deal of study over a long period of time before chlorhexidine is utilized to any great extent.

The search for the perfect solution continues. As a company, we are interested in having the best procedure, one that patients will use because they receive a direct benefit from daily use. This is one of the most important aspects of peroxide that I have personally experienced. I have observed that many patients find that when they use peroxide, their lenses always stay crystal clean. Proteins don't accumulate on it, and in the evening there is never any kind of visual hazing. If these same patients do not use the procedure routinely, they begin to notice, after 4 or 5 days, hazy vision late in the evening. Thus, they develop a Pavlovian response. They know that if they clean their lenses, their vision stays perfect. This makes them stick to the regimen and not wander from it because of the direct benefit.

Much research remains to develop a perfect solution procedure. I believe everybody is working intensively on it, and that corporate goals, though important, should come second to a cooperative effort to reach the major goal.

Dr. Kaufman: I would like to summarize some of our feelings and experience.

At least the Griffin and the Bausch & Lomb lenses are impermeable to microorganisms. Their pore size is so small that we cannot get radioactive albumin, a relatively small molecule, to penetrate these lenses at all. Herpesviruses and other viruses therefore could not get into these lenses. In fact, Dohlman's group in Boston, have taken a fluorescein with a molecular weight of 800 (a molecule much smaller than any organism) and found that it can be used with lenses and does not penetrate to a significant degree. The only way microorganisms could invade these lenses is if something like fungus is in contact with the lens long enough to digest its way into the lens (Fig. D-1). This happens to be a Griffin lens, but I have observed fungus in Bausch & Lomb and other lenses. However, such fungal invasion while the lens is actually in use seems highly unlikely if it is sterilized daily.

MICROBIOLOGY OF CLEANING AND STORAGE SOLUTIONS

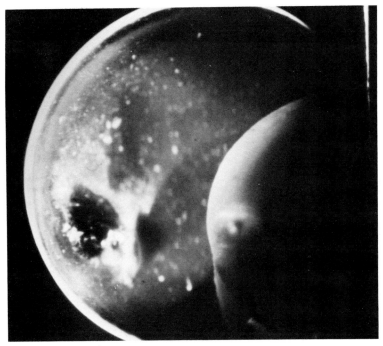

Fig. D-1. Fungal invasion of a Griffin lens.

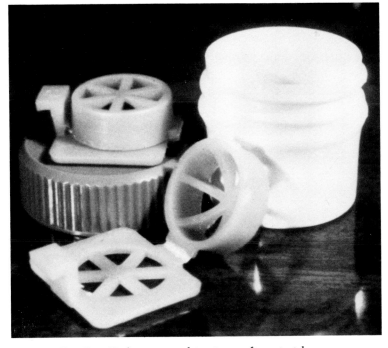

Fig. D-2. Early case used to store soft contact lenses.

Second, I think it is very important to emphasize that sterility is *more* than just solutions. Sterility is a case, the solution, and the lenses.

For example, if you push on the top of one of the early cases that some people used to store sterilized lenses (Fig. D-2), it acts like a diaphragm and sucks solution and microorganisms in from outside. It is really very difficult if not impossible to get lenses reliably sterile in this case. There was another popular case that had a rubber washer in the top, which could get debris and dirt under it, and it was also impossible to get that case reliably sterile. If you hear someone say, "I tried X solution and I couldn't get the lenses sterile," it suddenly becomes very important to know what kind of case he used.

For several reasons, we prefer glass vials (Fig. D-3) for soft lens storage. First, with glass vials and their impermeable plastic stoppers, it is very easy to sterilize the lenses with a variety of different solutions. Second, these vials are too small for patients to put their fingers inside. We found that when patients, especially economy-minded college students, can stick their fingers into the case, they remove the lenses and keep using the solution, with "essence of finger" added, over and over again. With the vials, they have to empty the solution to get the lens out, thus preventing the reuse of possible contaminated solutions. You must consider the type of case used when evaluating any reports on solutions.

In terms of asepsis, we have used peroxide for many years and have some experience with boiling. Although the three-step peroxide method is a nuisance in some ways, we have never seen any corneal damage from it. Boiling, although

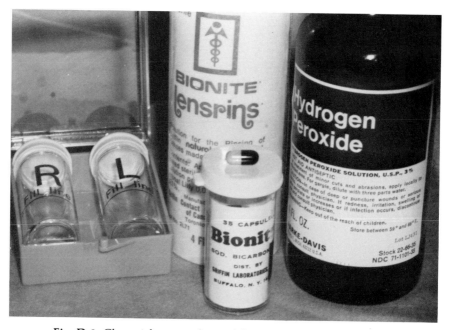

Fig. D-3. Glass vials currently used for soft contact lens storage.

effective, is also rather cumbersome. It would be nice if there were a one-step solution as effective as these methods.

I think we have to realize that the problems faced with soft lenses (Bausch & Lomb and Griffin) are really not a great deal different from those with hard lenses; that is, you have to worry about "bugs" on the lens surface. Are such organisms better able to hang onto the surface of soft lenses? There is no good evidence that this is the case.

Previous studies with hard lenses indicate that dry hard lenses are contaminated in from 65% to 100% of the cases. Wet hard lenses are also very frequently contaminated as ordinarily used. The point is that from a practical point of view, this is like sterilizing the fork before you use it. The eye, like the mouth, is a mucous membrane that is open to the outside. In fact, up to 25% of our eyes at random will have bacteria in them that could be considered pathogenic. Furthermore, if you are negative for *Staphylococcus* today, your odds are 25% that you will be positive tomorrow morning, or vice versa. Fortunately, the body handles superficial bacteria very well in the absence of injury if massive overgrowth does not occur.

The hygienic methods recommended for soft lenses, are probably superior to what is now available for hard lenses. Whatever standards are adopted for soft contact lenses should also be applied to hard contact lenses. Since the problems (surface contamination) are in effect the same, an evaluation of the existing hard lens solutions as ordinarily used and a comparison with soft lenses should be done, especially since with soft lenses there is less likelihood of epithelial damage, which is so common with hard lenses.

The most important point is that regardless of the theoretical problems associated with soft lenses, their safety has been established by clinical experience.

In summary, then, the risk of infection from soft contact lenses is, from a practical point of view, almost nonexistent in normal eyes and small in diseased eyes.

Dr. Rockert: I would like to report some experience we have had in Germany. We started fitting soft lenses at the end of 1970 and have since fitted about 20,000. We used several kinds of sterilization and have not seen one lens-related corneal disease. We observed lenses with an electron microscope to check for internal contamination and found none. We feel that the only problem is surface contamination, which seems to be handled adequately by present cleaning methods.

In essence, we would encourage you to continue fitting soft contact lenses as we plan to do.

Dr. Gasset: I would like to talk about peroxide sterilization, but because I developed this method and it is too close to my heart, I would like to call on several other people to give an unprepared, unrehearsed, 2-minute presentation on the methods they like and solutions they use.

Dr. Arias: We are using three methods (Flexsol, Hexaphen, and peroxide) to varying degrees. Some patients report stinging, burning sensations, and a haziness in vision with Flexsol. With Hexaphen, we noticed a drying of the lens and some patients are more susceptible to drying than are others. There was no fogging effect, but the lens did seem to dry and stick to the upper lid. We are very grateful to Barnes-Hind and Burton, Parsons for manufacturing these solutions, and we are using them when possible, giving the companies the feedback, and hoping that improvements or modifications will make them more acceptable. To date, however, the solution that works best with our patients is the peroxide regimen. In this procedure, we do insist that patients rinse the lenses several times with fresh saline solution before they insert them or store them overnight.

Dr. Moss: The procedure we now use in our office is to use Hexaphen or Flexsol solution and require that our patients use the peroxide cycle a minimum of 2 times weekly to ensure lens sterility. However, as Dr. Kaufman and Dr. Isen pointed out, patients seem to find their own level of using the peroxide cycle. In spite of my twice weekly instructions, they come in and say, "Well, my lenses got a little bit hazy; so I simply put them through the peroxide cycle, and they were perfectly clear again."

Dr. Arias: I found the same thing as Dr. Moss, but I don't let them do it when they wish. I feel daily peroxide sterilization is safer and find that this helps ensure maximum clarity of vision with the lenses.

Dr. Friedberg: My experience with the solutions is very similar to what was just reported. Contamination factors relative to Hexaphen, Flexsol, or hydrogen peroxide have been nonexistent in the years that I have been working with the soft lens. However, when we see a patient after a month or so or when a patient reports problems with smoky vision, we always have him go through the hydrogen peroxide procedure regardless of the type of solution he is using.

Dr. Katzin: We have had similar experience. From 400 or 500 lenses dispensed through our office, there were about a half a dozen cases of red eyes, and these were mostly mechanical. We did have one case of an invasion cornea in a patient who had a previous history of this. Routinely we used the hydrogen peroxide cycle every third day and soaked lenses in Flexsol I in the meantime. There have been no problems with this routine.

Dr. Black: Once upon a time a fellow came into my office and showed me some lenses Dr. Isen was making. In explaining the program, he took a bottle of wetting solution and said, "When you want to clean these lenses, just rub the front surface of the lens with a cleaning, wetting, or soaking solution."

With all the problems encountered cleaning Bausch & Lomb lenses, I often wondered what happened to that idea. Eventually I took that old idea and instructed my patients who seem to get dirty lenses to use Soaklens to clean their lenses. Soaklens was chosen because data suggest that its preservative thimerosal, is not picked up by the lens as much as other chemicals. In many cases, I think we should have included this method in the protocol for the Bausch & Lomb study. The daily use of this method before the lenses are boiled could well have prevented the problems with protein deposits.

Let me stress, however, the difference between washing the lens and soaking it. Soaking creates problems in that you can pick up the preservatives. On the other hand, cleaning by putting the solution on the lens, rubbing it, and rinsing it off does not allow enough chemical uptake to be a problem.

Dr. McCormick: I agree with everything that has just been said. In all of our work, we have seen no infections, and of all the cleaning solutions available, we found peroxide generally the best. We are also working with Flexsol I or IV or

Hexaphen, but find we need to periodically augment the cleaning cycle with peroxide.

Dr. Rogenthien: I also agree with what the other investigators have mentioned and particularly Dr. Moss's comment that the patient finds his own level of what is required from the peroxide ritual as I call it. I find some patients need to clean their lenses once a week in peroxide whereas others require every other day or every third day of all the solutions we have tried. I prefer peroxide and the majority of my patients are using it.

Dr. Hartstein: In my experience with solutions, the main factor to consider is the human one. The peroxide ritual as it has been referred to is an excellent procedure except for the human factor. The trouble that I have run into is, for example, if a person leaves the lenses in peroxide too long while answering the telephone, etc., then it may take 3 or 4 days of soaking to get the "burniness" out of the lenses.

I have used Flexsol I on a series of patients, and the eyes have been white and comfortable. I really had no problems, and thought that was the answer. Then I received new solutions to try out. In testing Hexaphen, I thought that it was ideal, being a single solution. However, eyes became red and irritated with this solution. With Flexsol IV, which apparently has chlorhexidine in it, patients again developed red eyes minus the irritation.

Dr. Kaufman: Did your peroxide patients have any damage that you could see?

Dr. Hartstein: The patients who left the lens in peroxide too long showed no damage. They just were not able to put on their lenses until they soaked out the peroxide.

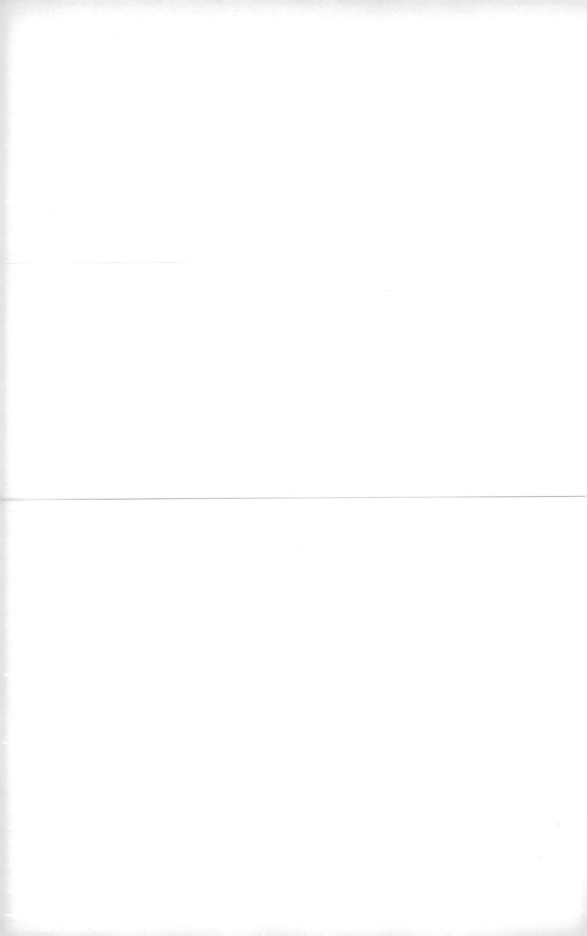

PART VIII

Miscellaneous

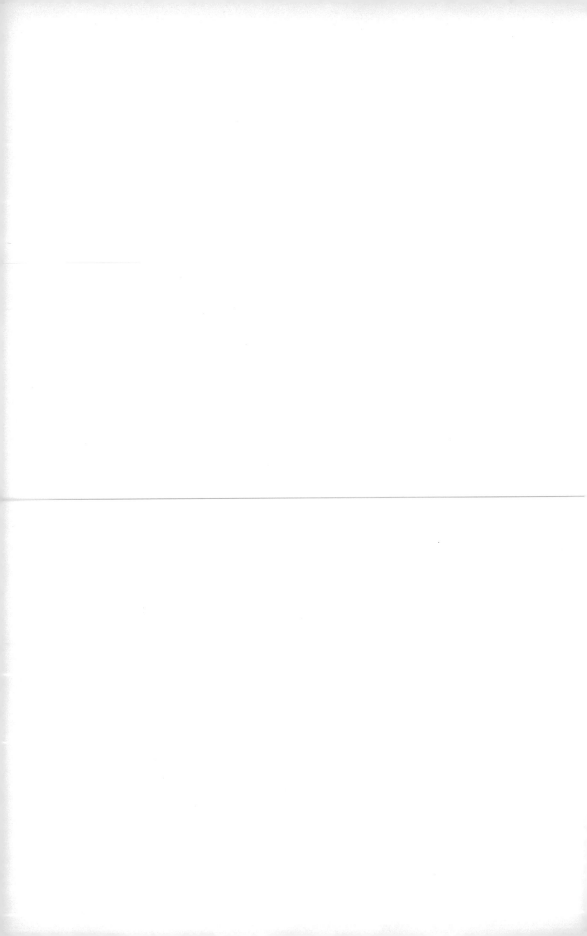

Chapter 32

Prescribing hard plastic corneal lenses

Harold I. Moss, O.D.

HARD PLASTIC LENSES

This section is purposely simplified and concise to enable the reader to familiarize himself with the general routine for the prescribing of conventional (hard plastic) contact lenses.

Important subjects such as corneal topography and physiology are covered briefly. Specialty prescriptions such as toric and bitoric lenses, lenses for aphakia, bifocal lenses, lenses for keratoconus, ellipsoidal lenses, and prism ballast lenses for the correction of residual astigmatism are covered but not in the depth required for the reader to become fully familiar with the intricacies involved.

Lens history. History reveals that the first corneal lens appeared in the 1880s but was never very successful. The first successful corneal lens appeared in 1948. The lens was large (11.5 mm.) and quite thick (0.3 to 0.4 mm.) and was prescribed about 0.3 mm. flatter than the cornea. It was basically a single radius lens. Somewhat later a bevel was placed on the edge of the lens.

The next step in the evolution of the corneal lens was the introduction of the microlens in 1951. This lens was about 9.5 mm. in diameter and about 0.2 mm. thick. It, too, was a single radius lens and was prescribed considerably flatter than the cornea.

Introduction of the contour (bicurve) corneal lens came about in 1955. The multiple inside radii permitted the practitioner to prescribe a lens with its base curve substantially the same as that of the cornea.

Many different lens constructions appeared after the contour lens, but they were all basically bicurve lenses and bicurve lenses with added edge curves.

Lens material. The lens material used since 1938 for both scleral contact lenses and the conventional hard plastic corneal lens is methylmethacrylate. The principle characteristics of this plastic are as follows: it is hydrophobic, has a low specific gravity, excellent light transmission, an index of refraction of 1.49, and little or no toxicity associated with its use, and lends itself quite readily to the fabrication of lenses. This plastic has very little, if any, oxygen permeability, and is commonly known as acrylic plastic, or plexiglas.

Other plastics have been used through the years with either higher or lower indices of refraction, but either the laboratory and other researchers invariably gave up on the new material or it was used so little as to make its contribution very insignificant.

Laboratory procedure

The lens is cut from a button of methylmethacrylate. The button is usually one half inch in diameter and about one fourth inch thick. The inside (base) radius is lathe cut and, in most instances, pitch polished. Some laboratories used buttons with cast radii. The outside curve of the lens, as determined by the lens power, is also lathe cut, but is usually rouge polished. The peripheral inside radii are ground by diamond-impregnated tools and are either rouge or pitch polished. Pitch polishing the base and secondary inside radii results in a more accurately fabricated lens, which lends itself to more accurate duplication. The size of the optical zone of the lens is controlled by how deep the secondary curve is ground into the lens. The thickness is controlled by how much stock is cut off the button when the front surface is cut. The lens is cut to size on a spindle and the edge is polished.

Lens construction

The average lens has, at least, the following seven variables:
Base radius
Secondary inside curve
Edge curve
Optical or visual zone
Power
Overall diameter
Color
Added to this list, there may be outside edge chambers, lenticular cuts to reduce edge thickness, and other variables. The frontal view and a cross section of the lens may be seen in Fig. 32-1.

Corneal topography

To enable the reader to fully understand the lens construction, a short discussion of the corneal topography is now essential.

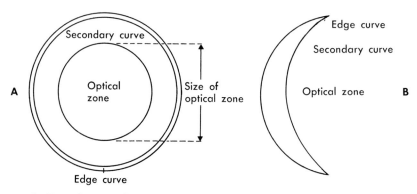

Fig. 32-1. A, Frontal view of methylmethacrylate (hard) contact lens; B, Cross-sectional view of hard lens.

The cornea has a near regular apical zone measuring about 3 to 5 mm. The fact is generally accepted that the cornea flattens as it approaches its periphery. This flattening may be spherical, toroidal, or ellipsoidal. Instrumentation is now available to aid the prescriber in analyzing the corneal contours and, from these findings, have a lens fabricated. For the average practitioner this fine instrumentation is not essential, provided that an analysis of the cornea can be carried out with control (trial) lenses.

Remembered that the steeper the apical corneal zone, the less the flattening of the peripheral cornea. Conversely the flatter the apical corneal zone, the greater is the peripheral flattening. In other words a cornea that measures 7.5 mm. in its central area has less peripheral flattening than a cornea that measures 8 or 8.5 mm.

Corneal physiology

The contact lens prescriber must be aware of the fact that the cornea requires oxygen. Any corneal lens prescription that does not permit the cornea to receive its adequate oxygen supply will cause corneal edema and the eventual breakdown of corneal epithelium. In all cases a lens prescribed so that it does interfere with the oxygen supply to the cornea will eventually become intolerable.

An adequate corneal contact lens prescription must therefore be prescribed in such a way so that (1) there is no interference with the interchange of gases at best or as little interference as one can achieve, and (2) it allows for an adequate tear flow under the lens to bathe the entire corneal area covered by the lens.

With the advent of the contour lens many laboratories attempted to make it easier for their customers by advocating either standard optical zones in the lenses, which, even when varied in size, were much too large. Rather than advocate knowledge they advocated expediency with the eventual result that great numbers of people lost their ability to wear lenses. To this date great numbers of prescribers and so-called experts do not understand why this occurred. The cause, as will be demonstrated in greater detail later in the paper, was that the periphery of the optical zone of the lens was too steep for the area of the cornea on which it rested. This resulted in a vaulting of the optical zone of the lens over the corneal apex, and binding at the periphery of this zone with the resultant tear stagnation and interference with the oxygen supply to this area of the cornea.

Prescribing the lens variables

To determine the proper base curve, the prescriber may start with the flattest corneal meridian as determined by the keratometric readings. The first lens chosen from the control set would therefore have its base curve the same as the flattest corneal meridian. We are indeed fortunate that research has provided us with a series of lenses, with known values, to utilize as a guide to aid us in determining the full lens prescription. A simple series of lenses is shown in Table 32-1.

We are aware of the clinical evidence that the corneal optical zone is smaller than 6.5 mm. (the smallest optical zone of the control lenses). As a result the periphery of this zone of the lens will be resting on a zone of the cornea somewhat flatter than the base radius of the lens. This will result in raising the optical zone of the lens off the central cornea, providing for the essential minimum clear-

Table 32-1. A simple series of lenses (in millimeters)

Base curve	Secondary curve	Overall diameter	Optical zone
7.2	7.8	8.3	6.5
7.3	7.9	8.3	6.5
7.4	8.0	8.5	6.5
7.5	8.2	8.5	6.5
7.6	8.4	8.6	6.5
7.7	8.5	8.6	6.5
7.8	8.6	8.8	7.0
7.9	8.7	8.8	7.0
8.0	8.8	8.8	7.0
8.1	8.9	8.8	7.0
8.2	9.0	9.0	7.0
8.3	9.3	9.0	7.0
8.4	9.4	9.0	7.0
8.5	9.5	9.0	7.0

ance in this area. There must, however, be only minimal clearance because any exaggeration of this clearance will result in pressure surrounding the cap. This pressure will prevent the proper tear flow and interfere with the oxygen transmission to the cornea, resulting in corneal edema and possible asphyxiation (Fig. 32-2).

It is imperative to understand that the construction of the control set must be infinitely accurate. The secondary corneal lens radii must be as accurate as the base radii. The optical zones of the lens must be accurate to 0.1 mm. Variation from this accuracy will prevent the prescriber from making an accurate analysis. Refusal of certain laboratories to make the bicurve corneal lens as accurately as it should have been made resulted in the considerable confusion as to the proper lens construction. Their refusal led to lenses that had secondary curves three and four times flatter than they should have been. The optical zones of the lenses were, on the average, 0.5 to 1 mm. too large. The result was that initially the patient was wearing comfortable but ill-fitting lenses. The ill-fitting lenses eventually caused the problems previously mentioned and the patient gradually but surely lost his wearing time. To resolve these problems, laboratories, rather than produce a lens of infinite accuracy, started to produce toric lenses, ellipsoidal lenses, and other types. Greater apical clearance may be achieved in any one or a combination of ways. The base curve may be steepened in 0.05 mm. (0.25 D.) steps, or the optical zone of the lens may be increased in 0.5 mm. steps, or the prescriber may utilize a combination of both—a steeper base curve with a larger optical zone.

When determining the optical zone of the lens, one takes visual factors into consideration with primary attention given to the pupil size. If the size of the optical zone of the lens is not larger than the pupil, especially in reduced illumination, patient complaints of flare and reflection will be quite severe and some

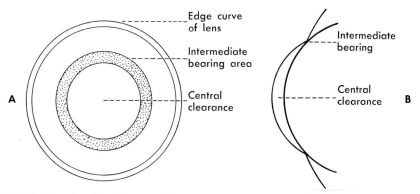

Fig. 32-2. A, Sketch of hard lens resting on cornea; note areas of intermediate bearing and central clearance. **B,** Cross section showing intermediate bearing and central clearance areas.

patients will find it intolerable. To resolve this problem, the prescriber should reconsider the corneal topography. As we increase the optical zone of the lens, the periphery of this zone rests on a continually flatter corneal zone. If we do not alter (flatten) the base curve of the lens, this will result in ever increasing apical corneal clearance. If, on the other hand, the base curve of the lens is flattened, as we increase the size of the optical zone, we remain with substantially the same lens-cornea relationship and a good clinical fit. Flare and reflection are considerably reduced.

A simple rule of thumb to follow is that the radius of the lens is flattened 0.1 mm. for every 0.5 mm. increase in optical zone size. There is a limit however, for if the optical zone of the lens is continually increased, a reversal of the clinical picture will result. We will begin to get apical touch and intermediate pooling. We want to avoid this almost as much as we want to avoid apical clearance with intermediate binding (Fig. 32-3).

The secondary curve of the lens must be flat enough to permit the proper tear flow, but certainly not so flat as to cause lens rocking or peripheral standoff or both, with resultant lid irritation. It is interesting to note, at this point, that when a lens is fabricated with its secondary curve lathe cut and pitch polished (optically correct), the secondary flattening required is considerably less than what one thinks is correct or required as a result of the lens not being made properly. It is essential, therefore, that the prescriber know how his laboratory is making the lenses and, based upon this knowledge, make the necessary allowances.

The junction between the base curve and the secondary curve is automatically blended when the secondary curve is polished. The prescriber may, however, ask the laboratory to provide a specific blend of curve. Care must be exercised, however, as to what one does in this area. It is essential that the transition area not be a sharp junction but it is also essential that the area not be eliminated completely. The net result of a severe blend is to effectively increase the optical zone area of the lens, resulting in a tighter rather than a looser fit (Fig. 32-4).

The edge or tertiary curve of the lens is primarily used for lens control as

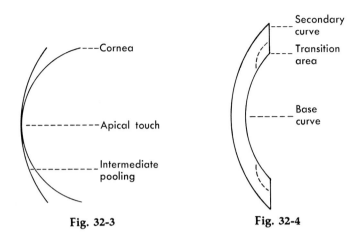

Fig. 32-3

Fig. 32-4

Fig. 32-3. Areas of apical touch and intermediate pooling seen with a hard contact lens.
Fig. 32-4. Junction between base curve and secondary curve of a hard contact lens.

well as for comfort. A well-rounded edge is essential for comfort. To enable a prescriber to have any lens properly duplicated, he should specify the radius of this zone as well as the depth it is to be ground into the lens. I prefer using an edge curve of 10.5 mm. radius and 0.15 mm. deep. This may be varied and comfort and effectivity may still be maintained.

The overall diameter of the lens should be as small as possible, with the lens variables as well as lid pressure, lens concentration, and so on, taken into consideration. One must keep in mind that the more the cornea is exposed to the atmosphere, the less the lens can possibly interfere with its metabolism.

As lenses have been made smaller, it has become less essential that the lens variables be as exacting as they could be. In other words, the smaller lenses permit a greater margin of error. I am certainly not advocating sloppiness in prescribing and still insist that lens specifications be arrived at through an exacting trial procedure; I am simply noting the reason why practitioners have been able to get away with some poorly prescribed lenses.

We have discussed the five basic essentials of the lens construction. The sixth variable is the power. To achieve maximum visual acuity, it is essential that refractive power be determined with the lenses in place. When prescribing hard lenses, one may possibly consider the spectacle prescription with minus cylinders and utilize only the spherical component as the power for the contact lens. This occurs because the spherical base curve of the contact lens neutralizes the front surface corneal astigmatism. What this latter procedure fails to take into consideration is the probability of residual astigmatism. Only a refraction performed with lenses in place can accurately determine this factor. When present to a degree that may reduce visual acuity or visual efficiency or both, the practitioner should prescribe prism ballast lenses with front surface cylinders.

When the spectacle prescription is used for corneal lens power determination, the tear lens formed between the inside lens curve and outside corneal curve (corneal flattest meridian) must be taken into consideration. A simple formula to follow is that for every 0.05 mm. steeper that the lens is, the tear layer has +0.25 D. effectivity. Conversely for every 0.05 mm. flatter that the lens is, the tear layer has a −0.25 D. effectivity.

Contrary to popular belief, the light shades of tint usually incorporated in hard lenses is not incorporated to reduce photophobia but rather to aid the patient in locating the lens should it displace. The light shades of tint have little or no effect on the reduction of illumination.

At this point a short discussion of photophobia, glare, and flare is appropriate. Most beginning patients with hard lenses report varying degrees of photophobia, which results from corneal irritation during the adaptation period. Thus one must make certain that there is minimal apical clearance with the prescribed lens. Glare is similar to photophobia. Flare, on the other hand, is caused by reflections from the edges of the lenses and/or the junction, or transition area between the optical zone of the lens and the secondary curve. Flare may be reduced by increasing the overall lens diameter, the optical zone of the lens, or both. Edge frosting may also be employed to help reduce flare.

Specialty lenses

Aphakia. I recommend the utilization of control lenses to determine both the clinical fit and the proper refractive correction. Lenses, similar in design to the control lenses herein described, may be employed, with the possible exception of the overall lens diameter. Less lens movement is necessary with these lenses, and to achieve slightly better lens stabilization, one may increase the overall lens diameter to 9.2 mm. All the control lenses should have, at least, +10.00 D. power in lenticular form. The outside lenticular cut should be as small as possible to keep the lens thickness to an absolute minimum. Refractions performed with these lenses in place are much more accurate than that of near plano lenses and the spectacle prescription. These lenses also permit a much more accurate procedure for the determination of the lens-cornea relationship.

Residual astigmatism. The correction of residual astigmatism, as previously mentioned, is achieved best through the use of prism ballast lenses. Control lenses should be employed to make the clinical determinations. Approximately 1.5 prism diopters are incorporated in each lens. This results in the area of the lens, at the base of the prism, to be the heaviest. The base of the prism will therefore be inferior on the cornea to achieve lens stabilization. In addition to all the previously described reasons for the employment of control lenses, the utilization of such lenses in cases of residual astigmatism is even more essential. Because of the prism ballast and resultant increased weight at the base of the prism, these lenses have a tendency to ride low on the cornea. If this tendency is excessive, visual disturbances could occur and often one needs to alter the lens variables such as the base curve, optical zone diameter, or overall diameter, or a combination of the three to achieve the proper lens-cornea relationship.

Bifocals. At the very best, bifocal corneal lenses have a great deal to be desired. I believe that each and every wearer of bifocal corneal lenses suffers from reduced visual efficiency. This statement does not mean that I do not advocate the prescribing of bifocal contact lenses. After every consideration is given to the patient's visual needs and a full analysis is made as to how much the patient's visual efficiency may be affected and the final determination is that "the end justifies the means," bifocal lenses may then be prescribed.

Bifocal corneal lenses fall into two basic categories. They may be classified as simultaneous vision lenses and bivisual lenses. Simultaneous vision lenses require that the patient look through both the near and distance sections of the lenses at the same time and select, visually, the portion of the lenses that gives maximum acuity. This type of bifocal, at the very best, reduces the wearer's visual efficiency considerably. At no time is the patient free of some visual blur. At night and in reduced illumination the peripheral blur is considerable and the flare almost intolerable. I consider people who wear lenses of this construction to be hazardous drivers.

The bivisual lenses, on the other hand, require lens translation for proper vision. The lens is constructed with prism ballast and the bifocal is located at the base of the prism. The form of the bifocal may be similar to the ophthalmic lens bifocals. Many different types are available. When the wearer looks at infinity, the bifocal is either below the pupil or does not encroach upon the pupillary area enough to cause visual distrubances. When he looks down to read, the lens moves up, by action of the lens bumping against the lower lid margin, bringing the bifocal over the pupillary area. When he looks up from the reading position, the bifocal drops down, permitting the distance portion of the lens to again be over the pupillary area. This latter bifocal form frequently provides the patient with as good a visual efficiency as is desired and is successfully prescribed.

Other forms of bifocals have been made through the years but, in the main, have proved to be unsuccessful either because they interfered too severely with the patient's visual efficiency or were extremely difficult for the laboratories to make and proved to be too costly. My bifocal development, based upon the contour principle described in this section, produced visually effective and optically good results. It is no longer being prescribed because of the inability of the laboratories to produce the lens accurately.

Keratoconus. Keratoconus is also known as conical cornea and is essentially a thinning and protrusion of the corneal apex. In advanced stages the prescribing of contact lenses is the only means available, other than surgery, that will restore reasonably good vision to the patient.

In the early stages of the disease the principles, as described in this paper, may be successfully employed to determine the lens variables. If, however, the condition is moderate to severe, one must utilize multicurve lenses to achieve a successful fit. It appears essential that if the lens is to aid in preventing the progression of the condition, there be a minimal amount of apical pressure. There must be, as with all lenses, no intermediate binding and there must be peripheral clearance. These lenses must move as little as possible in order to avoid rubbing on the corneal apex.

To achieve these goals, control lenses should be employed. They may be constructed with base curves of 6.0 to 7.0 mm. in 0.1 mm. steps. The visual zones of these lenses need be only 5.5 to 6.0 mm. The secondary flattening should be at least 1 mm., with the tertiary flattening 1 mm. flatter than the secondary. The edge curve can be 10.5 mm. in diameter and 0.1 mm. width. The zone of the lens, other than the optical zone, should be divided equally between the secondary and tertiary curves.

These lenses will, at the very least, provide the prescriber with a means to arrive at a prescription. In a good percentage of cases the lens specifications of the control lenses will prove to be accurate. In the balance of the cases they will provide the means by which additional control lenses, for a given patient, may be ordered prior to prescribing.

Toric and bitoric lenses. I have not found it necessary, except in extremely severe cases of corneal astigmatism, to prescribe toroidal lenses. However, in cases of moderate to severe corneal astigmatism, these lenses are usually employed. The problems associated with the prescribing of this lens form are many. There is usually an induced residual astigmatism created. The amount is approximately one third of the toroidal base curve. An outside cylinder, to neutralize the induced astigmatism, is now required. This creates an extremely difficult laboratory procedure—one very difficult to control accurately. Lens variables, such as optical zone size and thickness, often have to be sacrificed to permit the laboratory to fabricate the lens as best it could. There are instances where the induced residual astigmatism neutralizes the existing residual astigmatism. In this situation there is no need for an outside cylinder and the toroidal base curve becomes desirable.

For moderately severe astigmats, I prescribe the base curve that, with fluorescein, shows an H pattern. The curve of the lens is somewhere between the primary meridians, but is usually closer to the flattest meridian. When this clinical picture is achieved, we usually have a lens with good stability that causes less corneal distortion than the average toroidal lens.

Ellipsoidal lenses. When ellipsoidal lenses were first developed, they were ellipsoidal from edge to center. It first became necessary to provide a central spherical zone for visual efficiency; it then became necessary to provide for peripheral clearance by putting bevels on the lenses. The "glove fit" originally advocated proved to be intolerable for most patients. I do not object to the use of ellipsoidal secondary curves, provided that one understands that the same basic principles apply. There must be a good uniform central bearing with just minimal clearance, no intermediate binding, and peripheral clearance. It is interesting to note that when these objectives are achieved with lenses with spherical curves, the need for ellipsoidal curves becomes less necessary, if it is necessary at all. If, however, the prescribing of ellipsoidal curves helps achieve the proper lens-cornea relationship, then they should be employed.

Care of hard lenses. I advocate the following procedure:

1. Lenses should be cleaned with a contact lens cleaning solution after removal from the eyes regardless of how long the patient has worn the lenses.

2. Lenses, when not worn, should be stored in the wetting solution, with same brand name as the cleaner.

3. Since lenses have been cleaned prior to placing them in the storage case, they need not be cleaned upon removal from the case. Lenses should be removed

from the case and placed on the eyes without rinsing. The only exception to the latter procedure is if the wetting solution used caused any burning. In this situation attempts should be made to find a solution that does not burn. In the rare situation where one cannot find such a solution, the lenses may be rinsed lightly prior to insertion.

Contrary to popular belief, surface contamination of hard plastic lenses is possible. Since corneal abrasions are also possible with hard plastic lenses, especially if they are overworn or cause epithelial breakdown, lens care and sterility is very essential. It is advocated that the solutions in the storage cases be replaced frequently and that patients be instructed to keep their cases clean.

Discussion

I have attempted, in a very few pages, to review the prescribing of hard plastic lenses. All discussions have been as brief as possible, and elaborations on all subjects covered can be found in many other fine texts. Most institutions give postgraduate courses in hard lenses and I feel they are extremely worthwhile.

SOFT PLASTIC LENSES

With the advent of soft plastic lenses, a very new and extremely exciting innovation in the contact lens field, a short discussion and comparison between the soft plastic lens and the hard plastic lens appears appropriate.

The Bausch & Lomb Soflens has received full approval from the Federal Drug Administration (FDA) and is available to practitioners on a nationwide basis. The Griffin Naturalens is still undergoing clinical trials by several investigators in the United States. It is quite possible that by the time this article appears in print that the Griffin lens will, as well, have received its approval from the Federal Drug Administration. Many other laboratories have filed their NDAs (new drug application) with the FDA and are conducting their Phase I and Phase II studies. It is also quite possible that some have already entered upon their Phase III studies. My personal familiarity is with the Soflens and the Naturalens.

There is quite a difference in construction between these lenses. The Soflens is primarily a corneal lens about 12.5 mm. in diameter and 0.17 mm. thick. It has a central spherical zone with a peripheral aspherical zone. There is an edge bevel on the lens. The lens is made in two series, with outside curves of 7.2 mm. (N) and 7.7 mm. (F).

The Naturalens can be best described as a semiscleral lens. It can be prescribed in radii from 7.2 to 8.7 mm. in 0.3 mm. steps. These radii refer to the inside curves. The diameters can be had in most radii from 12.5 to 15.0 mm. in 0.5 mm. steps. In addition to the clinical investigation of this lens for refractive purposes, it is also used as a corneal bandage lens. Because of the distinctive properties of the plastic, the lens is being used in the treatment of many corneal diseases as well as glaucoma.

The soft plastic lenses may be compared to the hard lenses in many ways, some of which are the following:

1. Ease in prescribing. The Soflens, as now available, has as its only variable, in addition to the refractive power, two outside curves. The prescriber either

achieves a successful fit with one or the other or does not prescribe the lens. The two criteria are lens centration and visual acuity. The Naturalens, as described, has many more variables, which gives the prescriber greater latitude. Although care must be exercised in the prescribing and patient aftercare. I feel safe in stating that either soft lens is somewhat simpler to prescribe than the hard corneal lens is.

2. Patient adaptation. In adaptation there is no comparison. Either soft lens is much easier to adapt to than is the hard lens. Patient comfort with the Naturalens is almost immediate, whereas with the Soflens there may be momentary discomfort.

3. Sporting activities. Either soft lens is much superior to the hard lens in regard to sports. The lenses rarely if ever fall out. They rarely if ever are displaced off the cornea. Having foreign objects get under the lenses is also unusual.

4. Presence of photophobia, glare, and flare. Light annoyances, invariably present during the adaptation period with hard lenses, are almost nonexistent with the soft lens.

5. Afterblur or spectacle blur. Blur, one of the most vexing problems with hard lenses, is almost nonexistent with soft lenses.

6. Wearing of lenses. One should wear his hard lenses on a regular schedule if he is to be a successful contact lens wearer. With the soft lenses, one can wear them as conditions dictate, or as he prefers.

7. Care of lenses. Because the plastic is soft, extreme care must be exercised to maintain lens sterilization. Although internal lens contamination is virtually impossible because the soft plastic does not have any pore structure, surface contamination is possible. With the hard lenses the surfaces may be cleaned with a detergent, rubbed, and rinsed and the lens is clean. This procedure is more difficult and more exacting with the soft lens. Chemical sterilization and asepticizing are employed. The procedure is quite simple in either case, but it must be done. Patient laxity must not be condoned. Care must be exercised that hair spray, for example, does not get onto the soft plastic. The patient must be cautioned about the use of soaps. In this matter the care of the hard lens is somewhat easier than the soft lens.

8. Visual efficiency. In my opinion it is impossible to predict the visual outcome of any given case unless a refractive analysis is performed with the lenses in place. Generally speaking, however, the hard lenses will neutralize corneal astigmatism better than the soft lenses will. Again generally speaking, there will be more cases of residual astigmatism after soft lenses are prescribed than after hard lenses are prescribed. In my experience, however, if the optics in the soft lenses are as good as they should be, the visual results obtained provide the wearer with good to excellent visual efficiency. If the prescriber screens his patients carefully, the patient's visual results will be excellent.

Chapter 33

Computer-assisted fitting of soft contact lenses

Gerald L. Feldman, Ph.D., and John E. Carney, Sr.

The current procedure for the fitting of soft contact lenses is based on a trial-and-error technique. Regardless of whether a fitting set is used with lenses dispensed from inventory or a separate set to evaluate fit is employed, the basis for fitting is an educated guess based on central K values and the patient's spectacle prescription in minus cylinder. There is no accurate method of predicting the exact specifications for a given patient's lens requirements; hence this evaluation technique is the only practical way to approach fitting.

Our clinical experiences with soft lenses are based on the Bausch & Lomb Soflens and the Griffin Naturalens. The two lenses are sufficiently different so that their respective fitting techniques also differ. The Naturalens for example is larger and flatter and much more of a semihaptic lens than the Soflens is. Centering is not a problem with the Naturalens and the fitting is done strictly with visual acuity as the end point. After considerable frustration in fitting by the trial lens system with poor success, we learned to fit this lens to the spherical component in minus cylinder using an 8.4 mm. radius of curvature in the base curve of a 14.0 mm. diameter lens.[1] Such lenses usually act as though the lenses were too flat, but after several days of wear they settle down and display an optimal lens-eye relationship with clear, sharp vision. Fitting is thus not a problem with the Naturalens.

The Soflens however is not as easily fitted. Only two base curves are available,[2] but unlike the Naturalens these are anterior rather than posterior curvatures. Moreover, their posterior curvature is a function of power—the higher the minus power, the steeper the lens. Since all lenses have the same center thickness of 0.17 mm., this imparts considerable variation in posterior curvature. In addition, the small diameter of this lens requires that it center in much the same manner as a conventional corneal lens.

Our initial results in fitting the Soflens were poor. The recommended fitting technique requires that with a central K flatter than 44.50 diopters one fit with an F (flat) series lens whose base curve radius is 7.7 mm. When the central K reading is steeper than 44.50 diopters, one fits the N (nominal) series. But in many cases corneas steeper than 44.50 had to be refitted with F lenses and flatter corneas sometimes required N lenses.

The optical end points with the Soflens were frequently poor. In those patients, the visual acuity was reduced, and upon retinoscopy one could see that cylinder had been induced. Acting on the assumption that the cylinder was induced by apical compression of an overly steep lens, these wearers would be refitted with flatter lenses, which not only failed to solve the problem but also caused poor centering.

Thus, the basic fitting problem with the Soflens was a combination of several factors, which are poor centering, uncertain curvature requirements, and induced astigmatism with a reduction in visual acuity. All these factors point to a geometric problem in determining the shape of the eye and its relationship to lens fitting with the Soflens. Such geometric problems are nothing new. We have a similar type of problem with conventional corneal lenses, but it is uncomplicated by the pliability of the lens itself. We have, for example, seen cases in which lenses fitted as much as 1.0 diopter steeper than K were actually too flat for the eye, and conversely, we have recorded cases in which lenses fitted 0.5 diopter flatter than K were too steep to such an extent that extensive corneal steepening had been induced.

What is the basis for a similar problem occurring in both lens modalities? Obviously, we are dealing with the influence of the paracentral cornea. In the case of our conventional lens problems we learned that conventional keratometry was of limited value, since it only estimated the curvature of the apical K readings. We fit this type of lens with apical clearance so that fitting is actually done in the paracentral area. By using photoelectric keratoscopy and lenses designed by computer to fit the measured eye, we were able to resolve these problems.[3] Could the same technique be used to evaluate a soft lens fit?

BASIC CONCEPTS

Before the problem can be attacked, one must review several basic concepts regarding both the technique of photoelectric keratoscopy as well as the philosophy upon which soft lens fitting is based. Then we can explore the possibility of an interaction between these two concepts.

Photoelectric keratoscope (PEK). The commercially available instrument* that we use consists of a projector with concentric ring target mire and a camera that utilizes transparency film to photograph the image of the target mires on the corneal surface. The keratogram thus obtained is then enlarged fiftyfold so that the relative distances between the target rings can be measured. These data together with the spectacle prescription, lens diameter, and desired apical clearance are fed into a computer, which then determines the best lens design for a given eye. The computer readout also offers a calculation of the eccentricity of a given meridian. This value relates to the geometric shape of the cornea in its paracentral area. The eccentricity value is expressed as a decimal. At a value of zero, the mathematical consideration is that of a sphere, but with an eccentricity of 1.000 we are dealing with an ellipsoid.

In any given meridian the geometry of the cornea is generally ellipsoidal, although it is not necessarily equally so. Moreover, the degree of ellipticity is a variable from eye to eye both between individuals and between the eyes of an individual. Thus the values range between zero and 1.000. Obviously the wider the variation between the two meridians of a given eye, the more toric is the

---

*Wesley-Jessen, Inc., Chicago, Illinois.

paracentral area, and furthermore this toricity can occur even when the apical area is spherical.

It is the inability to quantitatively measure this parameter with conventional spherometers that frequently leads to poor fitting and tolerance problems with conventional lenses. One should bear in mind that in fitting conventional corneal lenses the apex is vaulted. The fitting is actually governed by the paracentral cornea, since it is eccentricity that determines the amount of this apical clearance. The clearance for any given base curve increases with increasing eccentricity. If, for example, one were to fit a lens "on K" with an eccentricity value of 0.800, the clearance would be over 0.05 mm. and might reach the bubble point of an excessively steep lens. On a spherical eye, however, the apical clearance is nil and even a lens fitted 0.5 diopter steeper than K would be too flat.

It thus becomes axiomatic with conventional lenses that if the lens fits within the limbal margin, its geometrical relationship is determined by the shape of the paracentral cornea. Consequently, the central keratometric readings contribute very little to accurate fitting. An eye with a spherical apex, but toric in the paracentral area, can cause problems from the rocking action of the lens as it moves over the cornea. Such an effect is particularly pronounced with tight lids, and such individuals complain of chronic overawareness with no apparent reason for their discomfort.

Such problems are attacked by empirical means. To arrive at a means of providing adequate apical clearance, some fitters utilize the amount of cylinder as an estimate of the amount of paracentral toricity. The nomogram method of Dyer[4] and the LD+2 technique[5] from which it is derived offer a rule-of-thumb procedure with this basis for the initial lens design. The lens is fitted by study of the fluorescein pattern and then rendering the appropriate modifications to obtain an optimal lens-corneal geometric relationship. Both methods are extremely useful, but it is still the fitter's skill in modification that determines maximum success. Moreover, these methods do not provide us with a quantitative determination of the shape of the eye, and in some cases a refitting is necessary to obtain the optimal geometric relationship.

The soft lens. The Bausch & Lomb Soflens is fitted in much the same manner as a conventional corneal lens. Its diameter of 12.3 mm. places it at the limbus, with much of the bearing surface fitting the paracentral cornea. Because of its size and design, the lens can pass over the limbus either as a result of lid pressure or because of the weight of the lens. This lens must center or its optical performance is compromised. In addition, the lens must be fitted with an apical touch because slight clearance will result in wrinkling during the blink thus causing fluctuating acuity.

The posterior geometry of the Soflens varies with power as previously mentioned, but it is sufficiently flexible so that the differences because of power may not be significant. Moreover, the lens conforms closely to the corneal geometry. This produces a unique optical situation. The lens power is determined by its posterior surface, but on the eye its geometry changes, which in turn changes its optics so that the power determinant is no longer the posterior surface, but the *anterior surface* of the lens.

This situation creates another problem. The posterior surface of the lens is aspheric. The cornea is ellipsoidal. The two fit fairly well, but when the lens is on the eye, the optical surface is spherical or nearly so, inducing some spherical aberration, which is another reason for blur in some wearers of this lens.

The fit of the Soflens determines its power. Therefore, corneal geometry is a highly significant factor in determining the optical performance of the lens on the eye. Moreover, since the lens is fitted to an apical touch, the paracentral cornea is important to the fitting just as it is in the conventional lens. It is for this reason that corneas with flat central K readings sometime require lenses with steep bases and vice versa.

But the real problem with the Soflens is induced cylinder. Patients with spherical central K readings and with spherical spectacle prescription will often present with 0.5 to 1.0 diopter of refractive cylinder that does not occur with a conventional lens. These wearers complain of poor acuity that is only partially improved with cylinder overrefraction. It is this phenomenon that led us to explore the feasibility of using the PEK to screen out patients who might not obtain satisfactory wear of the Soflens. In addition, we sought a method for ascertaining the optimal base curve without resorting to the trial-and-error technique, realizing that we still might require lens changes, but only for satisfying power requirements. If this goal could be fulfilled, it would save considerable time in fitting. The potential failure could be detected and fitted with something else that might provide a better result. This is a strong argument for more than one type of lens.

Use of the PEK. The PEK computer program is designed for hard lenses. How can it be utilized for the Soflens? We approached this with a consideration of a large lens fitted to zero apical clearance. This would give us an estimate of whether to use the N series or the F series, depending on the base curve given with the computer readout. The readout also provides us with the eccentricity in the two major meridians. From this we could estimate the amount of existing paracentral toricity that determines if it is sufficient to induce a cylinder when the lens is on the eye. The computer also provides us with an estimate of the amount of residual astigmatism that we should obtain with a conventional lens. With the Soflens this is actually a more meaningful value than with conventional lenses. We realize that the output is only an estimate. We would need a specific program for the Soflens so that the variations in posterior geometry could also be entered into the calculations. Indeed, with the proper program even the optimal power could be computed.

Let us examine a few actual cases to demonstrate how the computer data is utilized:

Case 1. Mr. J. C.
Prescription
O.D. -3.50 -0.50 cyl. axis 180
O.S. -3.00 -0.50 cyl. axis 180

Eye meridian	O.D.		O.S.	
	Horizontal	Vertical	Horizontal	Vertical
Central K	42.87	44.37	43.00	44.50
Eccentricity	0.339	0.407	-0.279	0.086
Residual astigmatism	1.01		0.92	

The inability of this patient to wear the Soflens is due to his residual astigmatism. The problem was not as bad with the right eye. A comparison of the meridian variation of the eye shows a difference of 0.078, indicating very little paracentral toricity. But the left eye shows considerable meridian variation. With the F series, the lens is centered poorly on this eye as one might predict with paracentral toricity. A lens of the N series centered better, but acuity was poor because of the blurring induced by a wrinkle passing through the optical zone whenever the patient blinked or even squinted. The patient was refitted with the Griffin Naturalens, but even with this lens the residual astigmatism produced a slight reduction in visual clarity. The left lens was displaced even with this larger lens, but with the Naturalens displacement was not a problem.

Case 2. Mrs. A. S.

Prescription

O.D. −3.50 sphere

O.S. −3.25 sphere

Eye meridian	O.D.		O.S.	
	Horizontal	Vertical	Horizontal	Vertical
Central K	42.87	44.00	42.50	43.50
Eccentricity	0.391	0.517	−2.09	0.506
Residual astigmatism		1.06		1.10

Centering was not a problem with this second patient; however, even the F series of lens was too tight. The best visual acuity attainable was 20/40 with the right eye and 20/60 with the left. Both eyes required a cylinder correction to improve acuity, especially in the left. Again, note that there is marked meridian variation in eccentricity, which together with the residual astigmatism is responsible for the poor acuity. The cylinder requirement with the left eye was greater than computed, indicating to us that the marked paracentral toricity added to the patient's astigmatism. This same patient wearing conventional lenses does not have reduced acuity even though there is indeed a residual cylinder. Therefore, one must conclude that the visual problem is probably a function of the paracentral toricity just as it was in the previous case. The lens probably does not fully conform to the corneal geometry, and this induces cylinder when significant differences exist between the two meridians of the paracentral cornea.

Case 3. Mr. H. W., Jr.

Prescription

O.D. −2.25 sphere

O.S. −2.00 sphere

Eye meridian	O.D.		O.S.	
	Horizontal	Vertical	Horizontal	Vertical
Central K	43.00	43.37	43.12	43.87
Eccentricity	0.565	0.392	0.662	0.599
Residual astigmatism		0.38		0.69

Our third patient illustrates the point that we are trying to make that it is the combination of residual astigmatism and meridian variations in the eccentricity that underlie the reduced acuity. This individual, a well-known entertainer, was unable to wear the Soflens. His acuity on the right was a blurry 20/25 requiring a 0.75 diopter of cylinder to correct. His left eye, however, was correctable to 20/20 even though we could anticipate over 0.50 diopter of residual astigmatism. Note that the meridian variation in eccentricity is less than 0.100 in that eye, whereas in the right eye the difference is 0.173. Again the most extensive reduction of acuity occurred with an interaction between shape and residual astigmatism, but in this case the interaction was marginal.

Case 4. Mr. D. M.

Prescription

O.D. −3.87 −0.25 cyl. axis 100
O.S. −2.75 −0.25 cyl. axis 45

	O.D.		O.S.	
Eye meridian	Horizontal	Vertical	Horizontal	Vertical
Central K	43.25	43.65	43.50	43.62
Eccentricity	0.406	0.373	0.502	0.219
Residual astigmatism	0.66		0	

The fourth patient is a successful wearer with visual acuity of 20/20 in both eyes. Residual astigmatism was anticipated in the right eye, but the meridian variation is small and the astigmatism did not occur. In the left eye there was a marked meridian variation, but no expected residual cylinder. Thus, successful wearing occurred in the absence of the interaction between residual astigmatism and the variation in meridian eccentricity.

Case 5. Mr. S. G.

Prescription

O.D. −1.25 sphere
O.S. −1.25 sphere

	O.D.		O.S.	
Eye meridian	Horizontal	Vertical	Horizontal	Vertical
Central K	42.87	42.87	43.12	42.75
Eccentricity	0.284	0.153	0.543	0.364
Residual astigmatism	0		0	

The visual acuity obtained by the fifth patient was 20/15 in both eyes. He obtained this with N series lenses even though with his central K readings an F lens is indicated. Note that there is a significant difference in meridian eccentricity in both eyes, but no residual astigmatism. Thus another successful wearer shows the pattern that equates poor vision with an interaction between residual astigmatism and paracentral shape.

In none of the cases that we have fitted is there a successful wearer who displays this interaction. A failure is seen whenever there is a marked interaction involving a meridian variation in eccentricity of 0.100 and residual astigmatism of 0.50 or more. Is astigmatism induced when only the meridian variation occurs? Apparently it is, but only when the difference is large does it become significant. When it does occur, the problem seems to be more of the physical relationship between eye and lens. The greater the difference between eccentricity values, the more the lens wrinkles with blinking.

The computer-assisted fitting is not absolutely effective. We occasionally have successes when a failure was predicted and failures when a success was predicted. But, these variants occur much less frequently than encountered by trial fitting alone. There are several reasons. First, of course, is the fact that we lack a suitable program for this system, as we mentioned earlier. But even with an inadequate program we can monitor such parameters as keratometric readings, peripheral flattening, and asymmetry of the cornea, and their interaction with residual astigmatism should any exist.

The second reason for variant behavior from predicted response is that there are parameters that we cannot monitor by computer. Such factors as disparity between optical and geometric axes, lid tension, ocular anatomical variants, tear osmolarity, the patient's blinking habits, and environmental exposure enter into the ultimate result but can only be monitored by the fitter's skill.

But these are not fitting problems and can be managed by changing lens design or other factors. The significant factors that influence fit can be computer monitored so that eventually a proper program will provide the best design for a given eye. In this present state of the art with empirical methods, we successfully fit 90% of the patients that should be successful with computer prediction. Without it our success rate is less than 75% based on optimal acuity as an end point. In other words, a patient is a success if he obtains the best acuity that the eye is capable of attaining and can wear the lens 12 or more hours. In addition, this improved result is realized with a considerable saving of time since fewer lenses are required for a fitting. Thus, the use of computer assistance is feasible and practical and actually may surpass the conventional trial lens as far as application to fitting is concerned.

But what about the failures? Why did they fail and what can we do about them? Most of the failures were caused by poor acuity rather than physiological intolerance. Their lenses did not center well and we were unable to fit them with either of the two base curves provided in the Soflens. Obviously a wider choice is needed. Most of these Soflens failures were successfully fitted with the Naturalens. Those that unsuccessfully wore both lenses might succeed if still another lens were available.

Thus soft lenses readily lend themselves to computerized fitting, especially when aphakic and astigmatic corrections become available. We also conclude that the maximum success with soft lens fitting requires a choice of lenses with various designs and materials. In view of the complexity of factors that influence soft lens performance, the fitter will need all the help he can get. Computer assistance will make his job easier and more successful.

REFERENCES

1. Feldman, G. L.: From the Editor's Desk, Contact Lens Society of America Journal 5(2):7-8, 1971.

2. Bausch and Lomb, Inc.: Seminar on the Fitting of the Soflens, Memphis, Tennessee, September 25, 1971.
3. Feldman, G. L.: Computerized corneal contact lens fitting. Bitonte, J. L., Keates, R. H., editors: Symposium on the flexible lens. In Proceedings of the Fifth Contact Lens Seminar, Ohio State University, St. Louis, 1972, The C. V. Mosby Co., p. 141.
4. Dyer, J. A.: A practical nomogram for fitting corneal contact lenses, Contact Lens Med. Bull. 1(4):8-11, 1968.
5. Soper, J. W., Sampson, W. G., and Girard, L. J.: Corneal topography, keratometry and contact lenses, Arch. Ophthal. 67:753-760, 1962.

Chapter 34

Instrumentation for flexible lenses

George M. Wodak

A successful contact lens fit depends on many factors and may be achieved in a variety of ways even on the same eye. Two conditions, however, must be fulfilled to enable the practitioner to deal scientifically with all fitting problems:

1. The lenses must conform strictly to the agreed or promised tolerances of physical and chemical qualities and quantities.
2. There must be methods and instruments available to the practitioner that enable him to quickly verify (measure) all, or at least the most important, of these specifications.

The physical fit of a contact lens is mainly determined by its base curve and its overall diameter, whereas the optical fit depends on front surface curvature, lens thickness, and its index of refraction.

The objective of this paper is to examine, discuss, and perhaps recommend a few methods and instruments with which the various parameters can be verified.

Since the polymethylmethacrylate corneal contact lens started its victory run almost 20 years ago, various instruments have been developed or adapted for measuring these lenses (such as the V diameter gauge and radiuscope). The lensometer and thickness dial gauges were easily adjusted from general optical laboratory work to contact lens measurements. Now, the new soft (hydrophilic) contact lenses present a new dimension in which the instruments employed successfully for hard lenses cannot be used. Since we do not wish to forego the security of judgment, we urgently need either new adaptations or instrumentation. Two factors necessitate a new approach to measuring soft lenses:

High lens flexibility

Hydrated lens state

Changes in soft lenses occur in two ways: either through the application of pressure, or through changes in the quantity of fluid either in the material of the lens itself or on one of its surfaces. Both of these factors make the handling of soft lenses more difficult and make it necessary for part of the measuring process to be switched over to visual evaluation or comparison rather than exact optical measurements.

BASIC MEASUREMENTS

In most of the present soft contact lenses, we have to consider four basic measurements: base curve, optical power, size or diameter, and thickness. For *quality* we must inspect both the concave and the convex surfaces of the lens, the material itself, and the edge of the lens.

INSTRUMENTATION FOR FLEXIBLE LENSES

Base curve. To measure the base curve in a rigid lens, the ophthalmoscope and later the radiuscope were used. Rapid evaporation changes in the fluid layer covering the surface of the hydrophilic lens prevent exact measurements with the radiuscope. Therefore, a new method of gauging by using a number of polished spheres of known radii (Fig. 34-1) has been utilized. The wet lens is put onto one after another of these spheres and its radius determined by an "alignment fit," meaning that the whole lens covers the sphere evenly in its complete area. An

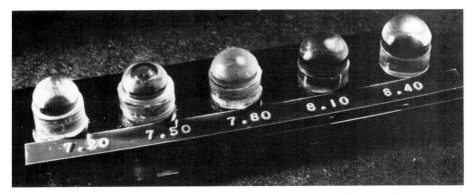

Fig. 34-1. Sphere gauges for measuring base curve of hydrophilic lenses.

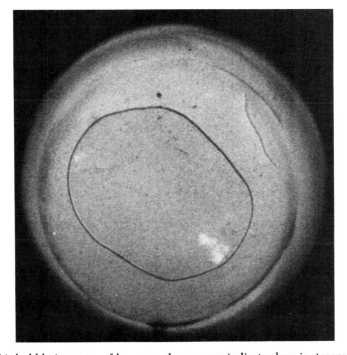

Fig. 34-2. Air bubble in center of lens on sphere gauge indicates lens is steeper than gauge.

MISCELLANEOUS

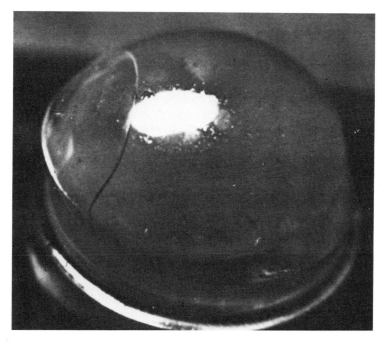

Fig. 34-3. Lens edges standing off from gauge indicate that lens is flatter than gauge.

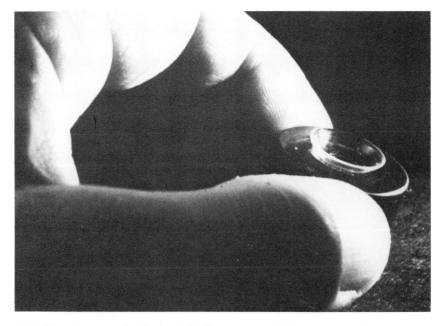

Fig. 34-4. New lens tray for hydrophilic lenses is used in measuring lens power with a standard lensometer.

air bubble in the center would indicate that the lens is steeper than the sphere underneath (Fig. 34-2) and edges standing off would mean that the lens is flatter than the gauge (Fig. 34-3). With a little practice, judging the size of the air bubbles can be developed into a very precise method. The spheres can be made of black material, which makes the bubbles more visible under direct illumination. Alternatively, the spheres can be made of a transparent material and set into an opaque base, which can then be illuminated from below and will also show the bubbles clearly.

Power. The lensometer is still the best instrument for power determination. However, the new lens is completely distorted when it is hand-held against the stop of the instrument. Therefore, we put the lensometer in an upright position and put the lens onto a small plastic tray with a hole in its center. This tray fits over the lens stop of the lensometer. It can be constructed so that the front surface of the lens rests in a hollow in such a way that it approaches the lens stop as much as possible. (Fig. 34-4). Since the eyepiece of the lensometer in the upright

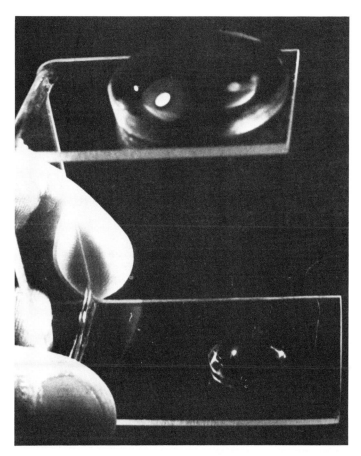

Fig. 34-5. Lens is placed on thin plastic tray with attached magnifier for determination of lens diameter.

position rises too high for comfort, the whole instrument can be lowered to a suitable height. This may be done by fastening it to the side of the working table.

After the lens is soaked thoroughly in standard physiological saline, its surface has to be dried carefully with a lintfree paper tissue without applying pressure and the lens must be centered well on the tray. Since we are interested in the measurements conforming to the state of the lens on the eye, the centering has to be done quickly in order to avoid excessive drying of the lens. This measuring process turned out to be a very awkward procedure because the space available on the lensometer is rather small for rapid handling and exactly centered positioning. Therefore, we made the tray easily removable and returnable with the lens centered on it. Since quality inspection is possible at the time of power determination, the hole in the tray should be as large as possible without causing the lens to sag, and the target or test mark in the lensometer should cover as much area as possible and should be of a stellate type.

Diameter. The next step is the determination of the diameter of the lens. Here the lens is compared with circles of progressively larger diameter in steps on 0.5 mm. To avoid excessive handling of the lens, we put it on a thin transparent plastic tray that is connected to a magnifier (Fig. 34-5). This permits at the same time an easy moving of the lens from circle to circle and exact obser-

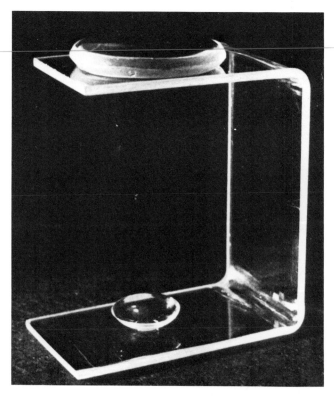

Fig. 34-6. Lens is placed concave side up on same diameter tray for surface inspection.

vation through the magnifier. A textile thread counter can be used for this purpose. The gauging circles can be inscribed on a sheet of transparent tinted plastic and illuminated from below. This arrangement permits at the same time a gross inspection of the surface and also of the material. A mask can be put between the illumination and the lens in order to exclude unnecessary light. For larger magnification, a focusing device can be added so that the lens and its inside material can be examined from the front to the back surface. The lens can then be turned concave side up (Fig. 34-6) and a spotlight can be used for additional surface inspection. The spotlight can be moved about so that different angles of illumination can be achieved, and the surface can be judged by reflex. Parallax can be overcome in the diameter gauge by the suitable proportioning of the circles.

Thickness. Lens thickness can be measured either optically, which is preferable, or physically. For optical measuring we use a radiuscope and a 7 mm. sphere. The radiuscope is focused first on the sphere and then on the lens surface. The difference in millimeters gives the thickness of the lens. A German firm (Carl Zeiss, Oberkochen, West Germany) has developed a thickness gauge on the slit lamp, but it does not seem to be available as yet.

Alternatively we measure the center thickness of our lenses with a very simple adaptation of the thickness dial gauge fitted with a highly polished re-

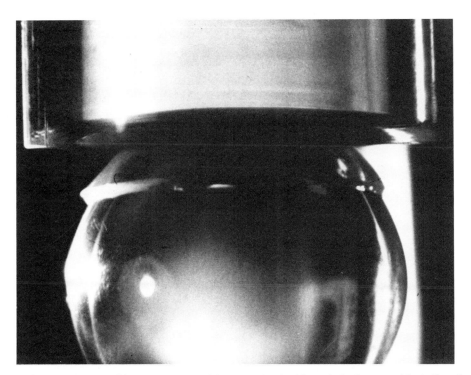

Fig. 34-7. Thickness of lens is measured by use of a highly polished removable ball-and-socket construction on the standard thickness dial gauge.

movable ball-and-socket construction instead of the two pins usually employed (Fig. 34-7). The two pieces are made of clear plastic, the lower one with a convex surface, the upper one with a concave surface. The lower one should have a radius smaller than the steepest available standard flexible lens, whereas the upper one has a concave radius of 10 mm. When they rest on each other with no lens between them, the gauge dial shows zero. Both are removable and can be cleaned easily before the measuring process. This must be done without fail because the occasional foreign body impressed into the lens surface makes all sorts of difficulties later on.

Quality control. In addition to the previously mentioned simple magnification device, a stereoscopic microscope is a must for efficient inspection. For surface and edge inspection two light sources should be employed for incident illumination. The material can be thoroughly examined by transillumination with the devices that usually come with the microscope. The inspection should include both surface for defects and an examination of the lens material between the two surfaces for foreign bodies, opacities, and other possible defects. Furthermore, the edge should be thoroughly inspected for unpolished parts and for exact roundness as well as an incipient splitting of the lens. These splits, starting normally at the edge, are possibly caused either on the manufacturing level or by excessive compression during handling. Lens inspection has always been an important part of every periodic or routine examination with rigid PMMA lenses. It becomes even more important with flexible lenses because of their greater vulnerability.

I hope that the methods and measuring devices described in this chapter will assist others as they have aided us in making our work easier and our patients happier.

Chapter 35

Soft contact lenses:
Past, present, and future

G. Peter Halberg, M.D.

Soft contact lenses made of hydrophilic plastic material became a reality when Czech researchers at the end of the 1950s proposed the use of 2-hydroxyethyl-methacrylate (HEMA) as a material for the fabrication of contact lenses. Thus the era of the soft or flexible contact lens was opened. Czech researchers were initially talking about disposable soft lenses sold over the counter in the price range of $1 or $2, and thus the era of boundless fantasies was also opened. Before long speculators and manipulators hitched on to the new idea, and in the canyons of Manhattan, rumors that very big profits are to be made on the soft contact lens became a common daily occurrence. Some of these rumors realized into fair-sized profits much before anybody could wear the new soft contact lenses in this part of the world. In the last 3 to 4 years, a very active competition developed between several firms who each claim to have the best of these new soft lenses.

The Food and Drug Administration stepped into the picture and investigational guidelines were set up for this material and classified it as a prescription drug, at lease de jure. De facto it continued to be handled like a device, but very strict manufacturing and packaging rules were imposed.

Early in the investigational phase of hydrophilic soft contact lenses, it became obvious that hygiene just as with hard contact lenses is a very important problem. Hydrophilic soft contact lenses showed specific affinity to some chemicals and, it was suggested, also to certain microorganisms and their by-products.

The Contact Lens Association of Ophthalmologists, although not a regulatory agency itself, nevertheless, through its many medical consultants, does assert a constructive influence by directing attention to the public interest in certain specific areas in which this new contact lens modality may show weaknesses and potential flaws. The major problem areas were visual acuity, hygiene, and durability of the lens.

Visual acuity is being gradually improved by introducing somewhat more rigid, but still soft, lenses and also by introducing a variety of base curves in which the lenses are being made available. This variety might frustrate some of the manufacturers who hoped to get away with a minimum number of curves, thus cutting across the difficulties by making available the simplest possible industrial product to the largest possible percentage of the potential contact lens–wearing population.

Hygiene remains a very important problem. It has to be examined from two points of view. First it has to be looked upon from the manufacturer's suggested hygienic management and, what is almost identical, the hygienic management suggested by the physician. But we also have to look at it from the patient's point of view and have to assess the potential for compliance on the patient's part. Those of us who have spent long years fitting hard contact lenses to the eyes of patients are quite aware of the degree of negligence to which the public can go, even though their own eyes are involved. We feel that a continued emphasis on this aspect of soft contact lenses is well justified.

In today's consumer-conscious society, I would like to bring out the third important area in which our Association shows concern. This is the durability, the life-span of these lenses. Because of a very high initial cost and also the time-consuming empirical fitting techniques, most ophthalmologists are forced to charge way above the hard contact lens fees when fitting soft lenses. In view of the high initial costs both to the practitioner and to the patient, the durability factor becomes even more important. It is believed that the HEMA materials, especially when subjected to meticulous hygiene have a relatively short life-span. We also know through the experience of many of our colleagues that irritating substances cake on some of these lenses, probably because of denaturation of proteins by heating. Other lenses show other difficulties and patients who tend to be neglectful with the hygiene of the lenses have shown in some cases disastrous consequences. The lenses have a tendency to become torn, especially when not cared for with the greatest of delicacy, and this is another important consumer point of view to be kept in mind.

The Association welcomes this and other new contact lens modalities onto the market. We feel that honestly investigated and classified into their proper place in our armamentarium they serve a very useful purpose and will allow the fitting of patients with a number of conditions that were in the past not satisfactorily accessible to fitting with hard lenses.

Soft bandage lenses, for instance, which provide crucial therapy for certain injured or diseased corneas, is a spectacular achievement and should be applauded by all of us who have to face these unfortunate patients in our daily practice.

Those of us who worked intensively with these materials in the past few years cannot altogether share the artificial enthusiasm generated in the market place. In between the lines extreme potentials were ascribed to these lenses. We nevertheless feel that these are very exciting new modalities that have already broadened the scope of contact lens ophthalmology, and we expect some further developments especially in the therapeutic field.

Our firm conviction is that meetings like this are major forums where investigators can compare notes and bring better understanding to this fairly new but nevertheless very important field.

APPENDIX

Fitting manual for

Bausch & Lomb
and
Griffin lenses

Maija H. Uotila, R.N.
Antonio R. Gasset, M.D.

THE ERA OF THE SOFT CONTACT LENS IS HERE

In fitting soft lenses, we must first file away the habits gained through 30 years of experience fitting hard lenses. For example, fluorescein cannot be used because it ruins the lenses and lens movement does not tell us much. Mastering soft lens fitting techniques is relatively easy, however, and once you have become skilled and learn to interpret the patient's symptoms correctly, fitting a patient will not take long. If the original fit is good, refits are rarely needed.

Of several soft contact lenses on the market; the Bausch & Lomb and Griffin lenses are the best known. This manual will deal only with these two types of lenses.

PATIENT SELECTION

Lately, soft contact lenses have received an inordinate amount of publicity in the lay press, which has given these lenses a panacea image. Consequently, many people, regardless of their needs, will want to try them. First the usual professional evaluation is necessary to determine if the patient is a good prospect for any contact lens. With soft lenses, another factor, astigmatism, must be considered.

The crucial question is, *How much astigmatism can be corrected with soft lenses?* The answer is, *None.* If you take keratometer readings on the cornea and then over the lens, you will notice that there is no difference between the two readings. However, this does not mean you should not fit anyone who has astigmatism. Your decision to fit or not to fit a particular patient should be based on several other factors. Some guidelines follow:

1. A patient can tolerate quite a large amount (up to 1.5 diopters) of astig-

matism, especially at 90° and 180°. Oblique astigmatism is harder to tolerate.

2. The more sphere lens power there is, the easier astigmatism is tolerated. For instance, a patient with a refraction of −8.00 +2.00 cyl. axis 90 would have acceptable visual acuity, whereas a patient with a −2.00 +2.00 cyl. axis 90 would not be happy with his vision.

The kind of astigmatism a patient has must be determined. Is he a candidate for any type of contact lens? Is his astigmatism corneal, lenticular, or a combination of both? The rule *"total astigmatism = corneal astigmatism + lenticular astigmatism"* must be kept in mind. The following are some examples:

1. Patient's refraction is −2.00, keratometer readings are 44.00/44.00. In this patient total astigmatism is zero. He is a good candidate for soft or hard contact lenses.

2. Patient's refraction is −2.00 +2.00 cyl. axis 90, keratometer readings are 44.00/46.00 cyl. axis 90. This patient has 2 diopters of corneal astigmatism. He would be a poor candidate for soft contact lenses. Fit him with hard lenses.

3. Patient's refraction is −2.00, keratometer readings are 44.00/46.00 cyl. axis 90. This patient has 2 diopters of corneal astigmatism at 90°, balanced by 2 diopters of lenticular astigmatism at 180°. He is an ideal candidate for soft lenses; with hard lenses he would do poorly.

4. Patient's refraction is −4.00 +2.00 cyl. axis 90, keratometer readings are 44.00/46.00 cyl. axis 180. This patient has 4 diopters of lenticular astigmatism at 90°, 2 diopters of which is balanced by the corneal astigmatism at 180°. This patient cannot be fitted with any kind of spherical contact lens. With soft lenses he will have residual astigmatism.

The visual acuity must be acceptable to the patient. There are patients who will not settle for less than 20/15 vision. On the other hand there are many who are perfectly happy with 20/30 visual acuity. However, you should be able to bring the visual acuity to 20/20 even if overrefraction is necessary. To clarify, let us look at this example:

The patient's refraction is −6.50 +1.00 cyl. axis 90. Keratometer readings are 45.00/46.00 cyl. axis 90. You fit this patient with 7.5 13.0 −6.00 soft lens. Overrefraction with spheres shows that the patient prefers +0.50 over the lens, which you change accordingly. Visual acuity is good and stable, however the patient has difficulty in reading the 20/20 line clearly. This is not caused by a poorly fitted lens or by a bad lens; it is simply caused by the fact that the patient has 1 diopter of residual astigmatism. This is easiest to determine by keratometer readings over the lens, which in this patient are 39.50/40.50, indicating 1 diopter of residual astigmatism. If you give him −1.00 +1.00 cyl. axis 90 in the trial frame, he could read the 20/20 line clearly or as well as with his glasses. Simply record this fact and send the patient home. On the next visit however, determine how satisfied the patient is with his vision. If he is perfectly happy and wears the lens 16 hours a day, you can stop worrying. If, however, the patient "loves" his lenses and wears them most of the time, but still prefers his glasses for close work or driving, suggest that he wear glasses with his astigmatic correction over the lenses when necessary. Suprisingly, in our experience patients readily accept this lens-glass combination.

INSERTION AND REMOVAL OF SOFT CONTACT LENSES

Before going into the actual fitting procedure we must learn soft lens insertion and removal techniques. The first rule is *do not use topical anesthetics in inserting the lens* even for the first time. Soft lenses are extremely comfortable and anesthetics are unnecessary.

Actual insertion is easy and can be done in two ways: simply pinch the lens between your thumb and forefinger (Fig. 1) and place it on the lower sclera as the patient looks up; or you can insert the lens the same way the patient does: place it on your forefinger (Fig. 2) and press it on the lower sclera. In either case you must *hear* the lens attach itself; it makes a sound when the air is released from underneath. When the patient looks down, the lens slips into place.

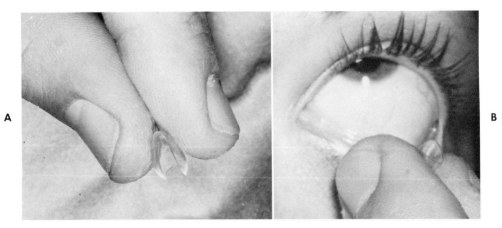

Fig. 1. **A,** When the lens is being inserted, it is first pinched between thumb and forefinger; **B,** The lens is then pressed on lower sclera while patient looks up.

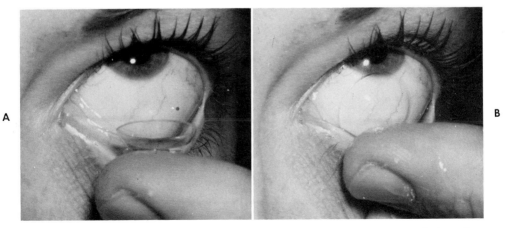

Fig. 2. Another method of insertion. **A,** Lens is balanced on forefinger first. **B,** It is then placed on the lower sclera while patient looks up.

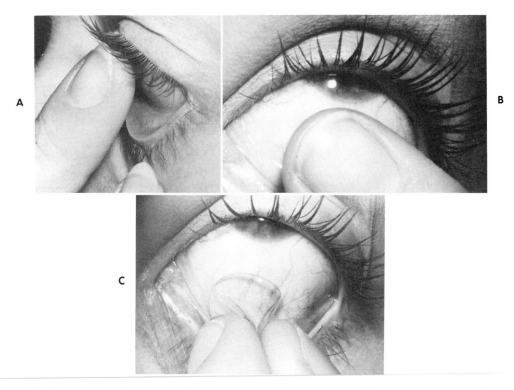

Fig. 3. Removing the lens. **A,** Forefinger is placed on the lens while patient looks straight ahead. **B,** The lens is pulled down while the patient looks up. **C,** The thumb is brought in to pinch the lens out of the eye.

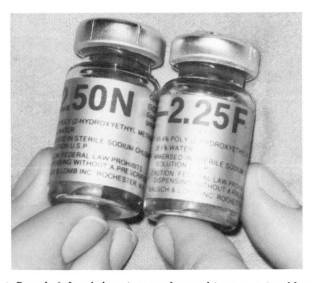

Fig. 4. Bausch & Lomb lens is manufactured in two series, N and F.

The doctor and the patient remove the lens the same way from the eye (Fig. 3): place your forefinger on the lens as the patient looks straight ahead, and then pull the lens down while the patient looks up at the same time. Then bring in your thumb and pinch the lens out of the eye.

The following simple rules must be followed while handling the soft contact lenses:

Your hands must be clean before handling the lenses. These lenses are like sponges and absorb solutions such as shaving lotion from your hands. You also have to be careful what soap to use, since some soaps can be a problem, Ivory and Neutragena soaps seem to be the least irritating to the patient.

Try not to touch the inside of the lens after it has been cleaned. Any small particle under the lens, or even perspiration from your fingers will be irritating to the patient.

If you do not get the lens in on the first try but drop it on the lashes, it is better to rinse if off with saline before trying again. This will remove any small particles the lens may have picked up from the lashes and, in the long run, will save time.

THE BAUSCH & LOMB LENS

The era of the soft contact lenses was officially blessed by the Food and Drug Administration's (FDA) approval of the Bausch & Lomb (B & L) lens in March 1971. This lens is manufactured in two series, N and F (Fig. 4), but only one size. It is shaped somewhat like a red blood cell and does not have base curves in the regular sense, but rather the series indicates different anterior curves. The posterior curve is the power curve.

The B & L kit supplied by the manufacturer includes a fitting set of 72 lenses, a boiler unit for office sterilization, crimpers for recapping the bottles, bottle caps, a few Aseptors, and forceps (Figs. 5 and 6).

The lens is very thin and therefore rather difficult to handle in the beginning. Forceps must be used to get the lens out of the vial; the easiest way is to pull the lens up one side with a fork of the forceps (Fig. 7).

Inspection, sterilization, and storage of the Bausch & Lomb lens

INSPECTION. The lens does not have regular base curves, which need to be checked. Lens power could be verified in a water chamber (Fig. 8). However the manufacturer carefully checks each lens and labels the bottles accordingly. The edges are easiest seen by slit lamp examination.

STERILIZATION. The lenses are sterile as they come from the manufacturer. However, after office use they must be resterilized. This is done by boiling the entire set in the Aseptor unit provided for this purpose (Fig. 9). If individual lenses are sterilized, sterilization is done in a small patient Aseptor unit. The lens vial is filled with normal saline (without preservatives), the small asepticizer unit is filled with one fourth cup of distilled water, and four vials are placed in a tray, which is then placed in the sterilizing unit (Fig. 10). The unit is activated, and when the lenses are ready, it shuts off automatically.

Patients sterilize their lenses daily. They insert the lenses in both caps of the

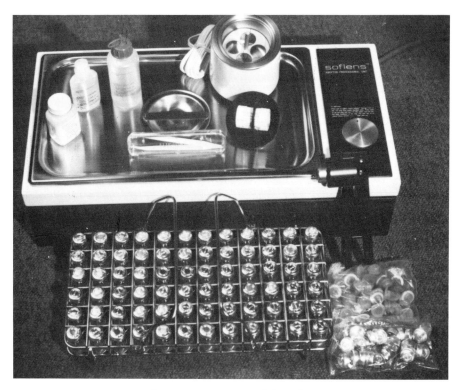

Fig. 5. Bausch & Lomb lens kit.

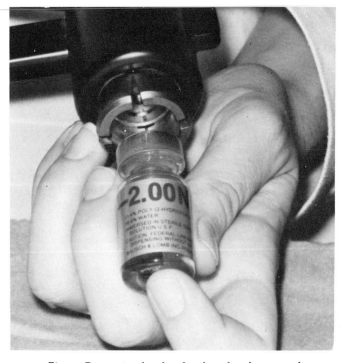

Fig. 6. Recapping bottle after lens has been used.

carrying case and fill the case with normal saline. The case is inserted in the patient Aseptor unit (Fig. 11) and sterilized as outlined previously. Lenses are left in the aseptor overnight and are ready for insertion in the morning.

At present there is no cleaner, available for use with the B & L lenses, that would remove all proteinaceous material that may coagulate on the surface when

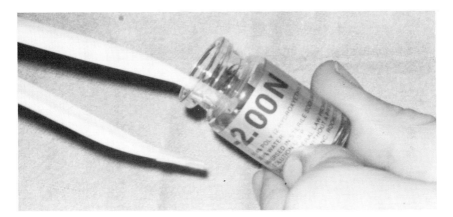

Fig. 7. Forceps are used in removing the Bausch & Lomb lens.

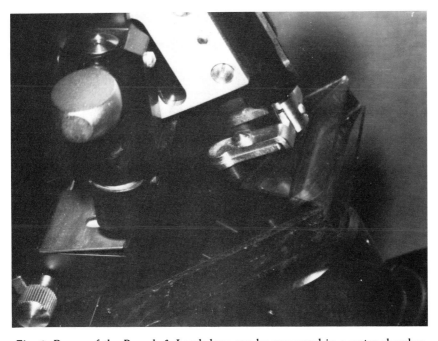

Fig. 8. Power of the Bausch & Lomb lens can be measured in a water chamber.

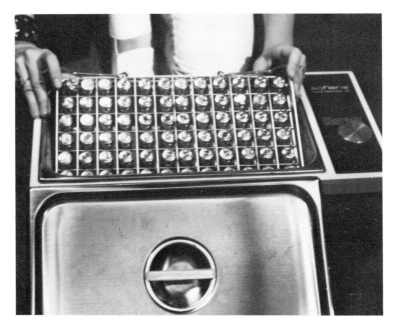

Fig. 9. Bausch & Lomb office sterilization unit.

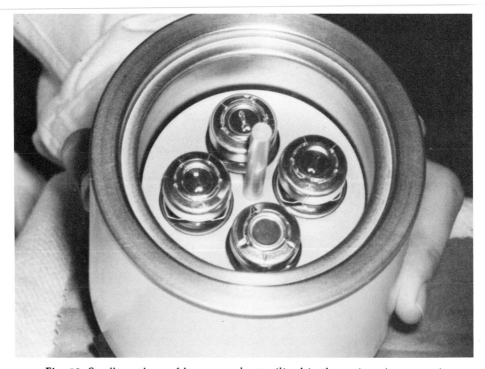

Fig. 10. Small numbers of lenses can be sterilized in the patient Aseptor unit.

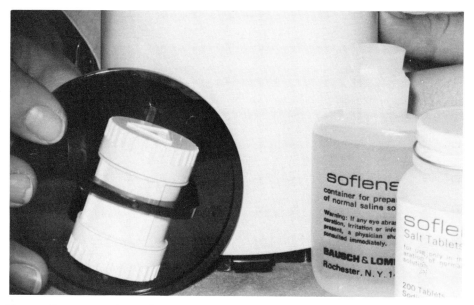

Fig. 11. Patient care kit includes Aseptor, carrying case, and salt tablets to make saline solution.

the lenses are boiled. Hopefully, this shortcoming will be remedied in the near future.

STORAGE. Trial lenses are stored in vials of sterile saline solution and remain sterile as long as the vial is unopened. Weekly sterilization, however, is recommended by the company.

Fitting of the Bausch & Lomb lens

The fitting technique for the B & L lens is relatively easy. You obtain the *lens power* by refracting the patient's eyes and using the spherical equivalent for the lens power. Vertex distance is noted if lens power is larger than −4.00. The horizontal and vertical keratometer readings are obtained and averaged. With this number you select the lens power compensation (Table 1). As a rule of thumb, if the average is flatter than 44.50, try F series lens; if it is steeper than 44.50, try N series lens. If the first series does not work, try the other series.

> **Example:** A patient has a refraction of −2.00 +0.50 cyl. axis 90 and keratometer readings 42.00/42.50 cyl. axis 90. The power of the lens would be −2.25, and since the average of the keratometer readings (42.25) is flatter than 44.50, the series should be F. Power is calculated as follows:
>
> | | |
> |---|---:|
> | Refraction is −2.00 +0.50 cyl. axis 90 = spherical equivalent | −1.75 |
> | Corneal power compensation at 42.25 | −0.50 |
> | Lens power | −2.25 |

In overrefraction the patient takes a plano lens, and keratometer images are clear over the lens. Prescribe the −2.25 lens in the F series for the patient and he probably will do extremely well.

The preceding example is greatly simplified. Let us make the problem a bit more complicated:

Example: You have the same patient as in the preceding example; however with the lens you have tried on him, his vision is not quite clear. You send him home, hoping that in a week or so his lens will equilibrate with his tears. However, when he returns for his checkup, he still complains of watery vision. You try N series in −2.25 lens but can tell immediately that this lens is too steep. You know that you need to make the lens flatter in order for the patient to see. Now the only way to do this is to go back to the original flatter (F) series and try to change the base curve by adding plus power to the lens. In other words, you try F series in −1.50 to −1.75 lens, hoping that you have created sufficient minus tear layer to give the patient the additional minus power that he needs. And similarly, if you need to make the lens steeper, add minus power to the lens and create a compensating plus tear layer.

Overrefraction is done after the patient has worn his lenses for a while (minimum of 20 to 30 minutes) and the lens has had a chance to equilibrate with tears. However, since the base curve is the power curve, the necessary changes in refraction cannot always be implemented.

Slit lamp examination is done to determine the movement and centering of the lens. It should remain centered at the vertical meridian but may ride low by as much as 2 mm. Remember that you cannot use fluorescein for this procedure. Bausch and Lomb recommends the wearing schedule as shown in Table 2.

Table 1. Bausch & Lomb lens power compensation

| Corneal radius | | Corneal power |
Millimeters	Diopters	Compensation (in diopters)
6.50	52.00	+1.00
6.75	50.00	+0.75
7.00	48.25	+0.50
7.25	46.50	+0.25
7.50	45.00	00
7.75	43.50	−0.25
8.00	42.25	−0.50
8.25	40.87	−0.75
8.50	39.75	−1.00

Summary

Follow these steps to fit Bausch & Lomb lens:
1. Refraction for lens power
2. Keratometer readings for cornea power compensation
3. Selection of lens series
4. Overrefraction
5. Slit lamp examination

Table 2. Suggested wearing schedule for Bausch & Lomb lenses

Day	Wear time (hours)	Rest period (hours)	Wear time (hours)	Rest period (hours)	Wear time (hours)
1	3	1	3	1	3
2	3	1	3	1	3
3	4	1	4	1	4
4	4	1	4	1	4
5	6	1	6	1	4
6	6	1	6	1	4
7	8	1	8		
8	8	1	8		
9	8	1	8		
10	10	1	Balance of the waking hours*		
11	12	1	Balance of the waking hours*		
12	14	1	Balance of the waking hours*		

*Lenses should never be worn 24 hours a day.

THE GRIFFIN LENS

The Griffin Lens is manufactured in several combinations of base curves and sizes, which are conveniently color coded (Fig. 12 and Table 3). The lens power is available in 0.25-diopter increments from −15.00 to aphakic corrections. Additional powers are made by request. These lenses can be manufactured in almost any thickness. The average thickness is 0.35 to 0.45 mm., but thinner or thicker lenses are available. Although a very thin lens may be extremely comfortable, some optical quality will be lost.

Inspection, storage, and sterilization of Griffin lens

Although the quality control in the laboratory is adequate, we recommend that you inspect your lenses before inserting them in the patient's eyes. Inspection takes only a few minutes and may save time later on. Our routine is as follows.

BASE CURVE. A simple ball gauge is available for measuring the base curve of the lens (Fig. 13). The lens is dropped on one plastic ball. If there is an air bubble under the lens, the lens base curve is steeper than that of the ball (Fig. 14, A). If the edge does not align itself with the gauge but shows convolution, the lens base curve is flatter than the ball (Fig. 14, B). Simply find the ball on which the lens fits perfectly and read the base curve from that ball.

DIAMETER OF THE LENS. Lens diameter can be measured simply with a magnifying reticule by reading the diameter from outer edge to outer edge along the scale (Fig. 15).

LENS POWER. Lens power measurement is the most difficult procedure, but with a little practice it can be done within a 0.25-diopter accuracy. The lens is cleaned well then blotted dry with lint-free tissue and placed concave side up under a lensometer (Fig. 16). After a few seconds the image becomes clear and lens power

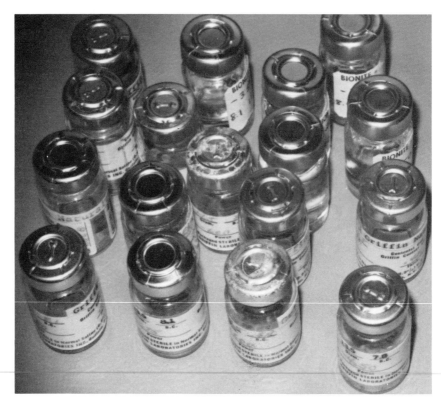

Fig. 12. Griffin Lenses come in a variety of sizes and base curves.

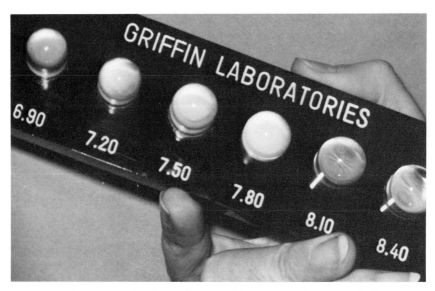

Fig. 13. Base curve of a Griffin lens can be measured by simple ball gauge.

FITTING MANUAL FOR BAUSCH & LOMB AND GRIFFIN LENSES

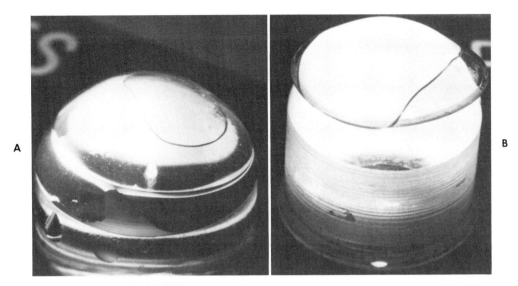

Fig. 14. A, If lens shows an air bubble underneath, lens is steeper than gauge. **B,** If lens shows convoluted edge, lens is flatter than gauge.

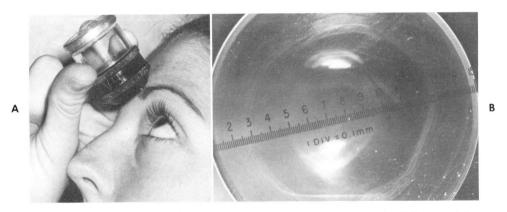

Fig. 15. A, Lens diameter can be measured by simple magnifying reticle. **B,** It is read from outer edge to outer edge along the scale.

can be read off easily. You must, however perform this maneuver rather fast since the lens becomes impossible to read if it dries too much. The Zeiss or Nikon lensometers are easiest to use for this purpose.

INSPECTION OF EDGES. Edge inspection is easily done under slit lamp magnification.

STORAGE. When out of the eye Griffin lenses must always be stored in saline solution containing weak thimerosal preservative, never in plain distilled water. If the lens dries out, it becomes brittle and is easily broken. Remember that the Bausch & Lomb lens is stored in saline without preservatives.

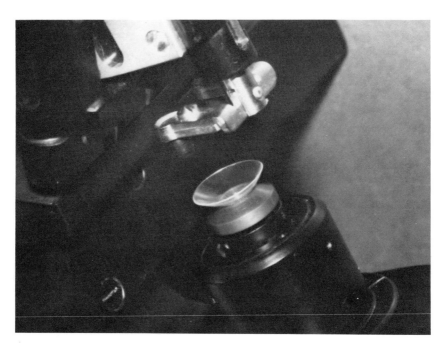

Fig. 16. Power of the Griffin lens can be read easily.

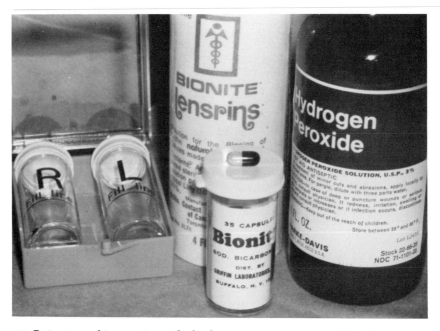

Fig. 17. Patient care kit contains vials for lenses, a carrying case, 3% hydrogen peroxide, premeasured sodium bicarbonate capsules, and thimerosal preserved saline (Lensrins).

CLEANING. Cleaning the surface dirt from the lens is important and must be done before sterilization and insertion of the lens into the eye. Simply set the lens on your forefinger, drop a couple of drops of soft lens cleaning solution, such as Flexsol or Barnes-Hind's cleaner, on the lens and rub it between your thumb and forefinger before rinsing it with saline.

STERILIZATION. Lenses fitted for optical purposes should be removed and sterilized once a day, usually at night. The preferred method of sterilization for Griffin lenses is the peroxide-bicarbonate method. Other methods, however, such as boiling or simple chemical one-step procedures are presently being investigated. With the peroxide method the patient cleans his lens as mentioned before and then soaks them in 3% hydrogen peroxide for 5 minutes. Although this sterilizes the lenses, it also changes lens dimensions and shaking the lenses 1 minute in bicarbonate solution is needed to return them to normal. After this step is done, the bicarbonate solution is discarded and the cases are filled with sterile saline solution (Lensrins) and shaken again for 1 minute. Then this saline is replaced with fresh saline and stored overnight (Fig. 17). In the morning the lenses are ready for use. If the lenses burn after this procedure, the patients quickly learn to regulate soaking time or give the lenses an extra saline rinse to fit their own individual needs.

THE GASSET "TACO SIGN." Sometimes it is difficult to tell whether the lens is inside out. To determine this, the Gasset "taco sign" is helpful. The lens is dropped into the palm of one hand and picked up between the forefinger and the thumb of the other hand. If the lens is correct and ready for insertion, pressing the edges of the lens together will make it look like a Mexican taco with edges touching and a space in the center (Fig. 18, A). However, if the lens is inside out, the edges do not touch, but the center will, and it will thus resemble a fireman's helmet (Fig. 18, B).

If you wish to practice this test, it is better to select a lens with normal thickness, because the shapes are difficult to distinguish with a very thin lens.

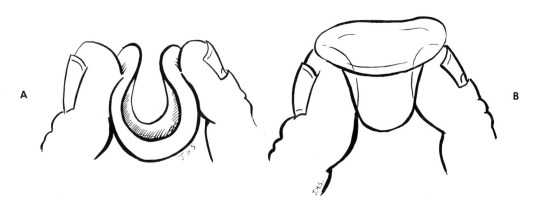

A   B

Fig. 18. A, If the lens is right side in, it looks like a taco when edges are pressed together. **B,** If it is inverted, it looks like a fireman's helmet.

Table 3. Griffin lenses

Base curves	Sizes	Color code
8.4	15.0	White
8.1	14.5	Yellow
7.8	14.0	Blue
7.5	13.5	Green
	13.0	Red

Table 4. Selection of Griffin lens base curves

Keratometer readings	Base curve
40.00–41.50	8.4
41.50–43.00	8.1
43.00–44.50	7.8
44.50–46.00	7.5

Table 5. Selection of Griffin lens size

Base curves	Sizes
8.4	14.5
8.1	14.0
7.8	13.5
7.5	13.0

Fitting of Griffin lens for optical purposes

To fit the Griffin lenses you need two parameters—refraction and keratometer readings. *Refraction* is done in minus cylinder form and only the sphere portion of that refraction is used to determine the lens power.

> **Example:** The patient's refraction is −3.50 −0.50 cyl. axis 180. The lens power you select is −3.50. Similarly, for a patient whose refraction is −4.00 +1.00 cyl. axis 90, you would select a −3.00 lens.

The *base curve* of the lens is determined by keratometer readings. After obtaining vertical and horizontal measurements, take the flatter reading and select a base curve from Table 4.

The majority of the patients fall between the 41.50 and 44.50 keratometer reading category and therefore the most commonly used base curves are 8.1 and 7.8.

> **Example:** For a patient whose keratometer readings are 42.50/43.50 cyl. axis. 90 you would select an 8.1 mm. base curve lens, the flatter reading, 42.50, being

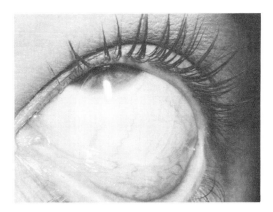

Fig. 19. Lens lag is an indication of a too flat lens.

in between 41.50 and 43.00. And similarly, for a patient with readings of 46.00/ 46.50 cyl. axis 90, you would select a 7.5 mm. base cirve lens.

The *diameter of the lens* is important for proper adherence. The soft lens is heavier than a hard lens and tends to decenter. It should fit approximately 1 mm. beyond the limbus for good adherence. We do not, however, recommend the measurement of the corneal diameter because it is difficult and could be confusing. For all practical purposes the rule "small cornea is steep cornea, large cornea is flat cornea" is true, and therefore we use the following combinations of base curves and sizes (Table 5).

You have now selected the trial lens for your patient—by refraction, the power of the lens; by keratometer reading, the base curve and lens size. Next you must determine whether this lens fits well or needs some changes. This probably would be easier if in the beginning you let the lenses equilibrate for a while (simply insert a lens in both eyes and send the patient to the waiting room for about 10 minutes). However, equilibration is not necessary, especially after you have gained some experience.

The *movement and centering of the lens* is easy to observe. Simply ask the patient to look up and to each side. Lens lagging on each gaze is an indication that the lens is too flat (Fig. 19). A flat lens may be comfortable and give good visual acuity; however constant rubbing of the apex can produce hypertrophic epithelium with or without deep keratitis (Plate I, *A*). On the other hand, too steep a lens clings to the eye like a suction cup, but this is difficult to see (Fig. 20). The easiest way to tell if the lens is too steep is by the patient's symptoms. He will complain that vision is blurry but clears for a moment immediately after blinking. This is because on each blink the lid pressure brings the lens in contact with the cornea allowing for momentary clear vision.

How do we change these lenses to make them fit better? Consider the following example:

You have selected a lens of 7.8 mm. base curve and 13.5 mm. diameter lens for your patient; however the lens seems to slide too much and the patient com-

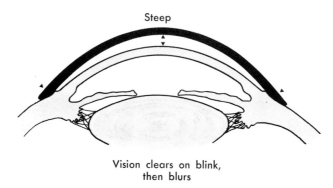

Steep

Vision clears on blink,
then blurs

Fig. 20. Cross section showing steep lens.

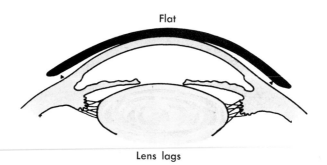

Flat

Lens lags

Fig. 21. Cross section showing flat lens.

plains that he can feel it moving. This means that the lens is too flat. To make it steeper, *either* make it larger (14.0) *or* go to a steeper base curve. On the other hand, if the patient complains of variable vision and you would like to make the lens looser, *either* go to a flatter base curve (8.1) *or* smaller lens. Do not change both parameters at once.

For final check of the fit of the lens, we check the *keratometer readings over the lens* and will accept as well fitted a lens on which mire images are as good as without the lens in the eye. By keratometer readings we also determine any residual astigmatism that may need to be corrected.

Refraction over the lens is necessary to make the final corrections in lens power. Using only sphere lenses, refract the patient's eyes and make final adjustments in the lens as in the following example:

A patient has refraction of −6.50 +1.00 cyl. axis 90 and keratometer readings 45.00/46.00 cyl. axis 90. You select a 7.5 13.0 −4.50 lens. Overrefraction shows that the patient likes −0.50 over the lens, and you change it accordingly. Your final lens is 7.5 13.0 −5.00.

Slit lamp examination is done for all patients. The edges of the lens should not stand off the eye; the edges do so if the lens is too flat (Fig. 21). On the other

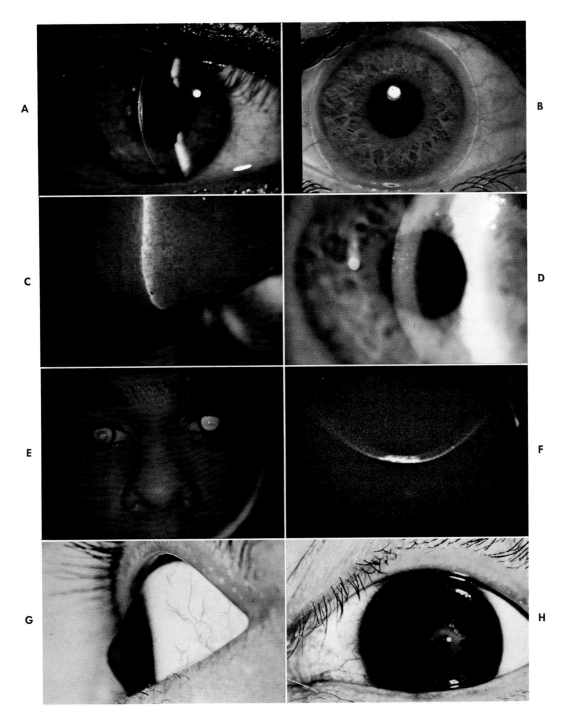

Plate I. A, Flat lens fit can cause "rubbing" on the apex. **B,** Limbal injection caused by steep lens. **C,** In keratoconjunctivitis caused by TRIC agent, mild follicular conjunctivitis is present. **D,** Subepithelial infiltrates in keratoconjunctivitis caused by TRIC agent. **E,** Shadow of cone in keratoconus is seen through dilated pupils and retroillumination with direct ophthalmoscope (taken with fundus camera). **F,** Thin cone in keratoconus with apical scar. **G,** Side view of keratoconus. **H,** Apical scar in keratoconus.

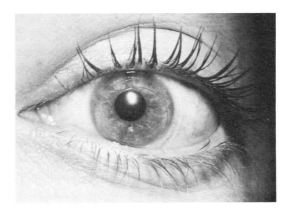

Fig. 22. On slit lamp examination there may be an air bubble under the lens indicating a too steep lens.

hand, if the lens is too tight, the edges may press against the eye or there may be air bubbles under the lens (Fig. 22). Ideally the lens should move about 0.5 to 1 mm. on blink while patient looks up. Remember never use fluorescein, it ruins the lenses.

In summary, follow these simple steps to fit Griffin lenses:
1. Refraction for lens power
2. Keratometer readings for lens base curve and diameter
3. Check lens movement for flat lens
4. Check visual acuity for steep lens
5. Keratometer readings over the lens for fit and cylinder
6. Refraction over the lens for final lens power
7. Slit lamp examination.

FOLLOW-UP VISITS

After fitting a patient, we check him first after a week and at monthly intervals until we are certain he has no problems. If the lens is well fitted and the patient is careful about sterilization, there should be no complications. However, improperly fitted soft lenses, although safer than hard lenses, can cause problems.

If the patient complains of smoky vision with rainbow-colored halos, look carefully for edema. This is sometimes hard to recognize since it is not the patchy edema seen with hard lenses but diffuse edema involving most of the epithelium. Such edema may occur in 4% to 5% of cases fitted but is very easily reversed (it disappears shortly after the lens is removed). If the patient is wearing Griffin lens, the lens is too tight and should be replaced with a smaller, flatter, and thinner lens. If the patient is wearing a Bausch & Lomb lens, start him again from the beginning of the wearing schedule.

When a patient has limbal injection (Plate I, *B*) or compression with some discomfort, this is probably due to either bad edges on the lens or too steep a lens. Correct this by replacing the lens with a smaller or flatter lens.

Burning can be due to a variety of reasons usually related to sterilizing solutions. However, as mentioned before, the lenses can also absorb liquids such as shaving lotion or perfume. In addition, they can become partially dehydrated and hypertonic. Care in handling and cleaning the lenses will usually alleviate this problem.

As a rule we see no bacterial infection caused by soft lenses. Although inclusion conjunctivitis caused by TRIC agent is not induced by soft lenses, it is made worse by their wear. It is very important to recognize this entity since it is common with both soft and hard lenses. In these cases, the patient usually complains of burning and discomfort whenever the lenses are worn. His condition is better without the lenses, but as soon as they are reinserted his eyes become red and very uncomfortable. On slit lamp examination, you see limbal injection with mild follicular conjunctivitis (Plate I, C) and very small, scattered subepithelial infiltrates (Plate I, D). In this case the lenses must be discontinued and the infection cleared with a sulfa drug and, if necessary, tetracycline before lens wearing can be resumed.

INSTRUCTION TO THE PATIENT

1. Insertion and removal must be properly taught. If the patient learns the wrong technique, he will break too many lenses. We must also emphasize that since the lenses are pinched out of the eye it is necessary to cut fingernails to avoid damaging both the cornea and lens.

2. The "taco sign" is important to the patient since he has just as hard a time telling whether the lens is inside out, as you do.

3. Patients who wear lenses for optical purposes must remove them once a day and sterilize them properly. This cannot be overemphasized, since the temptation is great to leave the lenses in and never remove them.

4. The patients must realize that the lenses must be stored in saline while out of the eye, never in distilled water, and that commercially available medications are not approved for use with the lenses.

5. Soft lenses are ideal for sports and can be used for swimming even in chlorinated pools. Usually the patients remove lenses after swimming under water and rinse off the chlorine before reinserting them. In fast sports such as motorcycle riding or skiing, air pressure may dry the lenses. but patients can regulate this by blinking.

6. If the patient has Bausch & Lomb lenses, the wearing schedule must be explained to him. With Griffin lenses no wearing schedule is necessary, and patients simply insert their lenses in the morning and wear them as long as they wish (usually 12 to 15 hours a day). If they wish to remove the lenses and wear spectacles, they have no difficulty in doing this. Keratometer readings do not change with soft lens wear and no spectacle blur occurs.

SIMPLIFIED TECHNIQUE

The fitting technique for Griffin lenses outlined in the previous chapter is only one of many. There is nothing wrong with trying any technique outlined in this book and selecting the one with which you feel most comfortable. We believe that the one we are using is safest to the patient, and by taking keratometer readings over and under the lens and trying to make sense out of the numbers, we gain understanding to the patient's problems. However, if you want a really simple technique, we recommend the following Gasset's "dial-a-lens" method:

1. *Modify your keratometer* by painting the horizontal and vertical dials as follows:

	Corresponding base curve
40.00 to 42.00 Yellow	8.4
42.00 to 44.00 Blue	8.1
44.00 to 45.50 Green	7.8
45.50 to 47.00 Red	7.5

2. *Refract patient's eyes and determine the power of the lens.* Take the spectacle refraction in minus cylinder form. Ignore the cylinder. When necessary, correct for the change in effectivity due to the vertex distance. Refine the lens power by overrefraction.

3. *Take keratometer readings.*

4. Select the color indicated on the keratometer. Vertical and horizontal readings will match in most cases. If the colors are different, order the color of the flatter meridian.

5. *Check lens movement.*
   Slight movement (0.5 to 1 mm.) on blink.

6. *Biomicroscopy.*
   a. Relationship between the lens edge and the sclera (1 to 1.5 mm. override of limbus)
   b. Appearance of the lens surface (free of "waves")
   c. Evaluation of the cornea (integrity remains unaltered)
   d. Lens centering (on center to slightly down)
   e. Lid pressure (lens must not be moved excessively by lids)

7. *Retinoscopy*
   The retinoscopy is used to evaluate the quality of the reflex and the amount of residual astigmatism.

8. *Keratometry*
   The quality of the image should be as good as the quality of the reflected image from the cornea itself.

FITTING OF SOFT LENSES IN PATHOLOGICAL CONDITIONS— GRIFFIN LENSES

One of the most significant developments in the ophthalmic field has been the use of soft lenses in the treatment of pathological conditions. Many of these conditions, previously regarded as untreatable, are now manageable with soft lenses. Most corneal surgeons who have used soft lens therapy will testify that it is hard to imagine what it was like to practice ophthalmology before their advent. For the purpose of this manual we are forced to limit ourselves only to fitting with Griffin lenses. We have very little experience with the Bausch & Lomb lenses in pathological conditions and those who do cannot repeat their initial good results since the company discontinued their early lens. So please keep in mind that pathological conditions should be fitted *only* with Griffin lenses.

Fitting patients with pathological conditions is more difficult than fitting patients for simple refractive errors; therefore experience in fitting refractive errors is mandatory for fitting pathological cases.

Keratoconus

Management of keratoconus patients represents an important and often difficult problem. Because keratoconus is still a much misunderstood condition as far as etiology, progression, and evaluation of the disease, proper and intelligent use of our diagnostic tools is of the utmost importance (Plate I, E, and Fig. 23), not only for the diagnosis, but also for the management and follow-up of these patients. For example, direct ophthalmoscopy can be used to determine the location, diameter, and shape of the cone.

Management of keratoconus usually parallels the severity of the disease. The early or mild form of keratoconus manifests itself by the development of myopia with astigmatism, which is usually oblique. Occasionally spectacles may correct this to a satisfactory level, but often contact lenses are needed because of secondary irregular corneal astigmatism. As the weakening of the corneal architecture progresses, the cone becomes steeper, larger and thinner (Plate I, F and G). These severe cases are usually unmanageable by nonsurgical techniques. Fortunately, penetrating keratoplasty is highly successful in this group of patients.

Our main goal in the management of keratoconus patients is to obtain satis-

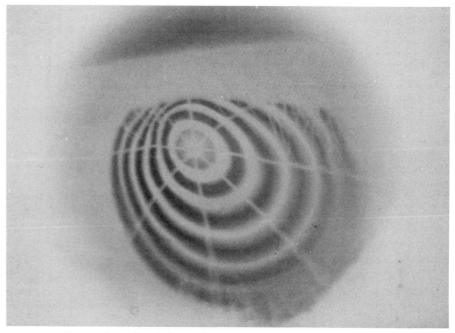

Fig. 23. Irregular circles in keratoconus as seen with keratoscope.

factory vision and comfort. For this purpose spectacles and contact lenses can be used as an alternative to surgical treatment. Patients with severe keratoconus generally cannot see without contact lenses, and the fitting of hard acrylic contact lenses for these patients has produced serious problems. Corneal ulcers, scarring, and vascularization may result from hard lens wear, thus accelerating the need for surgery (Plate I, *H*). These undesirable complications are not likely to be related to the skill of the fitter, but rather to the fact that a hard lens is not of optimal value in these cases.

Our present fitting technique is as follows, and again let me emphasize that this is only for use with Griffin lenses.

KERATOMETER READINGS. First of all we like to know the approximate size of the cone with which we are dealing. Therefore we start with keratometer readings. This step, however, does not give us the base curve of the lens; as in fitting optical lenses, it is for the record only. Often, it is impossible to obtain the keratometer readings on a steep cone. We then insert a −10.00 lens in the eye and then measure the cone. This technique may not be exact, but it is close enough to give an idea of the size of the cone.

> **Example.** Keratometer readings on the patient are off the scale. Insert a −10.00 lens on the eye and the readings over the lens are 48.00/52.00 cyl. axis 130. Therefore the size of the cone is approximately 58.00/62.00 cyl. axis 130. This is for the records only.

LENS BASE CURVE DETERMINATION. We do not use keratometer readings to determine the lens base curve, but select the largest, flattest lens available in plano power as the starting point. When we insert the lens in the eye, we use the eye as we use the ball gauge—if there is a bubble under the lens, it means that the lens is too steep; if it shows a convoluted edge, it is too flat (Fig. 24). We then change it as necessary.

> **Example.** For the patient in the previous example, you select an 8.4 14.0 plano lens. Immediately on insertion the lens feels very uncomfortable and the

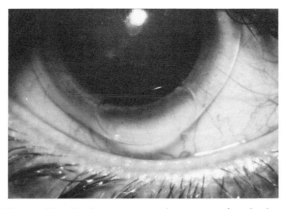

Fig. 24. Too flat lens on cone shows convoluted edge.

eye starts tearing. On examination you note that the lens edge is wrinkled, causing discomfort. This lens is too flat, and you have to make it steeper. You do this by increasing the lens diameter first to 14.5 and then, if necessary, to 15.0 mm.

KERATOMETER READINGS OVER THE LENS. Keratometer readings are helpful in determining the fit of the lens. Mire images over well-fitted lens in keratoconus patients should not be good. If the images are clear, the lens conforms to the eye too well and does not flatten the cone.

Lens power determination is done by refracting the patient over the trial lens. Refraction is done as in any patient with substandard vision; using only spheres, switch from plano to −4.00, then from −4.00 to −8.00, etc., until at the end you are able to refine the sphere power of the lens.

> **Example.** The patient is wearing an 8.4 15.0 plano lens. Refraction over the lens shows that the patient needs −11.00 over the plano lens. You now fit the patient with this power lens, keeping the lens diameters the same, that is, an 8.4 15.0 −11.00 lens. Mire images are somewhat poor.

Your next step is the *refinement of the visual acuity and the cylinder axis.* On checking your patient's vision, you notice that he can see a 20/30 line without difficulty. This vision will be sufficient for most of the things he will do, but for near vision and driving, he will need more accurate vision. He still has a large amount of astigmatism that needs to be corrected, and that is determined by keratometer readings over the lens.

> **Example.** The same patient as in the previous example. Mire images over the lens are not quite clear; however, you are able to determine that the keratometer readings are 43.00/47.00 cyl. axis 130. This indicates that the patient has 4 diopters of corneal astigmatism at 130 degrees.

The total amount of astigmatism present in keratometer readings must be accepted by the patient. This is one of the last checks of your fit; if his overrefraction is something other than what keratometer readings indicate, there is a mistake somewhere in your fitting. The total astigmatic correction may not be given to the patient all at once, but eventually he should wear in his spectacles all the K readings indicated.

> **Example.** With his soft lenses your patient is able to see 20/30. His K readings indicate 4 diopters of residual astigmatism. You now prescribe −4.00 +4.00 cyl. axis 130 (remember, your fitting is done in minus cylinder form), and he has good clear visual acuity.

The example shown in this chapter is greatly simplified and makes fitting of soft contact lenses for keratoconus patients sound very easy. The truth is that it is a very meticulous procedure and requires a great deal of patience and skill on the part of the fitter. But the end result is worth it—you may have saved another patient from corneal transplant and have fitted him with a totally comfortable contact lens.

In summary, these are the parameters in fitting soft contact lenses for patients with keratoconus:

1. Keratometer readings for size of the cone
2. Lens base curve determination
3. Keratometer readings over the lens for fit of the lens
4. Lens power determination
5. Refinement of cylinder axis by keratometer readings

With the entry of soft contact lenses into the field of keratoconus, we must reevaluate our indications for corneal surgery in these patients. No longer is failure to tolerate hard lenses because of discomfort, ulceration, and vascularization an indication for penetrating keratoplasty. However, we still must evaluate the size of the cone and the thickness of the cornea to determine when a patient should have surgery.

Bullous keratopathy

Bandage lenses have revolutionized the treatment of bullous keratopathy, one of the most common ophthalmic diseases that can be treated with these new lenses. Basically there are two reasons for using soft lenses in these patients—relief of pain and improvement of vision.

The pain in bullous keratopathy results mainly from lids rubbing on the bullae, rupturing them, and exposing corneal nerves. When a soft lens is inserted over these painful ulcers, it produces an almost instantaneous and usually very dramatic relief of pain. The fitting of the lens is relatively easy if keratometer readings can be obtained on the contralateral eye. However, trial lens fitting is often the only method by which these lenses can be fitted in patients with bullous keratopathy. Thus the first question is how to select a lens that will provide sufficient adherence to prevent movement without inducing too much apical clearance. If the patient's visual acuity is good enough, it is easy to determine when the lens is too steep by variable vision symptoms. If the vision is poor, however, you can use the eye as the ball gauge and determine the fit by air bubble and edge alignment. Too flat a lens also moves too much.

> **Example.** Keratometer readings are impossible to obtain on your patient, you must go by trial and error. You select an 8.4 14.0 lens, but that moves too much on the eye. On the other hand, a 7.8 14.0 lens seems to settle in like a suction cup and there is an air bubble trapped under the lens, indicating too steep a lens. You must select a lens that is in between; therefore you fit this patient with an 8.1 14.0 lens.

If the patient has only a mild amount of edema, his spectacle correction should determine the power of the lens. In more severe cases, however, the lens is fitted for comfort only. In the beginning, in either case the lens is worn full time, 24 hours a day for months at a time. Large single bullae usually disappear within a few days, and only diffuse epithelial edema remains. The constant wearing of these lenses also results in dehydration of the cornea and a significant change in corneal shape. In some cases several changes in the lenses, both base curve and power, are required before the cornea has stabilized.

Use of medication is extremely important since the soft lens alone will not take care of all accompanying problems. Because of concomitant iritis, pupils must be dilated with cycloplegics for the first few days, especially if epithelial defects are present. Atropine preparations without preservatives should be used if available, but one or two drops of regular atropine a day would probably be well tolerated. Again, the lens should be left in place as long as necessary and removed only by the doctor.

In many cases of chronic bullous keratopathy we have found it extremely useful to institute eyelid hygiene techniques. Lid scrubs for 5 minutes once or twice a day have virtually eliminated minor infection and unrecognized blepharitis, which are significant causes of patient discomfort. Antibiotics are used if secondary infection or chronic blepharitis is present at the time of fitting.

After the lens has been in place for several weeks and the eye has quieted down, an attempt can be made to fit the eye for vision. The results are a bit more unpredictable than in the relief of pain and will depend on the amount of folds in Descemet's membrane and corneal thickness. However, soft lenses will help the vision some just by removing the irregular astigmatism present in these patients.

The dimensions of the lens fitted for vision should be the same as the last lens fitted for comfort. Now power can be added by determining spectacle correction and selecting the proper power.

Five percent hypertonic saline without preservative is prescribed for improvement of vision only. It is impossible to dictate how often the patient should use this medication; simply give him the bottle and tell him to use it as often as necessary. For some reason patients seem to need it more in the morning than in the afternoon.

At this point you also should teach the patient the technique for insertion and removal of the lens, but this is for emergencies only. The patient should wear the lens continually. If the doctor feels that he wants the patient to sterilize the lens periodically, he should have it done in his office.

Summary

    1. Lens is fitted by trial and error method first for comfort.
    2. Iritis must be treated with cycloplegics.
    3. Lid hygiene must be instituted, if necessary.
    4. When edema subsides, lens can be fitted for vision.
    5. Five percent hypertonic saline is used as an adjunct for vision improvement.
    6. Lens is worn full time, 24 hours a day, for months at a time.

Syndrome of recurrent corneal ulcers and epithelial erosions

Corneas that tend to ulcerate can also be treated with soft contact lenses and ulceration can be prevented or healed. In normal corneas the corneal epithelium does not interdigitate with its basement membrane but rather sits on this membrane and attaches with electron-dense structures called "hemidesmosomes." If this basement membrane is damaged, the epithelium cannot spread over the surface properly and attach tightly (Fig. 25). It is this failure to attach that causes most recurrent erosions and inhibits healing of recurrent corneal ulcers. If the healing can be fostered by a protective shield, the attachment becomes possible and ulcers can heal (Fig. 26).

We fit the patients with recurrent erosions and corneal ulcers with a steep,

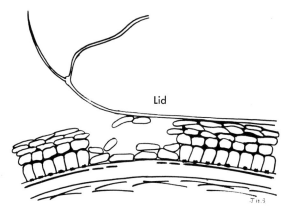

Fig. 25. Epithelium will not attach because of damaged basement membrane.

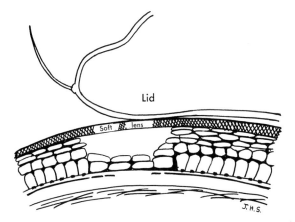

Fig. 26. Healing can be fostered by lens acting as protecting shield.

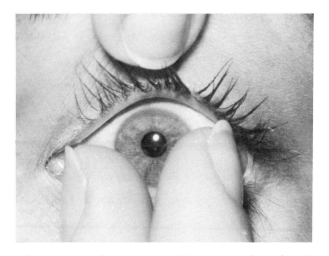

Fig. 27. In epithelium erosion, lens is removed by first gently rocking lens up and down.

thin lens to leave space for the epithelium to spread underneath. Lenses are worn continuously, and you need not worry about the edema that invariably will be present because of a steeply fitted lens; as a matter of fact by watching the edema spread over the cornea, one can note the progress of healing. Once the defect has healed we change to a properly fitting lens. Always remember to treat the accompanying iritis by dilating the pupil with cycloplegics, thus putting the iris sphincter to rest.

One very important point to remember in working with epithelial erosion patients is the manner in which the lens is removed from the eye. Do not attempt to pull the lens down as you would pull a lens from a normal eye. You are dealing with fragile epithelium and a lens that is very much attached to that eye. First flush the eye with saline drops and then place your forefinger and thumb on either side of the lens while it is still on the cornea (Fig. 27). Then gently rock the lens up and down until some air gets underneath and releases this suction. Now the lens can be lifted off the cornea.

Summary

1. Select a thin, steep lens.
2. Dilate pupil to treat iritis.
3. Lens is worn continuously, 24 hours a day, until defect has healed.
4. When removing lens, rock it off instead of pulling it down.
5. After defect has healed, fit patient for vision, if indicated.

Drying syndromes

KERATITIS SICCA. Soft contact lenses have proved useful in those cases of keratitis sicca, where routine treatment (such as artificial tears, wrap-around spectacles, sealing of punctum, and N-acetylcystine solutions) has failed. They provide a moist surface and good eye protection. An important point to remember when dealing with keratitis sicca patients is the fact that almost all of them have blepharitis of varying degrees. Insertion of a soft lens alone will not do anything for the blepharitis. Patients should be instructed to perform lidscrubs with baby shampoo and cotton swabs once or twice a day, and if meibomianitis is severe enough, antibiotics should be used.

Keratitis sicca without lid abnormalities is fitted, on keratometer readings, as if it were an optical case, and the lens is generally worn only during waking hours. Frequent administration of regular or hypotonic (0.45%) saline may be necessary to keep the lens moist. After initial adjustment the need for saline is diminished. Generally, after several weeks of lens wearing, saline therapy can be reduced.

Nonprogressive conjunctival cicatrization (Stevens-Johnson syndrome) and progressive conjunctival cicatrization (ocular pemphigus)

In no other condition is the result of soft contact lens therapy more dramatic than in the cases of severe dry eyes or conjunctival cicatrization. Here again, insertion of a soft lens is not going to take care of all problems; and each one must be dealt with separately.

In most cases severe blepharitis is present and must be treated. Lidscrubs once or twice a day are usually enough, but sometimes antibiotic drops must be added. In this case the chloramphenicol (Chloromycetin) drops that patients mix themselves are used.

A minimal degree of trichiasis is made tolerable just by lens wear. Significant amounts of trichiasis must be treated with conventional methods, such as frequent epilation, electrolysis, or lid surgery.

If small symblepharon is present in the fornix or in the periphery of the cul-de-sac, a soft lens can be inserted without difficulty. If the symblepharon is extensive, it needs to be surgically divided. Conjunctivalization of the cornea, if present, must be peeled off before the soft lens can be inserted.* After surgery is done, a contact lens is fitted by trial lens testing. Since it is impossible to determine the proper lens dimensions, the initial lens is selected almost at random from plano lens inventory.

Lenses are worn 24 hours a day. However they tend to dry out and fall off. To minimize this, one must very frequently administer normal or hypotonic (0.45%) saline or artificial tears manufactured especially for soft contact lenses. In severe cases this should be done as often as every 5 to 10 minutes.

After several days, lenses are changed by trial-and-error method until the best visual acuity is obtained. Less frequent administration of saline or Adapt is usually possible after the lens has adjusted to the eye.

Summary

1. Make space for lens if necessary by surgery.
2. Treat trichiasis.
3. Select initial lens at random.
4. Lenses dry out and must be replaced; therefore many lenses are required.
5. After several days, fit for vision by trial-and-error method.
6. Lenses worn full time (24 hours a day).
7. Medications:
    Special artificial tears for moisture
    Isotonic or hypotonic saline for moisture
    Lid hygiene for comfort
    Antibiotics for infection

These directions may make the fitting of drying syndromes seem very easy. In truth these patients are very time consuming and try your patience. In the beginning the lenses fall off daily and require constant replacement. The real summary for soft lens therapy in drying syndromes should be: lots of lenses and love.

---

*Gasset, A. R., and Kaufman, H. E.: Hydrophilic lens therapy of severe keratoconjunctivitis sicca and conjunctival scarring. Amer. J. Ophthal. **71:**1185-1189, 1971.

This study was supported in part by USPHS grants EY-52868 (Gasset) and EY-00446 from the National Eye Institute.

Index